ALZHEIMER'S DISEASE RESEARCH TRENDS

ALZHEIMER'S DISEASE RESEARCH TRENDS

A.P. Chan
EDITOR

Nova Biomedical Books
New York

For permission to use material from this book please contact us:
Telephone 631-231-7269; Fax 631-231-8175
Web Site: http://www.novapublishers.com

LIBRARY OF CONGRESS CATALOGING-IN-PUBLICATION DATA

Alzhemimer's disease research trends / A.P. chan (editor)
p. ; cm
Includes bibliographical references and index.
ISBN-13: 978-1-60021-712-8 (hardcover)
ISBN-10: 1-60021-712-5 (hardcover)
1. Alzheimer's disease. I. Chan, A.P.
[DNLM: 1.Alzheimer Desiase. 2. Aged. 3. Biomedical research--trends. WT 155 A478867 2007]
RC523.A3882 2007
616.8'310072--dc22

2007015413

Published by Nova Science Publishers, Inc. ✦ New York

CONTENTS

PREFACE

Dementia is a brain disorder that seriously affects a person's ability to carry out daily activities. The most common form of dementia among older people is Alzheimer's disease (AD), which involves the parts of the brain that control thought, memory, and language. Age is the most important known risk factor for AD. The number of people with the disease doubles every 5 years beyond age 65. AD is a slow disease, starting with mild memory problems and ending with severe brain damage. The course the disease takes and how fast changes occur vary from person to person. On average, AD patients live from 8 to 10 years after they are diagnosed, though the disease can last for as many as 20 years.

Current research is aimed at understanding why AD occurs and who is at greatest risk of developing it, improving the accuracy of diagnosis and the ability to identify those at risk, discovering, developing, and testing new treatments, and discovering treatments for behavioral problems in patients with AD. This new book gathers state-of-the-art research from leading scientists throughout the world which offers important information on understanding the underlying causes and discovering the most effective treatments for Alzheimer's Disease. This new book presents leading-edge research advances from around the world.

Chapter I - The modern era of Alzheimer's disease research really began with a series of important ground-breaking papers in the middle-to-late sixties by Kidd, Terry, Gonatas and Weiss on the ultrastructural aspects of the Alzheimer's disease lesions. In these studies neurofibrillary tangles were discovered to be twisted paired helical filaments, and complex amyloid-containing structures were found to be a major component of the insoluble senile 'miliary' plaques [7-10]. Shortly thereafter, Blessed, Tomlinson and Roth were the first to realize that microscopic examination of autopsied brains from the vast majority of all senile dementia/senile psychosis cases actually contained pathological features consistent with a diagnosis of the neuopathogical entity, which Alzheimer had originally described. Hence, it has only been about 4 or 5 decades since these discoveries have gradually brought interest in Alzheimer's disease to the medical research forefront.

Chapter II - Behavioral and psychological symptoms of dementia (BPSD), a term that has been applied to behavioral disturbance among elderly dementia patients in recent years, requires appropriate treatment and care intervention. BPSD not only increases caregiver burden, but also significantly reduces the quality of life (QOL) of elderly dementia patients.

Hall (1987) proposed the progressively lowered stress threshold model (PLST), which states that elderly dementia patients are at an increased risk to develop BPSD due to anxiety behavior resulting from a decreased stress threshold. In addition, using the PLST, Gerdner (2000) developed a mid-range theory as a hypothesis for the effects of music therapy on elderly dementia patients, and reported a reduction in the "agitation" symptom of BPSD due to stress reduction. However, neither Hall nor Gerdner performed measurements of stress hormones to demonstrate their relationship with the onset of BPSD.

Herein, the authors investigate the effects of music therapy and animal-assisted therapy on elderly dementia patients, with regard to levels of salivary Chromogranin A (CgA), a glycoprotein that is a more sensitive indicator of stress than cortisol, in addition to changes in BPSD before and after intervention. Salivary CgA was measured immediately before and after intervention for the intervention group and also for the control group. Following a total of 6 sessions of animal-assisted therapy conducted over a 3-month period for 7 elderly dementia patients residing at home and using daycare services, significant improvements in "aggressiveness" and "anxieties and phobias" of the behavioral symptoms in Alzheimer's disease (Behave-AD) were observed, in addition to a tendency toward a reduction in salivary CgA that was not significant. Similar results were obtained for pet type robot-assisted therapy, in which a pet-like robot was used instead of animals. Furthermore, following a total of 16 sessions of music therapy conducted over a 3-month period, significant improvements in "confusion", "irritability", "agony", and "inability to control bladder and bowel" on the GBS scale were observed, in addition to a significant reduction in salivary CgA.

These findings suggest that animal-assisted therapy and music therapy are effective for reducing BPSD in elderly dementia patients, and that stress reduction induced by intervention may result in BPSD reduction. In the future, it will be necessary to further develop care intervention for reducing BPSD in elderly dementia patients. Salivary CgA may be effective in studies of evidence-based care intervention due to its sensitivity to small changes in stress.

Chapter III - Although amyloid-β (Aβ) peptide production and clearance are crucial to understanding Alzheimer's disease (AD), the intervening events of misfolding and aggregation lead directly to toxicity and therefore require complete elucidation in order to develop comprehensive approaches to therapy/prevention. The authors analyzed the innate propensities of Aβ to assume diverse conformations by careful examination of predicted structure and previously documented solution structures. The authors comparisons of the solution structures of several Aβ fragments indicate the submissive nature of Aβ. The organizing effects of lipid-water interfaces, such as lipid rafts, and reticular networks of endogenous polymers, such as polyacrolein or melanoids, may direct the orientation of the Aβ chain segments. Secondary structure comparisons for the monomeric Aβ, protofibrils, and the predicted structures suggest that Aβ is susceptible to the organizing features of the microenvironment. Molecular models of polyacrolein illustrate the extensive two-dimensional properties of this organizing matrix. The authors discuss the potential significance of polymer templates as providing physico-chemical directives to Aβ peptides as they collapse to form stable aggregates.

Chapter IV - To date, acetylcholinesterase (AChE) inhibitors are clinically effective drugs for a palliative treatment of Alzheimer's disease, but their clinical efficacy is limited mainly due to their adverse effects on peripheral organs. Since patients of Alzheimer's disease often exhibit depression as well as memory impairment, dual inhibitors of AChE and serotonin transporter (SERT) would be a better therapeutic method. Anti-depressive effects based on SERT inhibition would reduce dose-related side effects of AChE inhibitors.

Such dual inhibitors were designed by the hybridization of rivastigmine and fluoxetine based on a hypothetical model of the AChE active site. Various derivatives were synthesized and evaluated for their *in vitro* inhibition, and then (*S*)-2j (RS-1259), which possessed balanced inhibitory activities of AChE (IC_{50} = 101 nM) and SERT (IC_{50} = 42 nM), was successfully obtained.

Molecular modeling studies of several compounds were performed to analyze their inhibitory activities against AChE. The results corresponded well with their potencies and provided some useful information about enzyme–inhibitor interaction.

An *ex vivo* experiment in mice indicated that (*S*)-2j (RS-1259) simultaneously inhibited AChE and SERT in the brain following an oral administration. The simultaneous elevation of extracellular levels of acetylcholine and serotonin in the rat hippocampus was actually confirmed by microdialysis. Both the cholinergic and serotonergic activation in the brain were confirmed by pharmacological tests such as the water maze test, and the merits of SERT inhibition were demonstrated.

Chapter V - The presence of Aβ-positive neuritic plaques with dense cores is considered an essential pathological marker of Alzheimer's disease (AD). However, there are atypical cases that have abundant non-cored plaques with surrounding minor dystrophic neurites. The atypical plaques are called 'cotton wool plaques', and AD with cotton wool plaques is thought to be one of the variants of AD. Cotton wool plaques are usually large, round, and eosinophilic, and appear to displace surrounding normal structures. Inflammatory glial response is mild. The authors here describe two autopsy cases of early-onset dementia with abundant eosinophilic non-cored Aβ plaques, the histopathological features of which are different. Patient 1 was a 44-year-old man at the time of death, with a clinical course of 8 years. Nine relatives in three generations had died in their thirties to forties, and some of them were verified to have had dementia. The proband presented clinically with spastic paraparesis at age 36 prior to the development of dementia. The brain weight was 1330 g. Macroscopically, only mild atrophy was found in the frontal, temporal, and parietal cortices. Histopathological examination revealed abundant, large, eosinophilic, non-cored plaques having the typical appearance of cotton wool plaques. The plaques were more strongly immunopositive for Aβ42 than Aβ40. A moderate number of neurofibrillary changes were found in the hippocampus and parahippocampal gyrus, but only a few in other anatomical regions, including the neocortex. The pyramidal tract was degenerated. Although moderate neuronal loss was found in the insular and entorhinal cortices, the other cerebral cortices were relatively spared. Genetic analysis demonstrated the G384A presenilin-1 gene mutation. Patient 2 was a 46-year-old man at the time of death, with a clinical course of 8 years. His family had no history of neurological diseases in the previous three generations. He presented with memory impairment at the age of 39. Subsequently, he showed disinhibition, impulsiveness, and paranoid ideation, but no neurological abnormality. The brain weight was 1700 g. Macroscopically, neither brain atrophy nor edema was observed. Histopathological examination disclosed abundant eosinophilic non-cored plaques in all cerebral cortices. The diameters were 40-100 μm, including plaques smaller than those in patient 1. The plaques showed little tendency to displace normal structures, but did not contain neurons. Intriguingly, the plaques in this case were were more strongly immunoreactive for Aβ40 than for Aβ42. In the cerebral cortex including the hippocampus, neurons were well preserved, and glial response was slight. In the pyramidal tract, glial proliferation was evident, although loss of myelin was not noted. No tau-positive lesions were found in any region. No mutations in presenilin-1, presenilin-2, or amyloid precursor genes were revealed by genetic analysis using formalin-fixed paraffin-embedded tissue. These findings suggest that factors besides neuritic plaques, neurofibrillary tangles, and severe neuronal loss play a pivotal role in the occurrence of cognitive decline in AD patients.

Chapter VI - Alzheimer's disease (AD) is a devastating and always fatal degenerative disorder of the brain, the most prominent form of dementia among the main types currently defined. Dementia itself is an acquired impairment in intellectual abilities that affects memory, language, visuospatial skills, cognition, emotion and personality. Although mild cognitive losses occur as part of the normal ageing process, the cognitive impairment observed in demented patients is both qualitative and quantitatively more severe. The AD process involves the progressive degeneration of synapses and neurons in brain regions that play fundamental roles in learning and memory, including the hippocampus, entorhinal cortex, basal forebrain, amygdala, frontal cortex, and inferior parietal cortex.

It has been estimated that approximately 50 million people around the world are currently affected by AD with a probable prevalence of 3% in subjects aged 65-74, 19% in those aged 75-84, and 47% in those over 85. Ageing itself is the most important risk factor for AD. Thus, with the continuing exponential increase of the aged population, the incidence of AD is expected to increase significantly in the next decades.

Chapter VII - Patients with Mild Cognitive Impairment (MCI) have the hallmark clinical feature of memory impairment beyond that expected for age and education, yet are not demented. Using fMRI, the authors studied differences in activation of bilateral mesial temporal structures between 9 MCI patients, 10 probable Alzheimer's disease patients and 11 healthy elders during a picture encoding memory task and a naming task at the level of random effects. A predefined masked region of interest including bilateral hippocampus, parahippocampus, posterior cingulate, and fusiform and lingual gyrus was applied for both paradigms. Within-group analyses showed main activations in the posterior cingulate, parahippocampus, and the lingual and fusiform gyrus for the three groups differently distributed during the memory encoding task; while the naming task showed its main activations in the fusiform gyrus among other activations throughout the occipito-temporal gyri in the lingual gyri and the mesial temporal lobe (MTL). Furthermore, the three groups differed in the magnitude of these activations with controls showing more activation than patients, and the MCI group presenting a higher activation than the AD group during both paradigms. These differences increased for the memory encoding paradigm when contrasts among groups were controlled by the hippocampal volume, but this did not occur during the naming paradigm. The authors may conclude that the differential brain activation in the MTL related to memory encoding among these groups of patients may be biased by hippocampal volumes. Therefore, individual volume differences may blur contrasts of functional activations depending on the functional task.

Chapter VIII - Oxidative stress (OS) and cytoskeletal changes may be a culprit in neuronal loss in Alzheimer's disease (AD), and that reactive oxygen species (ROS) are involved in the neuronal pathogenesis of this disease, as well as progressive loss of neuronal cytoarchitecture is an event that precedes neural death. Okadaic acid (OA) induces biochemical, physiological and morphological changes similar to AD such as OS, tau hyperphosphorylation, altered cytoskeletal and β-amyloid peptide plaques. Vitamin C is well known as a hydrophilic antioxidant in human cerebrospinal fluid. It is the antioxidant first consumed during the oxidation of plasma and cerebrospinal fluid. In this work the authors studied the effects of vitamin C on altered cytoskeletal organization and OS induced by OA in N1E-115 neuroblastoma cells. The authors demonstrated that exposure of cells to 50 nM OA for 2 h induced a reduction in cellular gluthatione transferase (GSH-Tr), glutathione reductase (GSH-Rd) and catalase activities and major axis length. Likewise, this acid prompted an increase in lipid peroxidation products. Treatment of cells with 0.5μg/ml vitamin C partially prevented the effects of OA. The vitamin C effects on altered cytoskeletal organization and OS induced by OA were time-dependent, showing its maximum effects when vitamin C was added to the incubation media 2h before OA. These results indicate that OA induces an OS imbalance and cytoskeletal alterations, while vitamin C prevents these changes. Likewise, these data indicate the great importance of OS and the morphological changes in both experimental model and in the development and course of neurodegenerative diseases. These results support the hypothesis that a good level of vitamin C can help to prevent or delay the appearance of neurodegenerative disease; especially AD, as well as they can indicate the participation of vitamin C and micronutrients on oxidative imbalance.

Chapter IX - Parkinson's disease (PD) is a disabling, progressive condition, frequently complicated by a spectrum of cognitive deficits ranging from isolated impairment to severe dementia. The purpose of this paper is to provide an overview of recent findings of dementia associated with PD (PDD), that is increasingly being recognized as a major prognostic factor for progressive disability and nursing home placement. Cholinergic deficits are prominent in PDD and are associated with cognitive slowing, attentional deficiency, memory impairment, and psychotic symptoms, particularly visual hallucinations. The treatment of PDD is challenging. Antipsychotic drugs can precipitate a profound, even fatal worsening in the motor symptoms of patients. On the other hand, dopaminergic agents for parkinsonism frequently cause worsening of hallucinations and cognitive function. The loss of cholinergic functioning suggests a potential utility for cholinesterase inhibitors (ChE-Is) in the treatment of PDD and large studies have been carried out with rivastigmine. This agent appears to moderately improve cognition and to a lesser extent activities of daily living in patients with PDD. Efficacy in other domains requires confirmation. Tolerability, in particular nausea, vomiting, and tremor, appears problematic.

Chapter X - Writing is a complex process requiring visual memory, attention, phonological and semantic operations and motor performance. For that reason, it can easily be disturbed by interfering with attention, memory, by interfering subvocalization, and so on. Using 23 female third-year students (23.4 ± 0.78 years old) from the University of Trieste, the authors investigated the production of errors in three experimental conditions (control, articulatory suppression and tapping). In the articulatory suppression condition, the participants produced significantly more linguistic impairments (such as agrammatism, unrelated substitutions, sentence omissions, and semantically deviant sentences), which are similar to linguistic impairments found in aphasia. On the tapping condition there were more perseverations, deletions, and substitutions, both of letters and of words. The authors then have considered 50 patients suffering from Alzheimer's Disease (CDR average' score=1.76±0.56): the authors evaluated their writing production, in the spontaneous, under dictation and on copy tasks. The authors collected the samples and analysed their production, with the same schema of mistake' classification score. The authors compared the results, and try to find a correlation with specific items of the AD population.

These data suggest that writing is not an automatic skill. Only after many years of experience and practice of processing information (through cortical subcortical channels) can writing be considered an automatic skill. Limited experimental conditions can disrupt the writing system in normal subjects, probably interfering with the cortical subcortical loops, and link normality to pathology. In neurodegeneration, such as in Alzheimer' Disease, writing is precociously impaired and the disruption is early macroscopically evident.

Chapter XI - Late onset Alzheimer's disease (AD) is considered as a polygenic disorder resulting from the coincidence of a moderate number of genetic functional variants, located in candidate genes and others, each contributing small effects. Many studies focused mainly on identifying common risk alleles make it possible to predict the conversion from normal cognitive individual to Mild Cognitive Impairment (MCI), and from MCI to neurodegenerative dementia. The authors review the increasing literature about the genetics of AD under the light of their experience. The authors report a prospective study of apolipoprotein E (APOE) genotype in 89 patients diagnosed as MCI based on the Petersen criteria and supported by the MMSE, GDS scale and neuropsychological tests. After a median follow up of 49.6 months, 27 subjects remained with MCI and 62 subjects developed AD. This latest group was stratified again into two subgroups considering whether they converted to AD before (n=40) or after (n=22) 20 months of evolution. In order to assess the risk associated to each genotype, a control group (n=90) matched for age and sex and without memory impairment (MMSE≥28) was included. Patients who developed AD showed significantly lower values than MCI subjects in the CAMCOG (76% sensitivity and 67% specificity), for prompt detecting the onset of AD, with a 4.65-fold times increased risk of converting to AD ($p<0.001$). The presence of at least one APOE 4 allele was associated with risk of developing MCI (OR: 6,04; 95%CI: 2,76–13,23; p<0,001) but did not have an effect on the predictive cumulative hazard ratio (HR: 1.2; 95%CI: 0.73-2.1; p:0.32) of developing AD. Though it did not reach a statistically significant level, the presence of at least one APOE 2 allele showed a protective effect for the risk of developing MCI (OR: 0,57; 95%CI: 0,14–2.26). No patient was homozygous for 2/2 and no patient with rapidly progressive disease carried the 2 allele either (HR: 0.4; 95%CI: 0.05-2.7; p: 0.25). The authors data demonstrated a strong association of APOE 4 carrier status by itself with MCI, predicting a higher risk to suffer MCI. APOE 2 variant showed an interesting protective effect to MCI. Notwithstanding, the presence of at least an allele 4 when the patient is suffering MCI did not change the probability of progression to AD.

Chapter XII - Nitric oxide and free oxygen molecular species would constitute integral system components in the realization of a neuroinflammatory series of events damaging cerebral cortical neurons in the Alzheimer brain. The impact of such processes of reactive injury would be manifested particularly in the development of injury to cerebral endothelial cells as progressive amyloid deposition and amyloid angiopathy in these patients. The blood-brain barrier and the distribution of neuritic plaques would attest to the evolving onset dynamics of a process of cell injury culminating in death of neurons. Nitric oxide as a primarily locally diffusible agent in the progression of neuritic and neuronal injury would implicate microglia as active participants in the progression of the Alzheimer brain process. Recognition of the various pathways that would contribute to neuroinflammation in Alzheimer disease would attest to a multiplicity of events in onset and progression culminating in ischemia/reperfusion injury and of excitotoxity of both neurons and endothelial cells. Thus a coupled series of parallel pathways would evolve implicating a neuronal and endothelial cell series of interactive pathologic lesions in the Alzheimer disease onset and progression of injury.

Chapter XIII - The n-3 polyunsaturated fatty acids, particularly docosahexaenoic acid (DHA), exert certain effects on the spatial cognition of normal and Alzheimer's disease (AD) model rats. Spatial cognition-related memory refers to the ability to recall previously navigated cues oriented in a specific arrangement in the individual's environment. The ability to navigate the hidden platform in the water maze and to obtain a reward (food-pellet) at the ends of the arms of the radial maze is always greater in DHA-fed rats than in control rats. The enhancement of spatial cognition is associated with both an increase in the molar ratio of DHA to arachidonic acid (AA) and a decrease in the oxidative stress in the hippocampus and cortex regions of the brains of rats administered dietary DHA. Since the hippocampus plays a crucial role in the constitution of the cognitive map and in the concomitant navigation through memory to past events, the authors demonstrate that DHA exerts a positive effect on accurately constituting the hippocampal map, on the occurrence of related background cellular events at the synapse and on restoring spatial cognition. Moreover, the AD individual characteristically suffers from continued loss of learning and cognitive memory with concomitant neuronal dysfunction attributed to amyloid β (Aβ) peptide-induced formation of neuritic plaques and neurofibrillary tangles. Therefore, the effects of dietary DHA on memory loss in AD subjects have been estimated. Immunochemical studies on AD model animals produced by infusing $A\beta_{-401}$ peptide into the cerebral ventricle of rats have revealed that the infusion of the peptide injures the neurons of the hippocampus and cortex and increases the level of DNA fragments. The memory-related performance of AD model rats has been measured in the shuttle avoidance system apparatus or in the eight-arm radial maze. The infusion of the peptide results in the impairment of both active avoidance-related and reference and working memory-related learning abilities, well-known characteristics of AD. The administration of dietary DHA prevents the impairment of active avoidance-related learning ability in the shuttle avoidance system apparatus and ameliorates the impairment of reference and working memory-related learning ability in the radial maze task. Both learning abilities correlate positively with the cortico-hippocampal DHA/AA molar ratio. Oxidative stress, believed to initiate deposition of Aβ peptide and to raise the levels of lipid peroxide and reactive oxygen species in the brains of AD subjects, is significantly lower in DHA-fed AD model rats than in AD model rats. Data suggest that DHA plays a positive role in constituting/restoring memory-retrieving neuro-connections involved in the associative functions of the cortex and the hippocampus, and that animals administered DHA perform better than controls.

Chapter XIV - Normal episodic memory and navigation require intact hippocampi and surrounding structures. Both are damaged in the early stages of Alzheimer's disease (AD). Specific cognitive dysfunction during early stage AD and the progressive course of AD offer an opportunity to understand the neural bases of higher cortical function and dysfunction both in human memory and in human spatial cognition. Understanding how residual cerebral functions compensate and cope with the progressive neural compromise – and associated cognitive impairment – also helps the authors to pinpoint the neural substrates of complex cognitive processes.

After a brief review of the literature concerning navigational disorders in patients with AD, the authors introduce their previous and current studies.

First, the authors describe a study investigating navigational skills in community-residing early AD patients. Following an average 37 months of disease duration, more than 50% of the participants had easily detected navigational problems, and 18% reported getting lost (GL) – a complete spatial disorientation requiring escort from others to return home – at least once. Second, the authors describe results from interviews of individuals caring for AD patients who had been lost at least once. These interviews focused on the settings in which GL occurred. Most of the patients first got lost in the early stage of AD in familiar places. Most had a definite destination at the beginning of the GL episode; some exhibited stereotypical search behaviors shortly after becoming disoriented. Third, the authors describe results from three experiments designed to test a retrogenetic account of navigational capacities in early AD patients. These theoretically driven experiments included measures of learning and recognition of novel landmarks, egocentric route learning, and allocentric map formation. The results confirm that navigational disorder appears in early stage AD and follows a sequence reverse to the topographic abilities a human develops over childhood.

The authors conclude that specific forms of navigational problems appear early in the clinical course of AD. Whether these demonstrable failures in cognitive mapping are based on progressive hippocampal damage, and whether the authors are studying a variant of AD in which navigational disorder manifests an incipient symptom, remain open questions.

In: Alzheimer's Disease Research Trends
Editor: A.P. Chan, pp. 1-10
ISBN 978-1-60021-712-8

Expert Commentary

ALZHEIMER'S DISEASE: THE CALMODULIN CONNECTION AND β-AMYLOID

Danton H. O'Day[1,*] ***and Michael A. Myre***[2]
[1]Department of Biology, University of Toronto at Mississauga, Mississauga, Ontario L5L 1C6, Canada;
[2]MassGeneral Institute for Neurodegenerative Disease, Harvard Medical School Massachusetts, MA 02129-9142, USA.

ABSTRACT

The calcium hypothesis of Alzheimer's Disease (AD) invokes the disruption of calcium signaling as the underlying cause of neuronal dysfunction and ultimately apoptosis. Since the intracellular effects of calcium are mediated by calcium binding proteins, the next logical step in this model is to define the targets that calcium is regulating. We have been interested in the role of calmodulin, the primary calcium binding protein in eukaryotic cells, as a potential regulator of the effects of calcium in the onset of AD. To this end, we have identified a large number of potential calmodulin-binding proteins linked to the formation, degradation and turnover of amyloid-β (Aβ). It has recently been shown that the β-site amyloid converting enzyme 1 or β-secretase (BACE1) binds to calmodulin-agarose *in vitro*. Furthermore, the β-amyloid precursor protein (βAPP) and its two closely related homologs, the amyloid precursor-like proteins 1 and 2, (APLP1/APLP2) are also retained on Ca^{2+}-dependent calmodulin-agarose. These interactions with calmodulin were also detected by co-immunoprecipitation experiments. These and other data suggest that follow-up research should explore the possible role of calmodulin in the development of familial and late-onset AD.

* Correspondence concerning this article should be addressed to Danton H. O'Day, Department of Biology, University of Toronto at Mississauga, Mississauga, Ontario L5L 1C6, Canada. Phone: 905-828-3896; Fax: 905-828-3792; email: doday@utm.utoronto.ca.

INTRODUCTION

The "amyloid hypothesis" is based upon the presence of protein aggregates called amyloid plaques in the brains of Alzheimer's patients. Amyloid plaques are fibrous aggregate of mis-folded proteins—predominantly fibrils of the peptide amyloid-β (Aβ) (Petkova et al, 2005). The amyloidogenic pathway predominantly produces Aβ40 and Aβ42 through the sequential proteolytic processing of βAPP. Evidence suggests that Aβ42 is the more toxic fragment of the two species with respect to AD pathology (Dobson, 2004). The amyloid hypothesis suggests that increased production of Aβ initiates the pathological cascade that leads to Alzheimer's disease (Hardy 1997, Selkoe, 1999). This cascade begins with the formation of amyloid plaques followed by neurofibrillary tangle (NFT) formation. These events lead to progressive neuronal dysfunction, locally increased inflammatory responses, and finally dementia due to the eventual death of neurons. Arguably, the amyloid hypothesis remains the dominant theory based upon the current understanding of how AD develops, and so most translational research has been focused on the development of therapeutic strategies aimed at reducing Aβ load (Annaert and De Strooper, 2002; De Strooper & König 2001). However, early Aβ detection methods have yet to be developed such that by the time AD symptoms appear, it's too late to reverse the amount of neuronal loss and subsequently halt the disease.

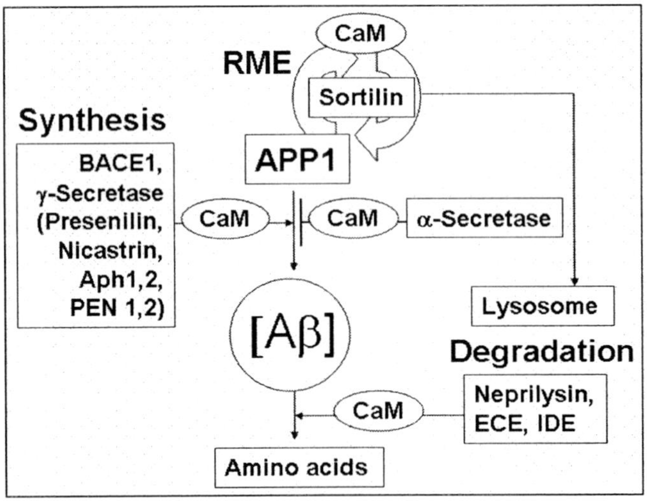

Figure 1. The synthesis, degradation and turnover of beta-amyloid. Beta-amyloid (Aβ) production from amyloid β precursor protein (APP) occurs through the action of BACE1 (β site-amyloid converting enzyme 1 or β-secretase) in concert with γ-secretase. γ-secretase is a tetrameric protein comprised of at least four different component proteins: anterior pharynx defective 1 a or b (APH-1a), nicastrin (Nic); presenilin enhancer protein 2 (PEN-2); and presenilin-1, -2 (PSN-1, 2). Alpha-secretase inhibits Aβ formation by producing non-amyloidogenic peptides from APP. APP trafficking involving sortilin-1 may reduce Aβ production by limiting APP-BACE interactions through the secretory system. Processing of APP to Aβ is also reduced by proteasomal degradation prior to entry into secretory vessicles. A number of Aβ degrading enzymes also exist including neprilysin, endothelin-converting enzyme (ECE) or the insulin-degrading enzyme (IDE). Calmodulin (CaM) is found and regulates a number of enzymes in each of the aforementioned pathways where Aβ production has been shown to occur.

The pathways leading to Aβ formation, endocytosis and degradation are summarized in Figure 1. The level of Aβ production in neurons requires an initial cleavage of βAPP by BACE1 which releases the large extracellular soluble βAPP fragment leaving a membrane bound C-terminal fragment (βCTF) 99 amino acids in length (C99) BACE1 has been shown to also cleave APP downstream at a second site to generate β'CTF (C89). The C99 transmembrane fragment is then cleaved by a presenilin-dependent γ-secretase to produce Aβ40 or Aβ42 (other Aβ species have also been shown to exist). The multimeric γ-secretase is comprised of at least four known transmembrane proteins including nicastrin, presenilin1/2, presenilin enhancer protein 2 (PEN-2) and presenilin stabilization factor-1 (or anterior pharynx defective 1; Aph-1) (Mattson, 2003). Cleavage of the bCTF requires a novel enzymatic reaction that takes place in the lipid bilayer that has been termed regulated intramembrane proteolysis (RIP; Xia and Wolfe, 2003). The more common pathway is the non-amyloidogenic cleavage of APP by α-secretases. Here, α-secretase cleaves within the Aβ domain precluding formation of Aβ (Kojro and Fahrenholz, 2005). After βAPP leaves the ER it enters the secretory pathway where it can be internalized by receptor-mediated endocytosis, where it is either metabolized or recycled back to the trans-golgi network (TGN) or cell surface for Aβ formation. βAPP may also be processed internally by the proteasome precluding Aβ production (Nunan et al, 2001). Aβ levels can also be reduced through the enzymatic degradation of specific proteases including neprilysin, endothelin converting enzyme, and the insulin-degrading enzyme. In spite of the excellent current state of knowledge, much remains to be learned about Aβ formation.

The Calcium Hypothesis of Alzheimer's Disease

An overwhelming body of scientific literature details the importance of calcium homeostasis and signal transduction in neuronal function. Homeostatic intraneuronal levels of calcium are maintained through fluxes across the cell membrane (e.g., via L-type, N-type Ca^{2+} Channels), by uptake and release from intracellular stores (e.g., endoplasmic reticulum, mitochondria) and from various calcium-binding proteins (e.g., CaBPs, calmodulin). Neuronal stimulation leads to increases in intracellular calcium levels that, in turn, lead to controlled neurosecretion, among other things. The "Calcium Hypothesis" of Khachaturian (1989) proposed that sustained alterations to calcium homeostasis, or as LaFerla (2002) puts it "calcium dyshomeostasis", are the underlying cause of Alzheimer's Disease (AD). In support of this there is evidence that increasing levels of intracellular calcium can drive the formation of some of the characteristic lesions of AD such as the accumulation of amyloid-β (Mattson and Chan, 2003). While increased calcium may affect amyloid-β (Aβ) peptide accumulation, Aβ itself can further perturb calcium homeostasis likely by forming unregulated pores in the cell membrane (Small et al. 2001). Since calmodulin is the primary calcium binding protein and effector of calcium signaling, any alterations in intracellular calcium levels would most likely impact the regulatory nature of this essential protein. In fact, AD brain tissue contains numerous examples of altered protein phosphorylation pathways (Jin and Saitoh, 1995). In keeping with this, the hyperphosphorylation of the microtubule-associated protein tau and production of NFTs, has been attributed to calcium/calmodulin-dependent protein kinase II (CaM kinase II; Wang et al, 2007). Our goal has been to understand the implications of the calcium hypothesis to downstream cell signaling and function mediated by calmodulin during the onset of AD.

Early Work on CaM and AD

Previous studies on the relationship between calmodulin and AD have been sporadic and few in number. Some of that work might at first glance seem to argue against the role of CaM in AD but careful consideration shows that this may not be the case. For example, using radioimmunoassay to quantify calmodulin levels, McLachlin et al (1987) found that the level of calmodulin protein in frontal, temporal, parietal cortex and sub-adjacent white matter of Alzheimer brains was two-thirds lower than that of normal, aged matched control brains in the brains of individuals with dementia and without AD pathology. In addition frontal cortex CaM was shown to be less efficient at activating Ca^{2+}/CaM regulated cAMP phosphodiesterase. The problem here is that only a single CaM-regulated enzyme was evaluated while other more relevant CaM-binding proteins that have been linked to AD were not studied, and the brain regions most affected including the hippocampus. Furthermore, the status of CaM signaling systems in AD brains has not been fully evaluated in lieu of the known Ca^{2+} dysfunction. CaM is known to undergo conformational changes affecting its function based on ion levels. CaM also shows differential target activation as a result of post-translational modifications (e.g., phosphorylation, prenylation). Since the potentially diverse roles of CaM in regulating AD proteins remain to be resolved, the significance of reduced CaM to AD neurons cannot simply be dismissed. For example, the absence of CaM may in fact serve to enhance the activity or protein-protein interactions that lead to Aβ formation and/or it may lead to excess intracellular Ca^{2+} simply by its absence or by affecting the ion channels linked to calcium homeostasis. Ca^{2+}/CaM signal transduction is not only regulated by the level of calcium ions or post-translational modifications but also by the presence and binding efficacy of various calcium binding and CaM-binding proteins. Recent work has shown that phosphorylation (e.g., Ser^{55}) of the regulator of calmodulin signaling (RCS) protein enhances its binding to CaM. This makes calmodulin unavailable for binding to other CaM-binding proteins such as protein phosphatase 2B which in turn affects the modulation of L-type Ca^{2+} channels in spiny neurons (Rakhilin et al, 2004). These are but a few of the factors that come into play when assessing the role of CaM and indicate the complexity of examining the role of CaM in AD neurons. In summary, no existing data rule out a role of CaM in the development or pathology of AD. Instead, there is accumulating theoretical and experimental data that suggest potential regulatory roles for CaM in the pathogenicity of the disease.

Neuronal Calmodulin Binding Proteins (CaMBPs)

Mammalian neurons are rich in calmodulin-binding proteins with at least 4 dozen present in differential amounts in different brain regions under different behavioral and physiological conditions (O'Day, 2003; O'Day et al, 2001). Many of these have been well characterized (e.g., neurogranin, neuromodulin, PSD-95, CASK, dynamin I, RACK1 and AKAP79) while others remain to be identified. CaMBPs, comprise a diverse group of proteins solely related by the fact that they interact with calmodulin, an interaction that usually is regulated by the intracellular level of calcium ions. In keeping with the vital role of CaM in all eukaryotic cells, CaMBPs are linked to many aspects of cell function. An unusual characteristic of CaMBPs is their lack of a conserved amino acid sequence for CaM-binding—the calmodulin binding domains show considerable variation in their amino acid sequences. Many Ca^{2+}-dependent CaMBPs have one or more CaM-binding domains (CaMBDs) approximately 20 amino acid residues in length that are characterized by a basic amphipathic helix which, when presented as an alpha-helical wheel, displays a segregation of hydrophobic residues on one side and basic charged residues on the other (Cohen and Klee, 1988; James et al, 1995; O'Neil and DeGrado, 1990). Calmodulin also binds a smaller number of target proteins (Ca^{2+}-independent CaMBPs) in the absence of calcium via IQ or IQ-like motifs (Bahler and Rhoads, 2002). Recently additional "novel" mechanisms of CaM-binding have come to light (Crivici and Ikura, 2005; Hoeflich and Ikura, 2003). Yap et al (2000) have developed an algorithm for identifying calcium-dependent CaM-binding domains that has been shown to be over 80% accurate in determining potential binding motifs. This approach has been used by our lab to identify potential CaM-binding motifs which are then experimentally identified using a diversity of cellular and molecular methods (e.g., Myre and O'Day, 2001, 2004; O'Day et al, 2005). It has also been used by others to determine the CaM-binding motifs of a diversity of human proteins detected by a novel screening method (Shen et al, 2005).

CaMBPs and beta-Amyloid Production

The production of Aβ from βAPP occurs through the sequential action of β-secretase (BACE1) and γ-secretase which is comprised of four component proteins (Figure 1). Each of the proteins involved were scanned for the presence of potential CaM-binding domains (O'Day and Myre, 2004). Of those, strong, putative Ca^{2+}-dependent CaMBDs were identified in Amyloid β Precursor Protein 1 (APP, 1 CaMBD); β-Secretase 1 (β-site-amyloid converting enzyme 1 or BACE1, 1 CaMBD); Nicastrin (Nic, 1 CaMBD); Presenilin enhancer protein 2 (PEN-2, 2 CaMBDs); Presenilin-1, -2 (PSN-1, 2 CaMBDs; PSN -2, 3 CaMBDs). In addition, nicastrin had two Ca^{2+}-independent IQ-like motifs (O'Day and Myre, 2004). Since experimental analyses have shown that there is an 80% chance such predicted CaM-binding domains are valid, this argues that at least 8 of the 10 will be valid Ca^{2+}-dependent CaMBDs. Additional research supports this. BACE1 has long been considered a prime target for pharmacological intervention (Vassar, 2001). Recent work suggests that BACE1 binds to calmodulin-agarose *in vitro* in a Ca^{2+}-dependent manner and, furthermore, CaM increases the activity of the enzyme *in vitro* while CaM antagonists inhibit the enzyme (Chavez and O'Day, 2007). Myre et al (2005) have also shown that mature full-length APP, APLP1 and APLP2 can be retained on calmodulin-agarose. In keeping with this, anti-CaM antibodies immunoprecipitate full-length APP, APLP1 and APLP2, while anti-APP, anti-APLP1 and anti-APLP2 antibodies pull down CaM from total mouse brain protein extracts. The CTFs did not bind CaM in either assay suggesting CaM interacts with the APP family of proteins upstream of each transmembrane domain. The predicted CaM-binding motifs in all three proteins appear to be located within the same regional domains based upon global alignment. The significance of these findings should be explored further.

Putative CaMBPs Linked to Amyloid Degradation

While therapeutic intervention historically has focused on the upstream components leading to the formation of Aβ, work on amyloid turnover including the role of the amyloid degrading enzymes has gained recent attention (Turner et al, 2004). The major enzymes of interest are neprilysin, endothelin converting enzyme, and insulin-degrading enzyme (IDE; Figure 1). Neprilysin levels decrease with aging leading to, among other things, a decreased ability to degrade Aβ. In support of this, neprilysin-deficient mice show increased levels of Aβ accumulation, amyloid-like deposits and behavioral deficiencies reminiscent of AD pathology (Madani et al, 2006). Similarly, Eckman et al (2003) have shown that Aβ is increased in endothelin converting enzyme-deficient mice. Like many proteins linked to AD, the relationship between IDE and late onset AD is not as clear. While some studies have shown a direct link, Nowotany et al (2006) have carried out a detailed study suggesting little if any relationship exists between enzyme variants for IDE and the risk for late onset AD. However, as these authors point out, many other factors come into play and certain groups show a direct relationship between IDE levels and late onset AD. These conflicting results need to be pursued further in order to determine the significance of IDE and Aβ degradation.

Information continues to accumulate on the role of these enzymes in the development of AD, so we examined their potential as CaM-binding proteins. Screening of the amino acid sequences using the Calmodulin Target Database reveals that each of these proteins contain at least one potentially strong Ca^{2+}-dependent CaM-binding domain that conforms to known motifs linked to CaM-binding (Table 1). A single putative Ca^{2+}-independent binding domain was also identified. Human neprilysin (P08473) was found to possess a strong CaM-binding domain at amino acids 180-201 but no evident IQ motifs. Human endothelin converting enzyme-1 (P42892) appears to contain one valid strong CaMBDs (673-695; Table 1). A potential Ca^{2+}-independent IQ-like domain (89-102) was also found in this protein (Table 1). Human IDE (P14735) revealed one strong (346-366) and several weak calcium-dependent but no calcium-independent CaM-binding domains. These data suggest at least two, if not all, of these Aβ-degrading enzymes physiologically bind calmodulin.

Calmodulin May Also Function in βAPP Endocytosis

A new way of looking at the way Aβ overproduction can be regulated in AD involves learning more about the secretory system and the receptor-mediated endocytosis of APP (Figure 1). The multifunctional endocytotic sortilin-related receptor (SORL1) was revealed to be involved in APP recycling leading to internalization of APP which would direct this precursor protein away from Aβ formation (Jacobsen et al, 1996). Rogaeva et al (2007) have since shown not only that inherited variants in neuronal SORL1 confer risk to late onset AD, but when SORL1 is under-expressed APP enters compartments directed towards Aβ formation. Because calmodulin is involved in various aspects of endocytosis in many cell types including neurons, we scanned human SORL1 (Q92673) for potential CaM-binding domains. No calcium-independent IQ motifs were detected but one strong calcium-dependent CaMBD (aa 148-161) was predicted that possessed a valid CaM-binding motif (Table 1) while a second moderately strong region (aa 2151-2170) did not contain a classic motif.

Table 1. Identification of Putative CaM-Binding Domains in Other AD-linked Proteins

Calcium-Dependent CaM-Binding Domains

Neprilysin (P08473, 180-201)
1 8 14
SWTAEKAIAQLNSKYGKKVLI
1 14
SWTAEKAIAQLNSKYGKKVLI
1 10
SWTAEKAIAQLNSKYGKKVLI
1 10
SWTAEKAIAQLNSKYGKKVLI

ECE-1 (P42892, 54-74)
1 14
SGQRCWAARTQVEKRLVVLVV
1 10
SGQRCWAARTQVEKRLVVLVV
1 16
SGQRCWAARTQVEKRLVVLVV

IDE (P14735, 346-366)
1 14
LSELKSKGWVNTLVGGQKEGA
1 10
LSELKSKGWVNTLVGGQKEGA
1 10
LSELKSKGWVNTLVGGQKEGA

SORL1 (Q92673, 148-161)
1 10
SYDYGKSFKKISDKLNFGLGNRSE

Calcium-Independent IQ Motifs

ECE-1 (P42892, 89-102)
IQYQTRSPSVCLSE

IDE, Insulin-degrading enzyme; ECE-1, Endothelin converting enzyme-1; SORL1, Sortilin-related receptor

Conclusion

The identity of the pathogenic signaling mechanism(s) that regulate Aβ fibril formation and consequently neurodegeneration are still under active study. Any work that provides insight into the regulation of amyloid plaque formation may provide new therapeutic routes to treat and someday prevent such neurological diseases. We have identified the presence of classic Ca^{2+}-dependent and -independent CaMBDs in the major proteins linked to the formation, degradation and endocytosis of Aβ. This is supported by evidence that at least two of these proteins can bind calmodulin and that BACE1 activity is enhanced by CaM *in vitro*. However, the role of CaM in the specific *in vivo* function of these and the other putative CaM-binding proteins that we have identified remains to be shown. The more we learn about how CaMBPs may be linked to Aβ formation, the greater will be our ability to develop new and specific drugs for the treatment of specific aspects of the disease.

Acknowledgements

This project was supported by a grant from the Natural Sciences and Engineering Research Council of Canada.

References

Annaert, W. and B. De Strooper, 2002. A cell biological perspective on Alzheimer's disease. *Annu. Rev. Cell Dev. Biol. 18*: 25–51.

Bahler, M. and A. Rhoads, 2002. Calmodulin signaling via the IQ motif. *FEBS Lett. 513*: 107-113.

Chavez, S. E. and D. H. O'Day, 2007. Calmodulin binds to and regulates the activity of Beta-Secretase (BACE1). In: *"Current Research on Alzheimer's Disease."* Nova Science Publishers, Inc., Hauppage, New York.

Cohen, P. and C.B.Klee (Eds.), Calmodulin. *Molecular Aspects of Cellular Regulation, Vol. 5.*, Elsevier, Amsterdam, 1988.

Crivici, A. and Ikura, M. 1995. *Ann. Rev. Biophys. Biomol. Struct. 24*: 85-116.

De Strooper B and G. König, 2001. An inflammatory drug prospect. *Nature 414*: 159–60.

Dobson, C.M., 2004. Protein chemistry: In the footsteps of alchemists. *Science 304*: 1259, 1261–1262.

Eckman, E. A., Watson M., Marlow L., Sambamurti K. and Eckman C. B. (2003). Alzheimer's disease β-amyloid peptide is increased in mice deficient in endothelin-converting enzyme. *J. Biol. Chem. 278*: 2081–2084.

Hardy J. 1997. Amyloid, the presenilins and Alzheimer's disease. *Trends Neurosci. 20*: 154–159.

Hoeflich, K.P. and M. Ikura, 2003. Calmodulin in action: Diversity in target recognition and activation mechanisms. *Cell 108*: 739-742.

Jacobsen, L, P. Madsen, S.K. Moestrup, A.H. Lund, N. Tommerup, A. Nykjaer, L. Sottrup-Jensen, J. Gliemann and C.M. Petterson, 1996. Molecular characterization of a novel human hybrid-type receptor that binds the alpha2-macroglobulin receptor-associated protein. *J. Biol. Chem. 271*: 31379-31383.

James, P., T. Vorherr and E. Carafoli, 1995. *Trends Biochem. Sci. 20*: 38-42.

Khachaturian, Z.S., 1989. Calcium, membranes, aging, and Alzheimer's disease. Introduction and overview. *Ann. NY Acad. Sci. 568*: 1–4

Jin, L.W. and T. Saitoh, 1995. Changes in protein kinases in brain aging and Alzheimer's disease. Implications for drug therapy. *Drugs and Aging 6*: 136-149

Kojro E, and F. Fahrenholz. 2005. The non-amyloidogenic pathway: structure and function of alpha-secretases. *Subcell. Biochem. 38*:105-27.

LaFerla, F.M., 2002. Calcium dsyhomeostasis and intracellular signalling in Alzheimer's disease. *Nat. Rev. 3*: 862-872

Madani, R., R. Poirier, D.P. Wolfer, H. Welzl, P. Groscurth, HP. Lipp, B. Lu, M. El Mouedden, M. Mercken, R.M. Nitsch and M.H. Mohajeri, 2006. Lack of neprilysin suffices to generate murine amyloid-like deposits in the brain and behavioral deficit in vivo. *J. Neurosci. 84*: 1871-1878.

Mattson, M.P., 2003. Ballads of a protein quartet. *Nature 422*: 385-387.

Mattson, M. P. and S. L. Chan, 2003. Neuronal and glial calcium signaling in Alzheimer's disease. *Cell Calcium 34*: 385-397

McLachlin, D.R., L. Wong, C. Bergeron and K.G. Baimbridge, 1987. Calmodulin and calbindin D28K in Alzheimer disease. *Alzheimer Dis. Assoc. Disor. 1*: 171-179.

Myre, M. A. and D. H. O'Day, 2002. Nucleomorphin: A novel, acidic, nuclear calmodulin-binding protein from *Dictyostelium* that regulates nuclear number. *J. Biol. Chem. 277*: 19735-19744.

Myre, M. A. and D. H. O'Day, 2004. Calmodulin binds to and inhibits the activity of phosphoglycerate kinase. *Biochim. Biophys. Acta, Mol. Cell Res. 1693*: 177-183.

Myre, M.A., R.E. Tanzi and W. Wasco, 2005. Calmodulin binding to the APP and the APLPs. Presentation P020 at Molecular Mechanisms of Neurodegeneration: a Joint Biochemical Society/Neuroscience Ireland Focused Meeting, Dublin, Republic of Ireland.

Nowatny, P. et al, 2005.. Association studies between risk for late-onset Alzheimer's Disease and variants in insulin degrading enzyme. *Am. J. Med Genetics Part B (Neuropsych. Genetics) 136B*: 62-68.

Nunan J, Shearman MS, Checler F, Cappai R, Evin G, Beyreuther K, Masters CL, and DH. Small. 2001. The C-terminal fragment of the Alzheimer's disease amyloid protein precursor is degraded by a proteasome-dependent mechanism distinct from gamma-secretase. *Eur. J. Biochem. 268*: 5329-5336.

O'Day, D. H., M. A. Lydan, J. Watchus, & A. S. Fleming, 2001. Decreases in Calmodulin Binding Proteins and Calmodulin Dependent Protein Phosphorylation in the Medial Preoptic Area at the Onset of Maternal Behavior in the Rat. *J. Neuroscience Research 64*: 599-605.

O'Day, D. H., 2003. CaMBOT: Profiling and Characterizing Calmodulin Binding Proteins. *Cellular Signalling 15*:347-355.

O'Day, D. H. and M. A. Myre, 2004. Calmodulin Binding Domains in Alzheimer's Disease Proteins: Extending the Calcium Hypothesis. *Biochemical Biophysical Research Communications 320*: 1051-1054.

O'Neil, K.T. and W.F. DeGrado, 1990. How calmodulin binds it targets: sequence independent recognition of amphiphilic α-helices. *Trends Biochem. Sci. 15*: 59-64.

Petkova A.T., et al., 2005. Self-propagating, molecular-level polymorphism in Alzheimer's beta-amyloid fibrils. *Science 307*: 262–265.

Rakhilin, S.V., P.A. Olson, A. Nishi, N.N. Starkova, A.A. Fienberg, A.C. Naim, D.J. Surmeier and P. Greengard, 2004. A network of control mediated by regulator of calcium/calmodulin-dependent signaling. *Science 306*: 698-701.

Rogaeva, E. and 40 authors, 2007. The neuronal sortilin-related receptor SORL1 is genetically associated with Alzheimer disease. *Nature Genetics Online 14 January* 2007 (doi:10.1038/ng1943).

Selkoe, D.J., 2001. Clearing the brain's amyloid cobwebs. *Neuron 32*: 177–180.

Shen, X., C.A. Valencia, J.W. Szostak, B. Dong and R. Liu, 2005. Scanning the human proteome for calmodulin-binding proteins. *Proc. Natl. Acad. Sci USA 102*: 5969-5974.

Small, D.H., S.S. Mok, and J.C. Bornstein, 2001. Alzheimer's disease and Aβ toxicity: from top to bottom. *Nat. Rev. Neurosci. 2*: 595–98.

Turner, A.J., L. Fisk and N.N. Nlaivaeva, 2004. Targeting amyloid-degrading enzymes as therapeutic strategies in neurodegeneration. *Ann. N.Y. Acad. Sci 1035*: 1-20.

Vassar, R., 2001. The β-secretase, BACE. A prime target for Alzheimer's disease. *J. Mol. Neurosci. 17*: 157–170.

Wang, J., Grundke-Iqbal I, and K. Iqbal. 2007. Kinases and phosphatases and tau sites involved in Alzheimer neurofibrillary degeneration. *Eur. J. Neurosci. 25*: 59-68.

Xia, W. and M.S. Wolfe. 2003. Intramembrane proteolysis by presenilin and presenilin-like proteases. *J. Cell Sci. 116*: 2839-2844.

Yap, K.L., J. Kim, K. Truong, M. Sherman, T. Yuan, and M. Ikura, 2000. Calmodulin Target Database. *J. Struct. Funct. Genomics 1*: 8-14.

In: Alzheimer's Disease Research Trends
Editor: A.P. Chan, pp. 11-15

ISBN 978-1-60021-712-8

Chapter I

ALZHEIMER'S DISEASE – 100 YEARS OF RESEARCH *A HISTORICAL PERSPECTIVE AND COMMENTARY*

Walter J. Lukiw
LSU Neuroscience Center and Department of Ophthalmology, Louisiana State University Health Science Center, New Orleans LA 70112, USA.

In November 1906, in Tubingen Germany, Alois Alzheimer (1864-1915) first described his laboratory's clinical and neuropathological findings on a then novel neurological disorder in one of his female clinical cases named Auguste D. Alzheimer's first patient had been institutionalized by her concerned family at the age of 51 and died of a progressive dementia just four years later [1]. Although the clinical features of this disease of the aged were long known since ancient times, and referred to as a 'senile psychosis', or 'age-related madness', Alzheimer was probably the first to observe the association of senile plaque (miliary foci) and neurofibrillary tangle (fibrils) propensity within the association neocortex with disease diagnosis and severity [1-5]. Alzheimer's advances in linking the clinical symptoms with novel neuropatholgical findings in this disease were enabled by the concurrent development of highly sensitive silver-staining, and related techniques, applied to human tissue sections pioneered by Maxwell Bielchowsky (1845-1928), Franz Nissl (1860-1926), Gaetano Perusini (1879-1915), Rudolph Virchow (1821-1902), Camillo Golgi (1844-1926), Santiago Ramon y Cajal (1852-1934) and others. Interestingly, Alzheimer's and his colleagues' description of a biophysical and ultrastructural basis for 'senile psychosis' and disease pathology was highly controversial for that time, and at odds with other theories for these kinds of afflictions, such as the series of psychoanalytical hypotheses proposed by Sigmund Freud (1856-1939) and his colleagues [6]. Although 'Alzheimer's disease', an eponym for this now common affliction, was given by Alzheimer's colleague and mentor Emil Kraepilin (1856-1926) in about 1910, Alzheimer's findings remained somewhat of a medical and neurological curiosity for many years, and it was not until almost 6 decades later that any new significant developments were reported that further expanded our clinical, neuropathological and biological understanding of this serious neurological disorder.

The modern era of Alzheimer's disease research really began with a series of important ground-breaking papers in the middle-to-late sixties by Kidd, Terry, Gonatas and Weiss on the ultrastructural aspects of the Alzheimer's disease lesions. In these studies neurofibrillary tangles were discovered to be twisted paired helical filaments, and complex amyloid-containing structures were found to be a major component of the insoluble senile 'miliary' plaques [7-10]. Shortly thereafter, Blessed, Tomlinson and Roth were the first to realize that microscopic examination of autopsied brains from the vast majority of all senile dementia/senile psychosis cases actually contained pathological features consistent with a diagnosis of the neuopathogical entity which Alzheimer had originally described [11-12]. Hence, it has only been about 4 or 5 decades since these discoveries have gradually brought interest in Alzheimer's disease to the medical research forefront.

During this period, the 'amyloid beta (Aβ) peptide cascade hypothesis', that amyloid production, morphology, speciation, deposition and it's neuropathological consequences, such as being a trigger for brain-specific oxidative and neuron-inflammatory processes, lies at the very heart of the Alzheimer process, has progressed to the extent that the neurobiology and genetics of Aβ peptides are now probably one of the most thoroughly studied entities in all of modern cell biology [3-5,13-15]. However, despite massive research efforts, the precise role of amyloid peptides in the initiation and progression of Alzheimer's disease remains unresolved, and open to serious question; the biological role of neurofibrillary tangle formation has received considerably less research attention [2,15,16]. Significant advances in Alzheimer's disease and amyloid research are the subject of several excellent comprehensive reviews, this being the 100th anniversary of the first description of Alzheimer's disease, and interested readers are encouraged to study them along with the references contained therein [2-5,13-15].

Interestingly, several of these recent reviews have come to the common and gloomy conclusion that currently, a very great deal of work remains to be done in the second century of Alzheimer's disease research, and that if Auguste D. were alive today, 'her sad prognosis would be pretty much the same as in 1906' [3].

The socioeconomic costs of Alzheimer's senile dementia are a very serious and growing concern as our elderly currently represent the fastest growing segment of our aging population. Recent epidemiological studies show that globally, about 25 million people today have senile dementia, with approximately 5 million new cases of dementia occurring every year, and with one new case being reported every 7 seconds [17-19]. Worldwide, the total number of people affected by dementia is expected to double every 20 years to at least 81 million by 2040 with Western civilizations and developing countries at particular risk [17,18]. In the United States alone, the average annual cost of Alzheimer's disease patient care is soaring out of control, and has been currently estimated to be about 100 billion dollars [17-19]. Our deeper understanding of the neurobiology of aging, basic Alzheimer's disease molecular mechanisms, and the prevention of Alzheimer's disease, remains a primary medical research concern, and effective drugs to treat Alzheimer's disease are an urgent pharmacological goal [18-22]. Unfortunately, while many primary clinical trials for

Alzheimer's disease are ongoing, *no primary pharmacological-based prevention trial has yet successfully delayed the development of this prevalent neurological disorder* [19]. Whether our basic understanding of the Alzheimer's disease process is severely flawed, or if longer clinical trials, or alternative pharmacological strategies are required, is open to question and debate. What is not controversial is that, without question, new understanding, novel research methodologies and new clinical treatments are essential to more effectively address the Alzheimer's disease problem. Alternative treatment approaches such as those involving the use of omega-3 fatty acid supplementation, docosahexanoic acid (DHA) and its derivatives, cholesterol reducing statins, novel antioxidants and chelators, natural herbal treatments from the extensive Chinese pharmacopeia, and many others, are receiving a lot of current research attention [19-24]. Western medical approaches to age-related diseases more often than not favor 'quick fix' strategies for healing progressive diseases that take many decades to develop. Significant non-pharmaceutical-based protection against Alzheimer's disease can be clearly obtained from life-long lifestyle changes. Diets reduced in saturated fat, enriched in omega-3-fatty acids and antioxidants, appropriate weight maintenance, regular physical activity and Alzheimer health care education collectively represent statistically significant and highly cost effective long-term therapeutic solutions [17-21]. It is unfortunate that in the recent "Perfect Storm" of dwindling National Institutes of Health research support, and at a time of most critical need, when opportunities for scientific progress and advances in Alzheimer research have never been greater, that significantly less federal funding is available to support the eager battalions of highly qualified and research-ready Alzheimer's disease investigators and their medical and graduate students whose research will ultimately define the future progress and treatment of this expanding health care problem [25-27].

REFERENCES

[1] Alzheimer A, Stelzmann RA, Schnitzlein HN, Murtagh FR. An English translation of Alzheimer's 1907 paper, "Uber eine eigenartige Erkankung der Hirnrinde". *Clin Anat. 8*:429-431 (1995).

[2] Iqbal K, Grundke-Iqbal I. Discoveries of tau, abnormally hyperphosphorylated tau and others of neurofibrillary degeneration: a personal historical perspective. *J Alzheimers Dis. 9*:219-242 (2006).

[3] Hardy J. A hundred years of Alzheimer's disease research. *Neuron 52*:3-13 (2006).

[4] Mott RT, Hulette CM. Neuropathology of Alzheimer's disease. *Neuroimaging Clin N Am. 15*:755-765 (2005).

[5] Tanzi RE, Bertram L. Twenty years of the Alzheimer's disease amyloid hypothesis: a genetic perspective. *Cell 120*:545-555 (2005).

[6] Freud S. The origin and development of psychoanalysis by Sigmund Freud, 1910. *Am J Psychol.* 1987 Fall-Winter;100(3-4):472-88.

[7] Kidd M. Paired helical filaments in electron microscopy of Alzheimer's disease. *Nature 197*:192-193 (1963).

[8] Kidd M. Alzheimer's disease - an electron microscopical study. Brain 87:307-320 (1964).

[9] Terry R, Gonatas Nk, Weiss M. Ultrastructural studies In Alzheimer's presenile dementia. *Am J Pathol. 44*:269-297 (1964).

[10] Terry RD, Gonatas NK, Weiss M. The ultrastructure of the cerebral cortex in Alzheimer's disease.*Trans Am Neurol Assoc. 89*:12-16 (1964).

[11] Tomlinson BE, Blessed G, Roth M. Observations on the brains of non-demented old people. *J Neurol Sci. 7*:331-356 (1968).

[12] Blessed G, Tomlinson BE, Roth M. The association between quantitative measures of dementia and of senile change in the cerebral grey matter of elderly subjects. *Br J Psychiatry. 114*:797-811 (1968).

[13] Golde TE, Dickson D, Hutton M. Filling the gaps in the Aβ cascade hypothesis of Alzheimer's disease. *Curr Alzheimer Res. 3*:421-30 (2006).

[14] Hardy J. Alzheimer's disease: the amyloid cascade hypothesis: an update and reappraisal. *J Alzheimers Dis. 9*:151-153 (2006).

[15] Armstrong RA. Plaques and tangles and the pathogenesis of Alzheimer's disease. *Folia Neuropathol. 44*:1-11 (2006).

[16] Lee HG, Casadesus G, Zhu X, Takeda A, Perry G, Smith MA. Challenging the amyloid cascade hypothesis: senile plaques and amyloid-beta as protective adaptations to Alzheimer disease. *Ann N Y Acad Sci. 1019*:1-4 (2004).

[17] Ferri CP, Prince M, Brayne C, Brodaty H, Fratiglioni L, Ganguli M, Hall K, Hasegawa K, Hendrie H, Huang Y, Jorm A, Mathers C, Menezes PR, Rimmer E, Scazufca M; Alzheimer's Disease International. Global prevalence of dementia: a Delphi consensus study. *Lancet 366*:2112-2117 (2005).

[18] Zhu CW, Scarmeas N, Torgan R, Albert M, Brandt J, Blacker D, Sano M, Stern Y. Longitudinal study of effects of patient characteristics on direct costs in Alzheimer disease. *Neurology 67*:998-1005 (2006).

[19] Thal LJ. Prevention of Alzheimer disease. *Alzheimer Dis Assoc Disord. 20*:S97-S99 (2006).

[20] Lukiw WJ, Cui JG, Marcheselli VL, Bodker M, Botkjaer A, Gotlinger K, Serhan CN, Bazan NG. A role for docosahexaenoic acid-derived neuroprotectin D1 in neural cell survival and Alzheimer disease. *J Clin Invest. 115*:2774-2783 (2005).

[21] Lukiw WJ. Cholesterol and 24S-hydroxycholesterol trafficking in Alzheimer's disease. *Expert Rev Neurother. 6*:683-693 (2006).

[22] Kruck TP, Cui JG, Percy ME, Lukiw WJ. Molecular shuttle chelation: the use of ascorbate, desferrioxamine and Feralex-G in combination to remove nuclear bound aluminum. *Cell Mol Neurobiol. 24*:443-459 (2004).

[23] Ren Y, Houghton P, Hider RC. Relevant activities of extracts and constituents of animals used in traditional Chinese medicine for central nervous system effects associated with Alzheimer's disease. *J Pharm Pharmacol. 58*:989-996 (2006).

[24] Wang R, Yan H, Tang XC. Progress in studies of huperzine A, a natural holinesterase inhibitor from Chinese herbal medicine. *Acta Pharmacol Sin. 27*:1-26 (2006).

[25] Wadman M. Disappointment in slow-down for biomedical funding. *Nature 433*:559 (2005).

[26] Weinberg RA. A lost generation. *Cell 126*:9-10 (2006).

[27] Zerhouni EA. Research funding. NIH in the post-doubling era: realities and strategies. *Science 314*:1088-1090 (2006).

In: Alzheimer's Disease Research Trends
Editor: A.P. Chan, pp. 17-22

ISBN 978-1-60021-712-8

Chapter II

EVIDENCE-BASED CARE INTERVENTION AIMED AT REDUCING BEHAVIORAL AND PSYCHOLOGICAL SYMPTOMS OF DEMENTIA (BPSD) AMONG ELDERLY WITH DEMENTIA USING THE PROGRESSIVELY LOWERED STRESS THRESHOLD MODEL

Masao Kanamori[1,*] and Mizue Suzuki[2]

[1]Biwako Sport College, Seikei University, Kitahira 1204, Ohtsu-city, Shiga, 520-0503, Japan;

[2]Mie-prefectural college of Nursing, Yumegaoka 1-1-1, Tsu, Mie-pref. 514-0016, Japan.

ABSTRACT

Behavioral and psychological symptoms of dementia (BPSD), a term that has been applied to behavioral disturbance among elderly dementia patients in recent years, requires appropriate treatment and care intervention. BPSD not only increases caregiver burden, but also significantly reduces the quality of life (QOL) of elderly dementia patients. Hall (1987) proposed the progressively lowered stress threshold model (PLST), which states that elderly dementia patients are at an increased risk to develop BPSD due to anxiety behavior resulting from a decreased stress threshold. In addition, using the PLST, Gerdner (2000) developed a mid-range theory as a hypothesis for the effects of music therapy on elderly dementia patients, and reported a reduction in the "agitation"

* Correspondence concerning this article should be addressed to Masao Kanamori, MD, PhD, Biwako Sport College, Seikei University, Kitahira 1204, Ohtsu-city, Shiga, 520-0503, Japan. E-mail: kanamori@bss.ac.jp; TEL/FAX:81-77-596-8466.

symptom of BPSD due to stress reduction. However, neither Hall nor Gerdner performed measurements of stress hormones to demonstrate their relationship with the onset of BPSD.

Herein, we investigate the effects of music therapy and animal-assisted therapy on elderly dementia patients, with regard to levels of salivary Chromogranin A (CgA), a glycoprotein that is a more sensitive indicator of stress than cortisol, in addition to changes in BPSD before and after intervention. Salivary CgA was measured immediately before and after intervention for the intervention group and also for the control group. Following a total of 6 sessions of animal-assisted therapy conducted over a 3-month period for 7 elderly dementia patients residing at home and using daycare services, significant improvements in "aggressiveness" and "anxieties and phobias" of the behavioral symptoms in Alzheimer's disease (Behave-AD) were observed, in addition to a tendency toward a reduction in salivary CgA that was not significant. Similar results were obtained for pet type robot-assisted therapy, in which a pet-like robot was used instead of animals. Furthermore, following a total of 16 sessions of music therapy conducted over a 3-month period, significant improvements in "confusion", "irritability", "agony", and "inability to control bladder and bowel" on the GBS scale were observed, in addition to a significant reduction in salivary CgA.

These findings suggest that animal-assisted therapy and music therapy are effective for reducing BPSD in elderly dementia patients, and that stress reduction induced by intervention may result in BPSD reduction. In the future, it will be necessary to further develop care intervention for reducing BPSD in elderly dementia patients. Salivary CgA may be effective in studies of evidence-based care intervention due to its sensitivity to small changes in stress.

TEXT

The behavioral disorders associated with dementia were once referred to as behavioral abnormalities or problematic behaviors. In 1999, the International Psychogeriatric Association proposed the collective term "behavioral and psychological symptoms of dementia" (BPSD) [1]. BPSD is common among the elderly with dementia, and it not only increases caregiver burden, but also significantly reduces the quality of life (QOL) of elderly patients with dementia. Establishing nonpharmacological therapy for BPSD and clarifying the effects of such nonpharmacological therapy are important goals for research on elderly patients with dementia. According to the American Psychiatric Association Practice Guideline, care intervention plays a very important role in a nonpharmacological approach [2], and intervention methods focusing on behaviors, emotions, recognition, and stimulation have been reported. In clinical settings, various care intervention methods have been developed, but there has not been sufficient evidence to support their efficacy. The progressively lowered stress threshold (PLST) is a conceptual model based on stress and coping proposed by Hall, and it is used for care of patients with dementia [3]. We have been assessing the effectiveness of music and animal-assisted therapies, which are interventional methods based on stimulation to alleviate BPSD, using PLST in terms of behaviors and stress. The present study investigated care intervention to alleviate BPSD in elderly patients with dementia and introduced evidence for care intervention using PLST.

According to the PLST model of Hall and colleagues [3], even healthy adults exhibit anxious behaviors when experiencing strong stress, but such anxious behaviors can be alleviated through stress control. However, because the stress threshold for patients with dementia is low, slight stress can induce not only anxious behaviors, but also BPSD. The mid-range theory [3,4] is a model for music therapy based on PLST (a stress and coping model) proposed by Hall and colleagues [5], and Gerdner [4,5] documented the effectiveness of the music therapy for alleviating agitation that can be induced by slight stress in elderly patients with dementia. Of the various components of BPSD, agitation is one of the behaviors that cannot be easily treated [1]. Cohen-Mansfield [6] defined agitation as "inappropriate verbal, vocal, or motor activity that is not judged by an outside observer to result directly from the needs or confusion of the agitated individual", and factor analysis yielded three syndromes of agitation: aggressive behavior (such as hitting and kicking), physically nonaggressive behavior (such as pacing and inappropriate robbing or disrobing), and verbally agitated behavior (such as complaining and constant requests for attention) using the Cohen-Mansfield Agitation Inventory (CMAI).

Gerdner [7] studied the effects of individualized music in five elderly patients with dementia of the Alzheimer's type (DAT) who were in a long-term care facility and who showed agitation. A modified CMAI was used to measure the outcome. The immediate and 1-hour residual effects suggested the potential of individualized music as an alternative approach to the management of agitation in agitated elderly patients. In the next Gerdner study, 39 subjects were recruited from six long-term-care facilities [4]. The subjects consisted of 30 women and 9 men (mean age, 82 years) with severe cognitive impairment. Baseline data were collected for 3 weeks. Group A (n = 16) received individualized music for 6 weeks followed by a 2-week "washout" period and 6 weeks of classical "relaxation" music. Group B (n = 23) received the same protocol but in the reverse order. Music interventions were presented for 30 minutes twice a week. The analysis of statistical method showed a significant reduction in agitation during and following individualized music compared to classical music. While the 1993 report was a case study [7], the 2000 study examined reduction in agitation due to music therapy by objective techniques in a total of 39 subjects. Gerdner [8] focused on the relationship between elderly patients with dementia and their caretakers and clarified that agitation could be significantly improved with individualized music therapy administered by family members and trained caretakers. Gerdner reported that music therapy could alleviate agitation in elderly patients with dementia, but did not assess stress.

We further clarified the effects of nursing intervention by assessing BPSD, activities of daily living (ADL), and stress [9,10]. In collaboration with music therapists, we administered music therapy and assessed its effectiveness by measuring the level of salivary chromogranin A (CgA), a stress indicator. Salivary CgA is an acid glycoprotein (439 amino acid residues) isolated from chromaffin granules in the adrenal medulla. The concentration of CgA has a direct relationship to catecholamine in saliva; therefore, testing for catecholamine is a precise indicator of CgA levels [11].

In the first study of music therapy, the subjects were 10 patients with senile dementia who received music therapy; 6 had DAT and 4 had vascular dementia. The music therapy was performed twice a week for 8 consecutive weeks (16 sessions) [9]. As a result, the total scores of the Mini-Mental State scale did not significantly change, but the scores of a subscale, "language", were improved significantly. In the Multidimensional Observation Scale for Elderly Subjects, the scores of "irritability" decreased significantly. Regarding changes in salivary chromogranin A (CgA) levels, the average was significantly decreased before session 16 compared to after that.

In the second study, a music therapy group consisting of 8 elderly patients with dementia and a control group including 8 similarly matched patients received a total of 25 one-hour sessions of music therapy that were conducted twice weekly for three months [10]. The Gottfries-Brane-Steen Scale and the Behavioral Pathology in Alzheimer's Disease Rating Scale were used to evaluate behavioral changes. Saliva chromogranin A (CgA) and immunoglobulin A (IgA) were used to assess changes in stress and immunological status, respectively. On the Gottfries-Brane-Steen Scale, the mean score for "different symptoms common in dementia" improved significantly after music therapy. The mean Behavioral Pathology in Alzheimer's Disease Rating Scale score for "paranoid and delusional ideation" also significantly improved ($p<0.05$) after the intervention. While IgA was slightly increased prior to intervention, by the 25th session, the mean CgA was significantly decreased ($p<0.05$). Because music therapy has been reported to improve immune function, the level of IgA was measured in the second study, but no change was seen in IgA. Therefore, based on these two studies, music therapy as proposed by Gerdner alleviated stress, and this was supported by the decreased levels of salivary CgA. Furthermore, music therapy improved not only agitation, but also BPSD and some cognitive functions, and the second study clarified ADL improvements.

Moreover, we investigated the effects of animal-assisted therapy in terms of salivary CgA levels. After a total of 6 sessions of animal-assisted therapy conducted over a 3-month period for 7 elderly patients with dementia residing at home and using daycare services, significant improvements in "aggressiveness" and "anxieties and phobias" of the behavioral symptoms in Alzheimer's disease (Behave-AD) were observed, in addition to a tendency toward a reduction in salivary CgA that was not significant [12]. Pet-type robot-assisted therapy utilizes a pet robot instead of a live animal, and this therapy has been shown to significantly lower salivary CgA levels and improve role functioning [13]. The above findings suggest that besides music therapy, animal-assisted therapy is effective in alleviating BPSD in elderly patients with dementia, and that care intervention can reduce stress and subsequently BPSD. Studies on music therapy have shown improvements in ADL, such as language (MMSE) and bathroom management (GBS). These improvements are believed to be due to reduced agitation. Based on Hall's model and our studies on music therapy and animal-assisted therapy, stress reduction lowers agitation, thus improving cognitive function and ADL and alleviating BPSD. In the future, it will be necessary to further develop more effective and efficiency care intervention for reducing BPSD in elderly patients with dementia. Because our study did not involve many subjects, it will be necessary to analyze more subjects with even more objective assessment methods. Salivary CgA may be effective in studies of evidence-based care intervention due to its sensitivity to small changes in stress.

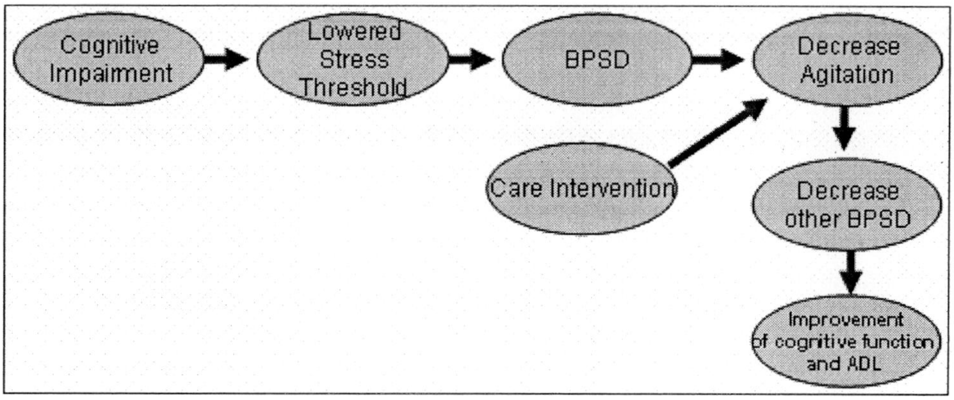

Figure 1. Hypothesis of Care Intervention Aimed at Reducing Behavioral and Psychological Symptoms of Dementia (BPSD).

References

[1] International Psychogeriatric Association (1999). *The BPSD educational pack.* First Japanese edition, Aruta Shuppan Co. Ltd., Tokyo

[2] American Psychiatric Association (1997*). Practice guideline for the treatment of patients with Alzheimer's disease and other dementia of late life.* first edition, Washington D.C.

[3] Hall, G.& Buckwalter K.C. (1987). Progressively lowered stress threshold: A conceptual model for care of adults with Alzheimer's disease. *Archives of Psychiatric Nursing, 1(6)*, 399-406.

[4] Gerdner, L.A. (1997). An individualized music intervention for agitation. *Journal of the American Psychiatric Nurses Association, 3(6)*,177-184.

[5] Gerdner L.A. (2000). Effects of individualized versus classical "relaxation" music on the frequency of agitation in elderly persons with Alzheimer's disease and related disorders. *International Psychogeriatric Association, 12(1)*, 49-65.

[6] Cohen-Mansfield J., Werner P., Marx M.S. (1989), An observational study of agitation in agitated nursing home residents., *Int Psychogeriatr. Fall, 1(2)*, 153-65.

[7] Gerdner, L.A.&Swanson, E.A.(1993). Effects of individualized music on confused and agitated elderly patients. *Archives of Psychiatric Nursing, 7(5)*, 284-291.

[8] Gerdner, L.A. (2005). Use of individualized music by trained staff and family. *Journal of Gerontological Nursing, 6* :22-30.

[9] Suzuki, M., Kanamori, M., Watanabe, M., Nagasawa, S., Kojima, E., Ooshiro, H., Nakahara, D. (2004). Behavioral and endocrinological evaluation of music therapy for elderly patients with dementia. *Nursing and Health Sciences, 6*, 11-18.

[10] Suzuki M., Kanamori M., Nagasawa S., Isowa T., Saruhara T. (2007). Music Therapy-Induced Changes in Behavioral Evaluations, and Saliva Chromogranin A and Immunoglobulin A Concentrations in Elderly Patients with Senile Dementia, *Gerontology & Geriatrics International, (in press)*

[11] Nakane H., Asai, O., Yamada, Y. (1998). Salivary chromogranin as an index of psychosomatic response. *Biomed Res, 19*, 401-406.

[12] Suzuki M., Kanamori M., Watanabe M., Nagasawa S., Kojima E., Ooshiro H., Nakahara N.(2004). *Behavioral and Endocrinological Evaluation of Music Therapy for Elderly Patients with Dementia Nursing and Health Sciences, 6(1)*, 11-8.

[13] Kanamori M., Suzuki M., Yamamoto K., Kanda M., Matsui Y., Kojima E., Fukawa H., Sugita T., Oshiro H.(2001).A day care program and evaluation of animal-assisted therapy (AAT) for the elderly with senile dementia. *Am J Alzheimers Dis Other Demen, 16(4)*, 234-239.

[14] Kanamori M, Suzuki M, Tanaka M.(2002). Maintenance and improvement of quality of life among elderly patients using a pet-type robot] *[Article in Japanese Nippon Ronen Igakkai Zasshi, 39(2), 214-218(in Japanese).*

In: Alzheimer's Disease Research Trends
Editor: A.P. Chan, pp. 23-56
ISBN 978-1-60021-712-8

Chapter III

POLYMER TEMPLATES HAVE AN ORGANIZING EFFECT ON Aβ AGGREGATION

Norbert W. Seidler and Randal C. Michelson
Department of Biochemistry, Kansas City University of Medicine and Biosciences, 1750 Independence Avenue, Kansas City, Missouri, USA.

ABSTRACT

Although amyloid-β (Aβ) peptide production and clearance are crucial to understanding Alzheimer's disease (AD), the intervening events of misfolding and aggregation lead directly to toxicity and therefore require complete elucidation in order to develop comprehensive approaches to therapy/prevention. We analyzed the innate propensities of Aβ to assume diverse conformations by careful examination of predicted structure and previously documented solution structures. Our comparisons of the solution structures of several Aβ fragments indicate the submissive nature of Aβ. The organizing effects of lipid-water interfaces, such as lipid rafts, and reticular networks of endogenous polymers, such as polyacrolein or melanoids, may direct the orientation of the Aβ chain segments. Secondary structure comparisons for the monomeric Aβ, protofibrils, and the predicted structures suggest that Aβ is susceptible to the organizing features of the microenvironment. Molecular models of polyacrolein illustrate the extensive two-dimensional properties of this organizing matrix. We discuss the potential significance of polymer templates as providing physico-chemical directives to Aβ peptides as they collapse to form stable aggregates.

INTRODUCTION

The amyloid-β (Aβ) peptide occupies the spotlight in Alzheimer's disease (AD) pathology and prevention of its formation represents the major therapeutic strategy. This small peptide is a product of selective proteolytic cleavage of the amyloid precursor protein

(APP), a ubiquitous single-spanning transmembrane protein [1]. There are three main isoforms of APP with 695, 751 and 770 amino acid residues. The 695-residue isoform, which is derived from a chromosome 21 gene that contains 16 exons, is predominant in neurons and interestingly lacks a protease inhibitor domain that is found on the other isoforms [2-4]. The multifunctional APP is held at the neuronal surface membrane and appears to be involved in processes that direct its lateral movement [5] proposing an APP-associated axonopathy. With about 90% of the protein projected extracellularly the N-terminal multidomain structure exhibits conformational agility [6].

Proteolysis is selective and the secretases along with their associated proteins regulate production of Aβ peptides. An initial proteolytic cleavage of the protein at a sequence that is projected just above the membrane surface releases the large ecto-structure. A second proteolytic event that cuts the transmembrane domain near the inner leaflet [7] releases the Aβ peptide, which is predominantly 40 residues in length. Peptides containing 38 to 43 amino acids are also released [8,9] with the Aβ (1-42) considered central to the disease process and found in extracellular plaques. The other major peptide, Aβ (1-40), which is missing the two C-terminal residues of Aβ (1-42), is associated with the formation of cerebrovascular plaques.

This chapter explores the innate propensity of the Aβ peptide to be submissive to the surrounding chemical milieu and describes the importance of interfaces in promoting conformational changes. Additionally, a novel conceptual framework is proposed in which biochemical scaffolds play a role in organizing the regular alignment of Aβ. In particular we discuss the evidence suggesting that plastic-like polymers may have an organizing effect on Aβ aggregation.

Innate Propensities of the Aβ Peptide

The sequence of amino acids in the Aβ peptide exhibits noteworthy features that may be ultimately useful in understanding the misfolding process of other amyloidogenic proteins. There appears to be an inherent propensity for conformational flexibility or wobble. Additionally, salient physico-chemical properties include hydrophobic patches which can form cores of residues with stable secondary structure. Concurrently, subsequently or prior to core formation, which involves β-strand stacking, the Aβ peptide can also form progressively stabilizing extended β-sheets.

Conformational Wobble

Understanding the factors involved in determining the secondary structure of Aβ remains an important research objective. A dominant theme in the etiology of AD positions a conformational event as foremost in the production of cytotoxic oligomers that contain β-sheets. What are the predispositions of the 40 or 42 amino acids in Aβ? The protein folding field provides us with algorithms that may be useful in predicting possible conformations. These predictions give an assessment of the intrinsic propensities of an amino acid based on their empirical predilections and their position relative to immediately surrounding residues.

We describe the properties of predicted structures using different algorithms. Secondary structure prediction has limitations, primarily because local secondary structure is often influenced by the context of the surrounding protein. In the case of small peptides without the context of tertiary structure, structural assessment depends on predictive modeling and solution structures in amiable media. Solution structures are reviewable in the Protein Data Bank [10], which lists the two major Aβ peptides (1-42 and 1-40) as well as several fragments (1-16, 1-28, 10-35 and 25-35). The solution structures of the peptides and their fragments were obtained under various conditions that are described below. The information contained in these experimental observations can be compared to intrinsic amino acid propensities. Careful analysis may help elucidate the impact that media components have on promoting specific adopted structures. We compared the solution structures among themselves and with predicted structures, yielding useful information. Lastly, the structure of the early Aβ aggregate, which is also available in the Protein Data Bank, was compared with the predicted structures and with the solution structures.

Predicted Structure

Web-based services exist for retrieving predictive analyses of submitted sequences. We used two websites: http://www.predictprotein.org and http://www.compbio.dundee.ac.uk to get predicted structures. These services employ algorithms described in published reports [11-14]. Four predicted structures were obtained through these services (Figure 1). Additionally, structures were prepared using the original algorithm established by Chou and Fasman [15,16] as well as a modified version [17]. The originally assigned values, which represent secondary structure propensities of the amino acids, are based on 29 proteins; the modified version is supported by a database of 1091 proteins. We present these predicted structures as having helical (H) regions, which include α-helices and 3_{10}-helices, β-strand (E) regions and loop (L) sequences, which include coils, bends and turns.

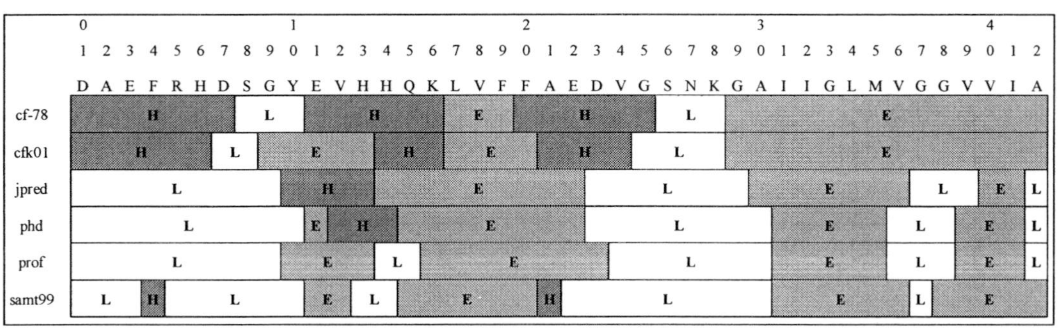

Figure 1. Secondary structure predictions. Designations are based on the original (cf-78) and modified (cfk01) algorithm of Chou and Fasman [15,16]. The other four predicted structures (jpred, phd, prof and samt99) are based on internet submission algorithms. The regions are defined as α-helical (H), β-strand (E) and loop (L) and aligned with the sequence of the Aβ (1-42) peptide.

The Chou-Fasman algorithm [15,16] for determining secondary structure allowed us to generate two predicted structures (Figure 1) that are useful in assessing amino acid susceptibility to conformational change. The first structure, cf-78, was generated from the original table of propensities, and the second structure, cfk01, was drawn from the updated list of amino acid propensities [17]. Both predicted structures, cf-78 and cfk01, have three α-helical regions and two loop sequences, which cover roughly the same areas. The second loop sequence (^{26}Ser-^{28}Lys) is likely a reverse turn, which is determined using the rules adopted by Rose where minimum hydropathy values occur in sequences not designated as having structure [18]. Both of the Chou-Fasman-derived predictions, cf-78 and cfk01, exhibit two β-strand regions that are in nearly identical positions. The cfk01 presents with another β-strand region (^{9}Gly-^{13}His). In fact, the middle region of the Aβ (1-42) peptide (^{9}Gly-^{25}Gly) appeared the most variable among the predicted secondary structures.

The propensities for α-helix and β-strand in this middle region seem equi-dominant. The algorithm assigns numerical values reflecting the propensities of amino acids to adopt an α-helix or β-strand. Values that are greater than 1.0 indicate a greater than average tendency for that amino acid to be found in an α-helix or β-strand. Each amino acid has two propensity values, one for forming α-helices and the other for forming β-strands. The rules include a method for assessing origins of nucleation, which then dictate the propagation of α-helices or β-strands. Using these rules we found three α-helical and two β-strand nucleation sites (Table I). Nucleation site A, which is in the N-terminus, only exists for α-helical formation. Potential secondary structure overlaps in site B, where nucleation can occur for both α-helical spreading and β-strand formation. In comparing the average propensities for α-helix versus β-strand formation in nucleation site B, which spans ^{9}Gly-^{24}Val, we observed near similar values: cf-78, 1.15 versus 1.13, respectively; cfk01, 1.09 versus 1.14, respectively. Both are greater than 1.0 indicating a favored conformation. The similarity in value suggests an either/or situation with no definitive dominance. Nucleation site C exists for both secondary structure types, but the propensities clearly favor β-strand formation.

Table I. Comparison of the average propensities within the designated secondary structure nucleation sites as defined by the Chou-Fasman algorithm

Type of Secondary Structure	Nucleation Site	Number of Amino acids	Location	Average Propensity cf-78	Average Propensity cfk01
α - helix	A	7	^{1}Asp - ^{7}Asp	1.18	1.09
	B	15	^{10}Tyr - ^{24}Val	1.15	1.09
	C	16	^{27}Asn - ^{42}Ala	1.00	0.95
β - strand	A	No nucleation site possible in this region			
	B	14	^{9}Gly-^{22}Glu	1.13	1.14
	C	13	^{30}Ala-^{42}Ala	1.25	1.27

The average propensities were calculated from the grouped propensities of the various tetrapeptides drawn within the respective stretches of amino acids. Note the similarity of the average propensity for the overlapping α-helical and β-strand nucleation site B, suggesting that these amino acids exhibit a nearly equal tendency toward the two types of secondary structure.

Let's further consider this middle region. We subtracted the β-strand propensity from the α-helix propensity ($P\alpha$ - $P\beta$ = Df), providing a determinant factor that assesses the committedness of the amino acid for a given secondary structure. A positive value indicates a strong commitment to forming an α-helix. A value close to zero suggests that the two propensities cancel each other with no residual propensity to either secondary structure. And a negative value indicates a strong commitment to forming a β-strand. When the propensity difference (Df) was plotted for the 42 residues (Figure 2A and 2B), the middle region (9-29) exhibited the greatest appearance of variability with values of alternating signs. The N-terminus appears α-helical dominant and the C-terminus, β-strand dominant with respect to their predicted tendencies.

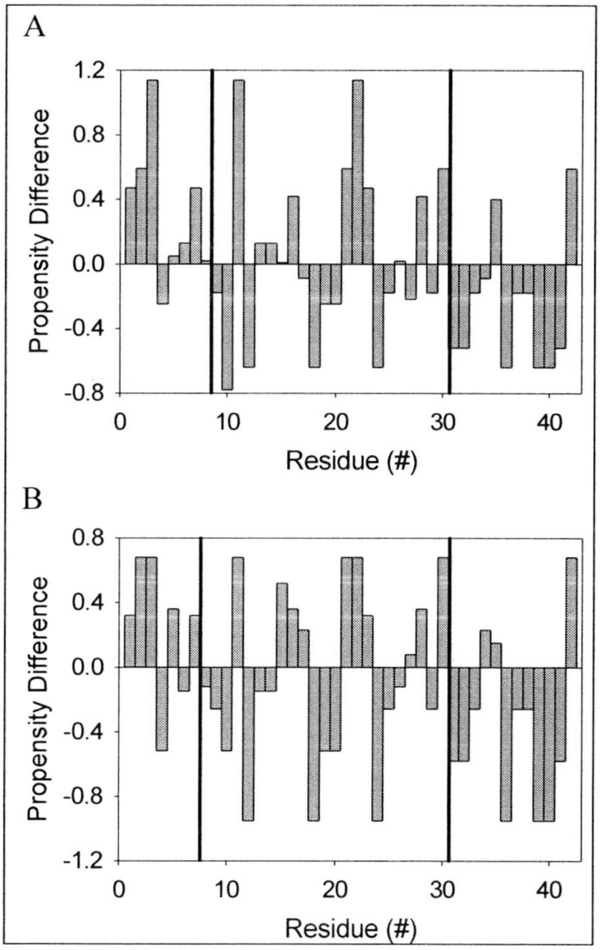

Figure 2. Propensity differences of each of the amino acids in Aβ. The Chou-Fasman-derived propensity to form a β-strand was subtracted from the propensity to form an α-helix in order to assess the preferred tendency of each amino acid. These values ($P\alpha$ - $P\beta$ = Df) are presented as a function of their positions in the peptide of the predicted structures, cf-78 (A) and cfk01 (B). Arbitrary vertical lines are drawn to demark a region that upon visual inspection appears potentially destabilizing in its ability to hold secondary structure.

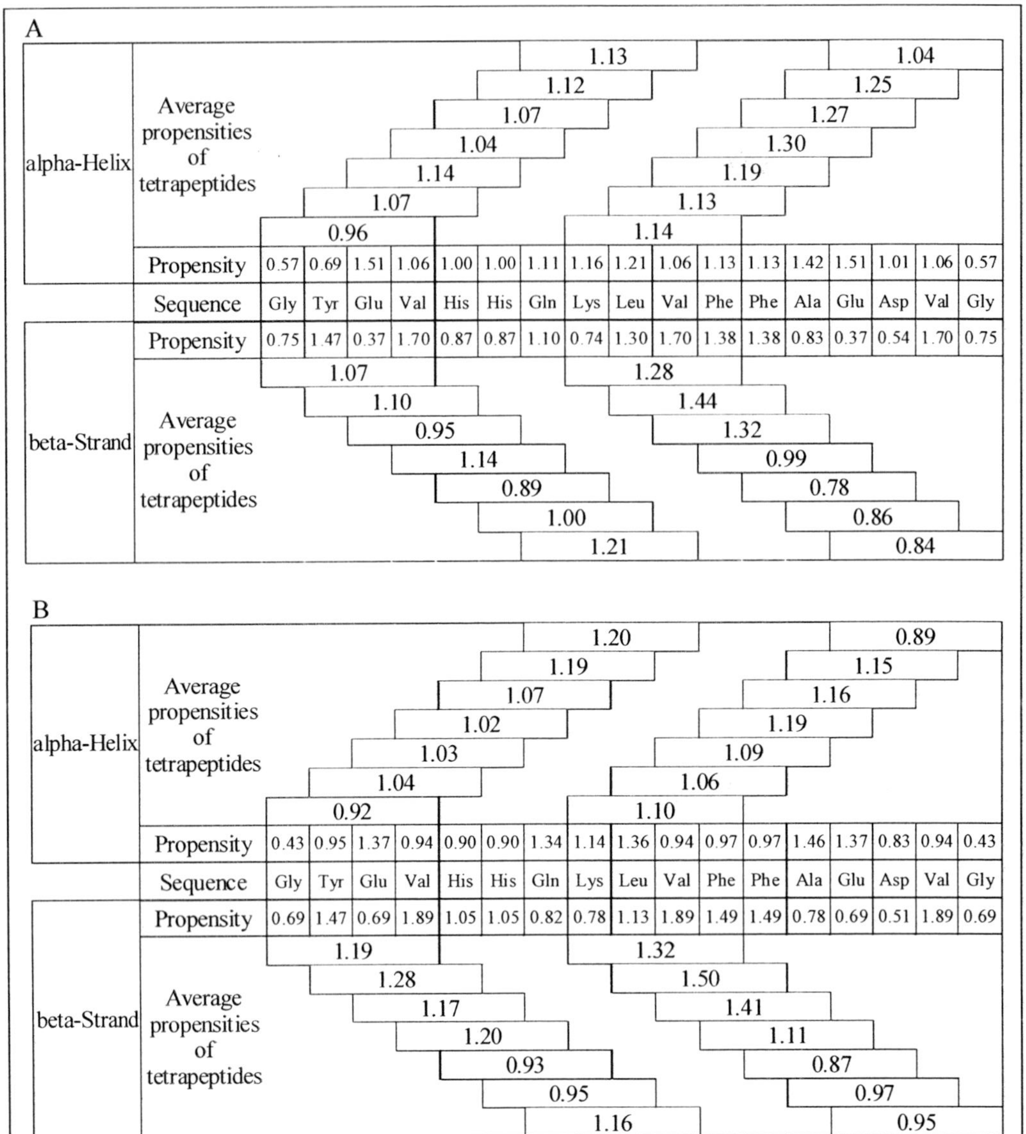

Figure 3. Propensities of individual amino acids and tetrapeptides in sequence ^{9}Gly-^{25}Gly. The α-helical and β-strand propensities were obtained from the original Chou-Fasman algorithm [15,16] that yielded the predicted structure cf-78 (A) and from the modified algorithm [17] that generated cfk01 (B). The indicated sequence contains a nucleation site (site B from Table I) for potential propagation of both α-helices and/or β-strands.

Looking more closely at this middle region (Figure 3), we see that the propensities of the individual amino acid residues as well as the grouped propensities of the drawn tetrapeptides provide little guidance as to the correct assignment of secondary structure. For the cf-78 prediction (Figure 3A), 14 out of 17 middle region residues show α-helical propensities above 1.0 with 93% of the tetrapeptides above 1.0, suggesting that this region favors α-helix. However, 57% of the β-strand tetrapeptides also exhibit propensities above 1.0, suggesting this region has no clearly predictable identity. The cfk01 confirms the findings of cf-78.

Although only 6 of the 17 residues in cfk01 (Figure 3B) show α-helical propensities above 1.0, 86% of the average α-helical tetrapeptides are above 1.0, suggesting a strong tendency to want to form α-helical structures. Juxtaposed to this predicted feature, 64% of the average β-strand tetrapeptides exhibit propensities above 1.1 (36% above 1.2), suggesting the contrary, that there's a strong tendency towards forming β-strands. These observations speak to an underlying structural conflict that may seek resolve in the environment.

We secured web-based predictions of Aβ peptide and compared them with the predictions (cf-78 and cfk01) derived from the Chou-Fasman algorithms (Figure 1). Consistently, the middle region exhibits the greatest variability. Nevertheless, some common features are apparent: a loop sequence centered on the ^{8}Ser; a β-strand centered on ^{18}Val; another loop sequence centered around the ^{26}Ser-^{27}Asn; and consistent β-strand dominance at the C-terminus. Additionally, a loop sequence centered on ^{37}Gly appears in four out of six predictions. Of the 42 amino acids residues only 14 show exact identities across the six predicted structures, 10 β-strand and 4 loop residues. This observation of poorly predicted concordance suggests an innate propensity for conformational plasticity.

The distribution of amino acids appearing as α-helices, β-strands and loops varies among the predicted structures (Table II). For α-helix content, we see a range of 0-19 amino acid residues. An almost equally expansive range exists for the loop sequences in these structures, ranging from 6 to 22. Interestingly, the range for residues in β-strands is rather narrow, fluctuating only from 17 to 23. Some of the predictions are tenuous in that they are likely not to appear. An example of this is in the samt99 prediction which twice shows a single residue existing as an α-helix. Despite the impossibility of the assignment this was the retrieved result, and we felt it justified to keep this anomaly in place in order to further illustrate the innate flexible nature of the residues that make up the Aβ peptide.

Table II. Number and percentages of amino acids in predicted secondary structures

		cf-78	cfk01	jpred	phd	prof	samt99
α-Helix	Number of amino acids	19	13	4	3	0	2
	Percent of total	45%	31%	9%	7%	0%	5%
β-Strand	Number of amino acids	17	23	18	17	20	19
	Percent of total	41%	55%	43%	41%	48%	45%
Loop	Number of amino acids	6	6	20	22	22	21
	Percent of total	14%	14%	48%	52%	52%	50%

Predicted Versus Solution Structures

The solution structures of the two major Aβ peptides (1-42 and 1-40) and their fragments (1-16, 1-28, 10-35 and 25-35) are compared with the predicted structure, jpred (Figure 4). The incompatibility can be used to assess a susceptibility to conformational fluctuation. Such an analysis was conducted on the prion proteins [19] and other diverse amyloid-forming proteins including Aβ [17]. By comparing predicted and experimentally determined secondary structures, sequences can be identified as being discordant. This mismatch can provide an assessment of the conformational wobble that may give rise chain alignments favoring amyloid formation. Aβ shows α-helices in regions that are theoretically predicted to be β strands, which is considered a harbinger for amyloid fibril formation [17].

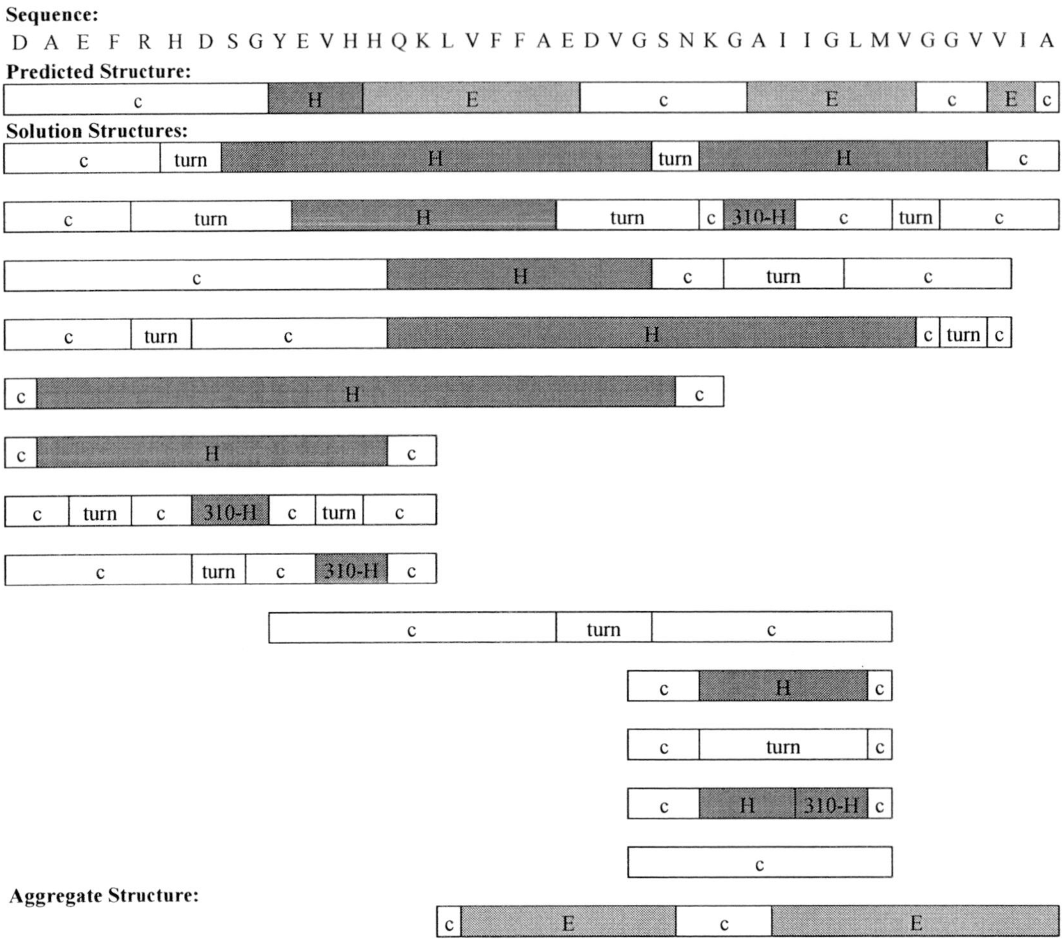

Figure 4. Comparison of predicted, solution and aggregate structures. The predicted structure, jpred, is compared with the various solution structures listed in Table III, in the order given in the table. The aggregate structure is from pdb.2beg. Secondary structure assignments are presented as in Figure 1 with the exception that coils, c, and turns are defined. 310H represents 3_{10}-helices.

The sequence ^{17}Leu-^{19}Phe is particularly worth noting. In all of the predicted structures (Figure 1), this stretch of amino acids occurs as a β-strand. To the contrary, solutions structure show α-helices in this region. Five of the six peptides and fragments that contain the ^{17}Leu-^{19}Phe sequence exhibit α-helices. Interestingly, these five solution structures were prepared in media containing fluoro-alcohols, either hexafluoroisopropanol (HFIP) or trifluoroethanol (TFE), or sodium dodecyl sulfate (SDS) micelles (Table III). The solution structure that does not show an α-helix in this region is the Aβ fragment (10-35), 1hz3, which presents with a coil. The structure of 1hz3 was obtained in water in the absence of fluoro-alcohols or SDS micelles.

Table III. Media conditions for determination of solution structures

Fragment	PDB	Medium	*p*H	Comments	Ref.
1 - 42	1iyt	80/20 (HFIP/water)	NA		[20]
	1z0q	70/30 (HFIP/water)	NA		[21]
1 - 40	1ba6	SDS micelles	5.3	^{35}Met is oxidized	[22]
	1ba4	SDS micelles	5.1		[23]
1 - 28	1amb	60/40 (TFE/water)	3.0		[24]
1 - 16	2bp4	80/20 (TFE/water)	3.0		[25]
	1ze7	Phosphate buffer	6.5		-
	1ze9	Phosphate buffer	6.5	Zn(II) ions are present	-
10 - 35	1hz3	Water	5.6		[26]
25 - 35	1qcm	LiDS micelles	4.0		[27]
	1qyt	SDS micelles	4.15		[28]
	1qwp	80/20 (HFIP/water)	4.5		[28]
	1qxc	20/80 (HFIP/water)	4.5		[28]

Additionally, the C-terminus is predicted to form β-strands (Figure 1) with a 57% to 100% concordance among the six predicted structures in the sequence containing ^{29}Gly-^{42}Ala. The solution structures tell a different story as no β-strands are observed in this region which has a range of helical content from 21% (1z0q) to 79% (1iyt). The other solution structures that overlap to this region exhibit diverse structures that include helices (α-type and 3_{10}-type), turns and coils. The secondary structural elements in this region appear to be dictated by the fragment investigated and the media conditions used.

The regions observed to be α-helical but are predicted as β-strands indicate intrinsic instability [17]. In the previous section we discussed the indeterminate features of the middle region including the predicted β-strand, which is observed as an α-helix sequence centered on ^{17}Leu-^{19}Phe. The duality of propensity of this region (Figures 2 and 3) is actualized in the solution structures. The discordance between predicted and experimental structures is also observed at the C-terminus, which is derived in part from the transmembrane helical domain of the protein of origin, APP.

The predicted structures, cf-78 and jpred, were compared quantitatively with the solution structures to assess the degree of discordance over the length of the peptide (Figure 5). We determined a concordance value as the number of similarities between cf-78 and each of the solution structures that contain a given residue. This value is a fraction that can reach 1 or zero at its extreme representing either all similarities or none, respectively. Concordance values were then calculated for each residue associated with cf-78 and jpred, averaged and plotted as a function of residue (Figure 5). Three concordance minima are observed at sequences ^{17}Leu-^{19}Phe, ^{30}Ala-^{36}Val and ^{40}Val-^{42}Ala, indicating maximum discordance. These regions are critical in amyloid fibril formation. A fragment of Aβ (1-42), which lacks the residues ^{14}His-^{23}Asp, does not form β-sheet containing fibrils as compared to the full-length peptide [29]. Additionally, alanine mutations at ^{16}Lys, ^{17}Leu and ^{20}Phe prevent fibril formation [30]. These findings support the significance of these discordant residues.

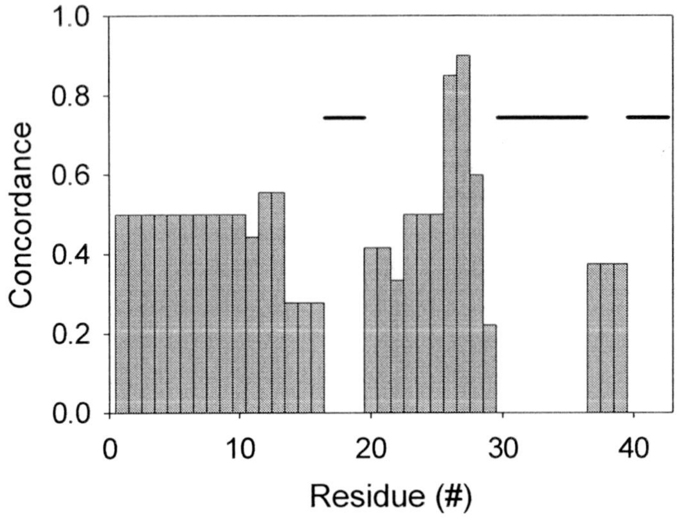

Figure 5. Middle and C-terminal sequences exhibit discordance. The predicted structures, cf-78 and jpred, were compared individually with the solution structures and then averaged. The average value assesses the degree of discordance over the length of the peptide. If all of the solution structures showed concordant secondary structure, the value would be 1.0. A score of zero indicates no concordance between the predicted structures and the solution. The bars represent discordant sequences.

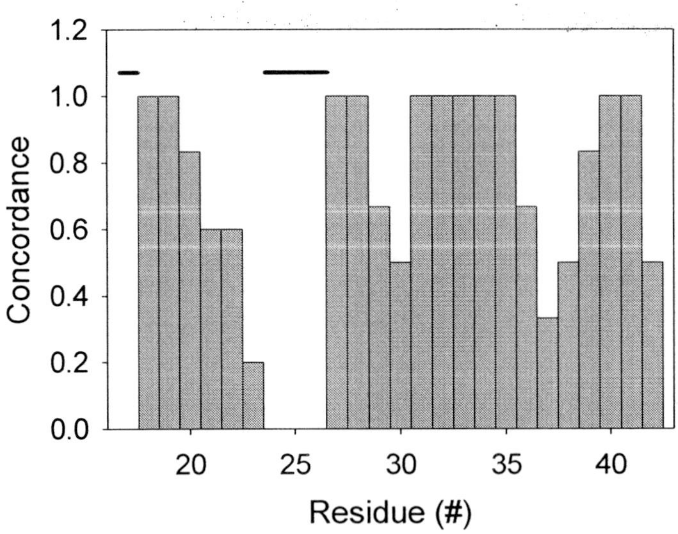

Figure 6. Sequences of minimum concordance are in the middle region. The aggregate structure, 2beg, were compared individually with the predicted structures, cf-78, cfk01, jpred, phd, prof and samt99, assessing concordance over the length of the peptide. Complete concordance in secondary structure gives a value of 1.0. A score of zero indicates no concordance between the aggregate structure and the predicted structures. The first 16 amino acids were not scored. The bars represent discordant sequences.

Predicted Versus Aggregated Structure

An aggregate structure (Aβ protofibril) is available in the Protein Data Bank under 2beg, which gives the structural assignment of 5 peptides in an aggregated state [31]. We compared the secondary structure of this aggregate and that of the predicted structures, which are presented in Figure 1. Concordance values were calculated for each residue associated with the predicted structures vis-à-vis the aggregate structure and plotted as a function of residue (Figure 6). Aside from ^{17}Leu, the only area of minimum concordance, and therefore maximum discordance, is the sequence ^{24}Val-^{26}Ser. Essentially, the region associated with a coil in the predicted structure is shifted relative to the coil seen in the aggregate structure. In the predicted structures the coil is centered around ^{26}Ser-^{28}Lys, whereas the experimental aggregate is centered around ^{28}Lys-^{29}Gly. The predicted coil is considered a turn since it contains very low hydropathy values [18]. The predicted turn is consistent with the bend that is created to allow for the inter-β-strand interaction of the side chains in the folded aggregate. The anticipated discordance would then be associated with the tightness of the turn, as the coil region in the predicted structures range from ^{22}Glu-^{30}Ala, which covers the tight coil seen in the aggregate structure, ^{27}Asn-^{30}Ala. A predicted large area that is unstructured would favor environmentally-directly changes to position the β-strands in the optimal orientation, promoting interaction and further β-sheet extension.

Solution Structures Versus Aggregate Structure

While it is interesting that the solution structures do not exhibit easily identifiable consistencies in their secondary structure, they have even less similarity to the aggregate structure (Figure 4). Concordance values were calculated for each residue associated with the solution structures relative to the aggregate structure. Aside from ^{17}Leu, which exhibited concordance with only the 1hze solution structure, the only area that exhibited concordance is the sequence ^{27}Asn-^{30}Ala. This unstructured coil or turn is a consistently important feature in all of these peptides and fragments, allowing the chain to bend. The two stretches of β-strand in the experimentally-derived aggregate structure show absolutely no concordance with any of the thirteen solution structures listed (Figure 4). Whether the conformation change occurs from coil to helix to strand or from coil to strand during Aβ aggregation, only the features of a coil or turn at ^{27}Asn are maintained.

Solution Structures

The intrinsic structural properties of Aβ can be assessed by examining the solution structures of the full-length peptides and their fragments, and by making comparisons within this group. Thirteen representations of secondary structure are presented here (Figure 4 and Table III). Differences are immediately noticeable. Among the solution structures, we see that many elements of secondary structure exhibit inconsistencies.

In looking at the two Aβ (1-42) solution structures (1iyt and 1z0q), we notice only a 52% homology in secondary structure despite that the conditions used to assess structure are fairly similar (Table III). HFIP/water mixtures were used with only a 10% difference in HFIP that contributes to the variability in secondary structure. Twenty amino acids deviate from their structural positions with most of the differences clustered by the C-terminal end of the peptide. The loss of structural homology due to changing HFIP concentrations suggests that the peptide is highly adaptable to the environment. In 80% HFIP, 30 amino acids out of 42 are in α-helices, whereas only 14 form helical structures in 70% HFIP. HFIP changes the dielectric constant of the medium making the solution more nonpolar. This may explain the C-terminal changes as this portion of the peptide (^{29}Gly-^{42}Ala) was derived from the transmembrane domain of APP. The more than 50% loss of α-helical content in going from 80 to 70% HFIP may be attributed to the α-helix stabilization effect of fluoro-alcohols [32].

Aβ (1-40) peptide structures (1ba6 and 1ba4) are only 60% alike with most of the deviations at the C-terminus. The lack of homology occurs around the ^{35}Met which is oxidized to methionine sulfoxide in 1ba6. Both Aβ (1-40) peptides were analyzed in a medium of SDS micelles, suggesting that the loss in hydropathy in that region may alter peptide-micelle interaction.

In comparing Aβ (1-42) in 80/20 (HFIP/water) to Aβ (1-40) in SDS micelles (1iyt versus 1ba6, respectively), we see a turn at ^{26}Ser-^{27}Asn with 80% HFIP that is abolished in the SDS medium. Clusters of HFIP with its bulky nonpolar group may allow for distant hydrophobic patches (^{17}Leu-Val-Phe-Phe-Ala and ^{30}Ala-Ile-Ile) to interact requiring a turn as seen in 1iyt and 1z0q.

The Aβ (1-28) fragment (1amb) exhibited a 46 to 69% structural homology with the Aβ (1-42 and 1-40) structures. The structure was determined in 60% TFE, and interestingly, the greatest homology is with Aβ (1-42) peptide, 1iyt, which was prepared in 80% HFIP. No turns are observed in the (1-28) fragment, 1amb. The absence of turns is likely due to the truncation of the fragment, which does not contain the C-terminal hydrophobic patches: ^{30}Ala-^{32}Ile, ^{34}Leu-^{36}Val and ^{39}Val-^{42}Ala. Furthermore, the α-helices in the (1-28) fragment, 1amb, extend almost to the N-terminus. Let's compare this to the previous peptides. Aβ (1-40) peptides do not propagate past the ^{13}His-^{14}His in the N-terminal direction and the Aβ (1-42) peptides do not propagate beyond the ^{6}His. While this may be in part due to the helical-stabilizing effect of TFE, the low *p*H may have contributed to α-helical formation by protonation of side chains. Aβ fragment (1-16), 2bp4, which was also in TFE at low *p*H, shows an 88% homology to 1amb over the same stretch of amino acids. The other (1-16) fragments, 1ze7 and 1ze9,which were at higher *p*H and in the absence of TFE, have helical content merely consisting of a 3-residue 3_{10}-helix. Deprotonation of ^{22}Glu and ^{23}Asp is associated with loss of the α-helical structure of the sequence ^{15}Gln-^{24}Val in the Aβ (1-40) peptide prepared in SDS [23]. Interestingly, by visual inspection it appears that the N-terminus of the larger peptides and fragments (1-42, 1-40 and 1-28) shows a large variability. When we compared the N-terminal fragments, Aβ (1-16), there is a paltry 29% homology suggesting that the N-terminal amino acids are highly promiscuous and easily influenced by media composition and *p*H.

The Aβ (10-35) structure, 1hz3, in contrast with those solutions structures determined in fluoro-alcohols or SDS, was analyzed in water. This fragment does not contain any α-helical regions. Interestingly, the (1-16) fragments prepared in aqueous buffer (1ze7 and 1ze9) were relatively devoid of helical content compared to 2bp4, which was prepared in 80% TFE. The loss of structure appears tightly dependent upon nonpolar components of the media. Consider the ^{10}Tyr-^{25}Gly stretch found in the Aβ (1-42) peptide, 1iyt, which was prepared in 80% HFIP and is 100% α-helix. The same stretch in 70% HFIP, 1z0q, or in SDS, 1ba6 or 1ba4, loses a third of its helical content. The same stretch in water, 1hz3, contains zero helical content. The Aβ (25-35) fragment, 1qwp, which demonstrates 60% helical structure in 80% HFIP contrasts with 1qxc, which does not exhibit any helical regions in 20% HFIP or the same stretch in 1hz3, also devoid of structure and which was prepared in water. These observations demonstrate the manipulative effects of the environment on Aβ.

Interior Packing

In addition to the conformation change from coil and helical structures to that of β-strands, the Aβ peptide appears to bend and fold such that the β-stands stack. The side chains project inward between the stacked stands as well as projecting outwards on the back side of the stack. From the stacked strands, the β-sheets propagate sideways. The stacking and sheeting are separate events with the stacking requiring side chain interaction. The stacking alignment is not perfect with a slight angle resulting in some inter-peptide interactions [31].

The interior packing of the stacked β-strands appears to involve hydrophobic residues. Patches of hydrophobic residues in a protein or peptide are prone to forming unproductive aggregates [33]. It is therefore understandable that patches of three or more contiguous hydrophobic residues are generally not found in globular proteins [34]. The Aβ peptide contains four hydrophobic patches: ^{17}Leu-^{21}Ala, ^{30}Ala-^{32}Ile, ^{34}Leu-^{36}Val and ^{39}Val-^{42}Ala, making this peptide quite susceptible to this hydrophobic aggregation. The folded aggregate shows a ^{23}Asp to ^{28}Lys salt bridge in the interior of the stack of β-strands [35]. Given this arrangement, it is likely that the interior contains ^{17}Leu, ^{19}Phe and ^{21}Ala from the one strand and ^{34}Leu, ^{32}Ile and ^{30}Ala from the other, forming a complementary hydrophobic core.

Interestingly, the last hydrophobic patch, ^{39}Val-^{42}Ala, in the Aβ (1-42) peptide does not exist in the Aβ (1-40) peptide. There are two additional hydrophobic residues (isoleucine and alanine) in the Aβ (1-42) peptide that create a stretch of four contiguous hydrophobic residues. The Aβ (1-42) aggregates much faster than the Aβ (1-40) [36], suggesting an added role for this hydrophobic patch. In reviewing the predicted structures (Figure 1), we see a possible turn or bend at the ^{37}Gly-^{38}Gly stretch, which is defined as a loop in several predicted structures. Were an additional stacking of another segment of β-strand (^{39}Val-^{42}Ala) to occur, then an interior packing would consist of ^{39}Val and ^{41}Ile from the terminal strand and ^{31}Ile from the previous strand. As sheets propagate, either prior to or after stacking, the adjacent interior cores would provide additional thermodynamic incentive toward extension.

Rules of β-Sheet Extension

Several diseases other than AD are associated with the misfolding and aggregation of specific proteins, each providing a signature for its disease. These diverse proteins likely follow a common path to aggregation that is regulated by intrinsic susceptibilities to misfolding. Additionally, proteins must carry structural barriers to unproductive protein-protein interaction. We even see that many proteins that are not directly related to specific pathologies can misfold and collapse to form aggregates. The common structural endpoint resembles amyloid fibrils.

Amyloid formation appears to be a general feature of protein misfolding. What are some of the barriers that must be in place to avoid peptide chain arrangements that are self-propagating and unproductive? We discussed at length the secondary structures changes that may arise, and we covered the issue of stacking of β-strands. Let's briefly discuss the process by which the resulting Aβ peptide β-strands extend into β-sheets. This is a process that must be allowable and favored by the intrinsic properties of the peptide. The propagation of β-sheets depends on the edge strand. The availability of backbone hydrogen bonds at the edge is crucial. In the case of Aβ, once the peptide conformation shifts to β-strands, the simplicity is such that β-sheet extension would appear unhindered and that the edge strand would be unencumbered by folded sequences from distant domains. Even in the stacked conformation the edge strands would provide available hydrogen bonds. Some hindrance may exist due to the slight misalignment of the stacking of the β-strands from the same peptide segment, causing some of the backbone hydrogen bonds of the edge strand to be in linkages with unstacked side chains.

The composition and structural orientation of the amino acids on the stacked β-strands determine β-sheet extension. We already discussed the presence of the hydrophobic amino acids in these strands and their importance in the stacking phenomenon. Consider the extension of those β-strands. This would require side-by-side connections through backbone hydrogen bonding that involves close association of like amino acids. The position and number of charged residues play a role. Centrally located the ^{22}Glu-^{23}Asp would provide a barrier to extension as this pair would not likely align with itself with any affinity. The aforementioned hydrophobic residues would, on the other hand, provide a driving force for β-sheet extension as their side-by-side alignments would be thermodynamically favored. Lastly, the planarity of the strand contributes to the vulnerability of the peptide to extend into β-sheets. This area of consideration is poorly understood as the only aggregate structure (2beg) shows rather planar β-strands. Nevertheless, this topic may be thought of as an area that may lead to breakthrough interventions focused on decreasing oligomerization. Given that the only well-defined barrier to β-sheet extension may be the ^{22}Glu-^{23}Asp sequence, the crucial step towards oligomer formation of Aβ is the conformational transition, which is thought to involve tying up the ^{23}Asp in a salt linkage with ^{28}Lys [37].

PROTEIN MISFOLDING AND INTERFACE CHEMISTRY

The term interface implies a heterogenous contact between surfaces that cover a large area and extends in two dimensions. While colloidal chemists rule this dominion, life scientists have much to gain in studying interface chemistry. The living tissues of the brain possess diverse interfacial areas. On a molecular level and to the Aβ peptide, these areas are enormous. Consider, for example, the blood brain barrier and cell surfaces (myelinated axons, clusters of cell bodies and complex dendritic processes). A traversing peptide may make contact with two-dimensional structures of various physico-chemical properties. The extensive amount of cell surface area in the brain is evident in the very high percent of lipid per tissue weight. Surface membranes are specialized protein-containing lipid bilayers. An adequate understanding of the processes associated with protein misfolding that occurs in neurodegeneration necessitates acquisition of knowledge on interfaces.

The cell interior provides a plethora of interfaces in the form of membrane-enclosed organelles and cytoskeletal systems that are both static and motorized. Cytoskeletal filaments and microtubules exist as a repetitive alignment of proteins which may offer docking points as would internal biomembranes. The curiosity here is in the manner by which the Aβ peptide behaves at these interfaces. And given the promiscuity of these peptides in adopting multiple conformational states, interfaces likely have an enormous effect on conformational decisions. Consider in this light the observation that inhaled anesthetics, which are known to act as interfacial regions in membrane proteins, promote Aβ aggregation [38].

While many types of interfaces exist, the lipid-water interface provides the most pronounced heterogeneity. Experimentally the air-water interface is a useful model to mimic the lipid-water interface where air represents lipid-like characteristics [39]. Behavior of proteins and polypeptides at these interfaces remains an area of considerable uncertainty. While the field of protein folding is founded on studies in bulk solutions, the dynamics occurring at interfaces represent an expanding frontier.

Lipid-Water Interface

Investigation of the lipid-water interface involves many experimental models. Monolayers, micelles and liposomes can be created and studied *in vitro*. The composition of these macromolecular entities can be controlled and specific endpoints can be measured. The cylindrical shape of di-acyl amphipathic lipids allows for the spontaneous two-dimensional arrangement of monolayers and bilayers that can be induced to curve and seal, forming microvesicles or liposomes. The cone-like architecture of monoacyl amphipathic lipids creates micelles. These experimental models provide opportunities to examine lipid-protein interactions. It is important to note that the Aβ peptide is excised from the region of APP that is embedded in the surface membranes of neurons.

Other lipid-containing structures that are areas of research focus are biomembranes and lipoproteins. Biomembranes define the boundary of cells and make up the internal organelles. Lipoproteins constitute the body's mobile lipids, which are extracellular and flux through the circulatory and lymphatic systems as well as the tissue matrix. Additionally, monolayers and micelles exist *in vivo*. The nasal cavity consists of epithelial cells, whose surface membrane is layered with mucopolysaccharides that are covered with a monolayer of phospholipid. The acyl chains are projected towards the cavity and interface with air. This structure provides an organizing entity for promoting the alignment of amyloidogenic peptides. Interfacial Aβ aggregation in two-phase systems (i.e. buffer/chloroform) reveals globular clusters that align linearly [40]. These structures occur rapidly but their morphologies are rather unstable. Interestingly, in very dilute HFIP, microdroplets form with the appearance of Aβ aggregation at the edge of these globular structures that over time result in a mesh or lattice of fiber-like elements [41]. The seeding efficiency of Aβ protofibrils, which are grown at HFIP interfaces, is less than that of soluble Aβ aggregates grown without HFIP.

Monolayers

Typical monolayer formers are polar lipids such as monoglycerides, long-chain fatty acids, phospholipids, lysophospholipids, cholesterol and sphingomyelins. They orient themselves at the air-water interface with the polar groups extended into the aqueous phase and the hydrocarbon chains into the air in order to produce a minimum amount of interference with hydrogen binding structures of water. A useful technique in studying protein-lipid interaction is to inject protein below the surface of the monolayer and monitor penetration into the monolayer. Penetration occurs when the polar and nonpolar parts of the protein interact strongly with complementary regions in the monolayer. The primary interaction of absorbed protein involves charged residues on both lipid and protein. Penetration attends marked irreversible unfolding of the protein.

The interface-mediated change in protein conformation causes insolubility and loss of biological activity [42]. The α-helix provides stability at oil-water interfaces [43]. The specificity of the interaction of proteins with monolayers remains in debate and likely is dependent upon the protein studied. Aβ's intrinsic malleability may undergo manipulative conformational changes at the interface. At monolayer interfaces, Aβ undergoes a conformational conversion forming β-sheets, the long axis of which is parallel to the surface [44]. The physical constraint of the interface may constrict the organization of Aβ into a planar arrangement. Monolayer deposition and fibril formation may be an integrated event [45]. Aggregates of the Aβ fragment (10-35) deposit on co-substituted alkanethiol monolayers [46]. While Aβ interaction occurs between positively charged amino acid residues and negatively charged polar headgroups [47], insertion is not dependent upon anionic phospholipids [48]. Studies of Aβ insertion into monolayers indicate that that there is strong interaction between Aβ and cholesterol [49]. Aβ increases monolayer permeability to proteins [50] and ions [51] and creates toxic non-fibrillar diffusible agents [52] presumably by mechanisms that involve lipid perturbations at the membrane interface [53].

Micelles

Water-insoluble amphiphatic lipids coalese into organized arrays of micelles in aqueous solutions. These micelles may be spherical, discoid, rodlike, hexagonal or lamellar in their topology. The polar groups are on the exterior surface of these structures forming contacts with water molecules. The nonpolar groups align themselves in the buried interior. Typically, equilibrium exists between free lipids and micelles. Free lipids must reach the critical micellar concentration before micelles can form. Micelles provide an excellent research model for studying the interaction of proteins at a lipid-water interface.

Fluoro-alcohols, which were long considered to be α-helix stabilizers, affect hydrophobic interactions in peptides providing a useful investigative tool. In TFE/water, a synthetic Aβ fragment presents mainly with α-helical content [54]. Concentrations are likely important as dilute solutions of HFIP allow for the formation of β-structure in Aβ (1-40) and promote soluble fibril formation [55]. Following a survey of stabilizing media, Crescenzi and coworkers [56] concluded that fluoro-alcohols enhance the formation of α-helical regions in Aβ. These fluoro-alcohols alter the dielectric constant of water and form clusters of various sizes [57]. Because of their topology, which is due to a large bulky hydrophobic group and a relatively small polar group, fluoro-alcohols would not form spherical micellar structures reminiscent of ionic detergents.

Aβ, which absorbed to SDS micelles at neutral *p*H (7.2), folds predominantly in α-helical structures that do not embed themselves into the hydrophobic regions of the micelle [58]. At a lower *p*H (5.1), the N-terminus appears unstructured (water-solvated) and the remaining two-thirds of the Aβ (1-40) exhibited helical structures that were SDS-solvated [23]. Lipid-solubility appears to be *p*H-dependent with more solubility at lower *p*Hs, and the susceptibility for β-sheet aggregation as the *p*H approaches 7.9 from 4.2. Both of these SDS-adsorbed Aβ structures exhibited a hinge domain at residues ^{25}Gly-^{27}Asn.

In addition to changes in protein protonation *p*H may affect the micellar dynamics of SDS. Interestingly, micellar dihexanoylphosphatidylcholine (DHPC) maintains the proper α-helical folds of apolipoprotein C-II while submicellar concentrations promote amyloid fibril formation [59]. The monomer to micelle equilibrium may help explain the observation that SDS enhances the formation of soluble fibrils of Aβ (1-40) [55].

An Aβ analog in solutions of micellar octyl-glucoside exhibits a high β-sheet content [54] suggesting that interaction with the micelles promotes the conformational change. Aβ fragment (11-25) exhibits micellar forms as well with the critical micellar concentration dependent on *p*H [60]. The dynamics of Aβ (1-40) with micellar components of various lipids demonstrate that an aggregated form of Aβ preferentially binds to micellar lipids with cholesterol being favored over phosphatidylcholine or fatty acids [61]. Using spin-labeled Aβ fragment (25-35) with probes at the termini, the fragments interact with micelles in a specific manner [62]. The C-terminus of the Aβ fragment (25-35) inserts into the lipid portion of the micelle while the N-terminus remains water solvated. The C-terminal two-thirds of the Aβ (1-40) was previously shown to be embedded in SDS micelles [23] though the degree of penetration is in question [58].

Lipoproteins/liposomes

Aβ peptides bind to lipoprotein particles and the binding is associated with changes in secondary structure [63]. Aggregation of Aβ fragment (25-35) is accelerated with vesicles containing negatively charged phospholipids compared with vesicles containing zwitterionic phospholipids, suggesting that interaction with vesicles is electrostatic [64]. The resulting aggregates alter the lipid-water interface. The interactions with the mobile lipid carriers as well as the contribution of apolipoprotein E variants contribute to the persistence and types of Aβ in brain.

Air-Water Interface

Proteins such as the Aβ peptide can spread at an air-water interface forming a layer that is one molecule thick. The process involves large conformational changes. The orientation of polypeptides at this interface is anything but fixed. Dispersion of hydrophobic and hydrophilic residues creates a dynamic instability. Many proteins irreversibly alter their conformation [42].

Insoluble planar aggregates of albumin [65], Aβ (1-42) [66] and Aβ fragment (31-35) [67] form at the air-water interface. The interface of air to water provides a practical approach to studying Aβ aggregation at the lipid-water interfaces in brain [39]. At the air-water interface, Aβ peptide reconfigures into β-sheets from soluble helical structures. The β-sheets are parallel to the surface. The physical constraint of the interface forces Aβ into a planar arrangement.

Unstirred Samples

Spherical particles (2-20 nm) may appear during fibrillogenesis [68,69]. Particles as large as 150nm are observed [66]. The differences in size of these early oligomers may be in part due to experimental conditions. In addition to using interfaces and adding acrolein, the experiments yielding the largest amylospheroids were those in which the samples were kept unstirred. Agitation clearly promotes fibrillogenesis [70,71], while larger spherical aggregates form during prolonged storage [72] and in the absence of vigorous stirring [68].

Agitation of Samples

Shear stress on a dissolved peptide occurs when a sample is aggressively mixed. A peptide can experience a considerable amount of shear in an agitating vessel. The ascribed stresses can be oriented to the three spatial dimensions (Figure 7). For example, two apposing flows along the x-axis would represent a shear stress (σ_{xx}). A flow along the x-axis that has an apposing flow perpendicular to it that is along the y-axis would represent an additional shear termed σ_{xy}. In a non-repetitive agitator nine different shear stresses may act on a protein sample being mixed: three parallel and six perpendicular. Basically, shearing forces in a vessel are (a) left-to-right, (b) top-to-bottom, and (c) front-to-back during agitation (Figure 7).

Solutions can be mixed several ways (Figure 8A). The repetitive process of drawing samples in and out of a pipette tip represents a mixing environment with rather clear dominant shear forces. The shear forces in a continuous vortexing sample would likely not include shear flows in the top-to-bottom axis. Nonetheless vortexing exerts parallel and perpendicular shear stresses on a peptide in solution. The strain acting on a peptide particularly in a coiled conformation causes tension (Figure 8B). The peptide chain stretches in the direction of the dominant stress [73]. In a vortexing test tube the wall is constantly moving and there is a gradient force on the molecule with an initial dominant shear force. With a magnetic stirring bar the walls are stationary but the solution rotates with a gradient force, which is strong in the middle and weaker by the walls. Rapid changes in speed bring about other dominant forces. The presence of dominant forces would stretch the peptide to achieve an orientation necessary for β-sheet formation. In the case of an agitator, where there is no constant established gradient, deviant forces dominate which would result in more rapid stretching of the polypeptide chain. Additionally, multiple passes through a narrow bore pipette results in extensional flows that stretch the peptide in the direction of the main sheer stress whether that be while drawing material into the pipette tip or during extrusion.

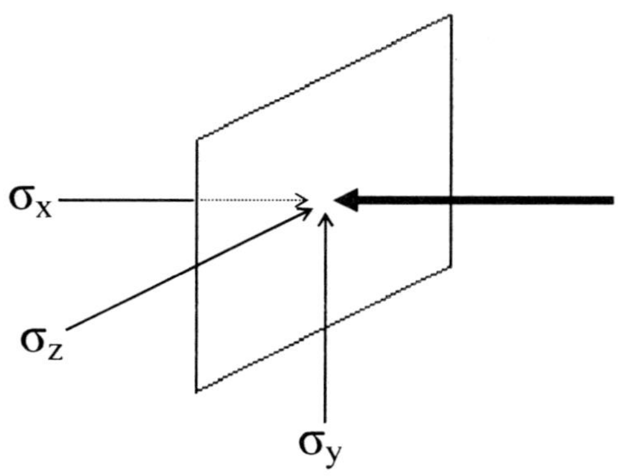

Figure 7. Opposing flows that exert shear stress. The bold arrow represents the flow of the solution containing the peptide. The other three arrows represent antagonizing flows that proceed along the three spatial dimensions with the designated symbol (σ) indicating degree of shear stress [redrawn from 73].

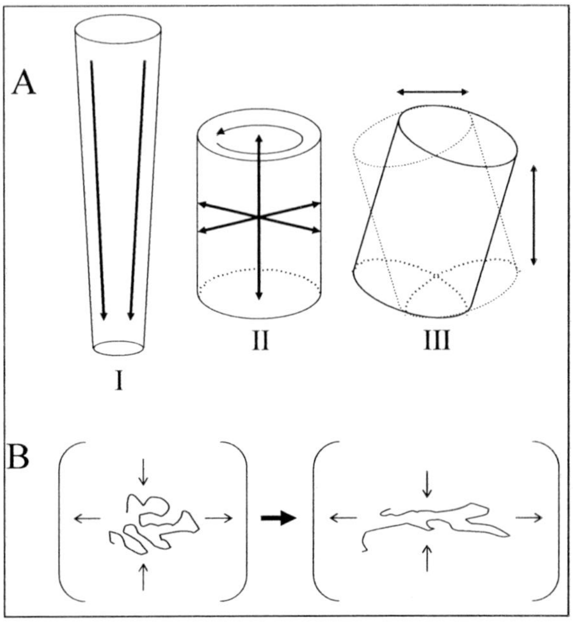

Figure 8. Proposed effects of mixing on the Aβ peptide in solution. Three types of mixing procedures are indicated in (A) with the drawn arrows representing the dominant flows: passing through a pipette tip, I; vortexing or using a magnetic stirring bar, II; and mixing on an agitator, III. The effects of mixing in which a dominant shear stress is exerted on the Aβ peptide showing the stretching of the polypeptide chain (B).

These conditions would allow for stretching of the Aβ peptide from a collapsed coil, 1hz3, to an extended β-strand (Figure 4). We calculated the compaction of the stretch of amino acids ^{17}Leu-^{26}Ser, which represents a β-strand in the stacked peptide in the aggregate structure, 2beg. The residues in 1hz3 are more tightly condensed than those in 2beg (Figure 9). Aβ protofibrils undergo progressive stabilization in the absence of Aβ monomers [41] suggesting that additional events such as shear-induced helical twisting of protofibrils or shear-induced curling of additional two-dimensional aggregates may be occurring.

Air-water interfaces promote Aβ peptides to form β-sheets [39]. Synthetic peptidolipids containing the Aβ fragment (31-35) form two-dimensional aggregates at air-water interfaces [67]. The β-sheets of Aβ peptides at air-water and lipid-water interfaces are oriented parallel to the interface [39,74], which provides an organizing constraint to Aβ aggregation. Shearing of aggregates that form at air-water interfaces, especially with the introduction of bubbles from high agitation, may physically fix structures in more stable tertiary conformations that would be consistent with a dock and lock mechanism that is proposed [75].

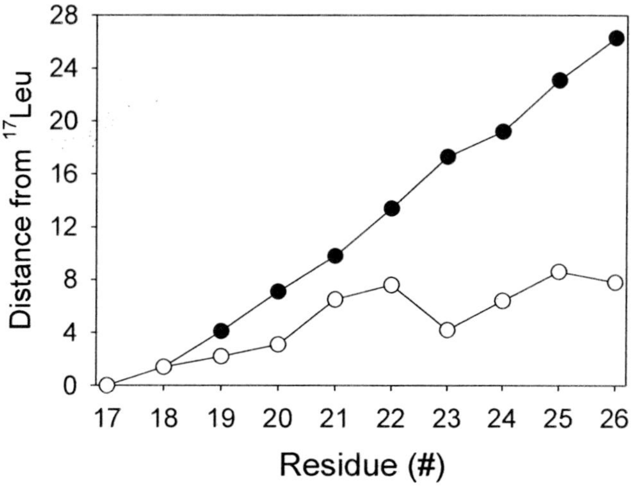

Figure 9. Distance comparisons of the middle regions in 1hz3 and 2beg. The distances (in angstrom) of each of the indicated amino acids from ^{17}Leu were obtained from the structure database (ncbi.gov) for 1hz3 (open circles) and for one of the chains in the protofibril in 2beg (closed circles).

Chemical Directives

Proteins, which have not been identified as fibril-formers *in vivo*, can be induced to form fibrils in media that promote secondary structure changes [76,77]. In addition to very acidic or basic *p*Hs and hydrophobic co-solvents, reactive agents such as oxidized lipids or sugars may play an amyloidogenic role. Oxidized products of cholesterol are implicated in AD [78]. They are cytotoxic to cells of the nervous system [79,80]. 3β-Hydroxy-5-oxo-5,6-secocholestan-6-al is isolated from the ozonation of cholesterol [81], and like other endogenous aldehydes, may contribute to Aβ aggregation, presumably by reacting directly to the peptide via the carbonyl group [82,83]. Glycation adducts that are formed from reactive carbonyls introduce hydrophobicity to a sequence that may alter solvent accessibility [84], creating localized or global compaction [85]. These chemical events may promote the dehydration of peptide sequences stabilizing them as aggregates.

Biochemical Scaffolds

The studies involving interfaces imply that biological structures may act as scaffolds upon which protein or peptide deposition can be organized. These skeletal frameworks may include cell surfaces or other internal biomembranes, and more specifically, lipid rafts. Additionally, we propose a novel class of biochemical scaffolds. This class of structures involves the formation of a polymeric underlayment that is spontaneously formed by the polymerization of small molecules.

Cell Surface

The surface of a cell, or the plasma membrane, may act as an organizing template that promotes fibrillar or non-fibrillar alignments of amyloidogenic peptides. Aggregates of Aβ (1-42) peptide assemble on biomembranes, and cholesterol content appears to modulate this membrane-dependent aggregation [86]. Furthermore, gangliosides at the surface membrane promote helix-to-strand conformational changes of Aβ [87]. It is curious to speculate that the sugar hydroxyls on the gangliosides (in perhaps specific chair or boat configurations) participate in stabilizing the elongated β-strand backbone hydrogen bonding that is required for extension into β-sheets.

The potentially deleterious effect of cell surfaces on protein integrity may be a general feature of the chronic diseases of aging. The ubiquitous nature of APP suggests that Aβ may be present in other tissues and could be playing a role in diseases other than AD. In age-related macular degeneration, drusen, which is the name given to these extracellular deposits, contain Aβ. The localization of drusen suggests deposition involved cell surfaces. Drusen exhibit a central core with one or more concentric rings; the outer layers consist of densely packed spherical structures composed of Aβ [88]. These studies suggest that cell surfaces may act as tissue-specific organizing templates upon which Aβ deposition and accumulation may occur.

Lipid Rafts

Lipid rafts are ordered sections of surface membranes. They serve to localize a wide array of processes. Acting as either large molecular platforms or smaller microdomains, lipid rafts segregate membrane components. They may be partly responsible for the aberrant processing of APP in AD. The unique lipid composition of lipid rafts includes cholesterol and saturated polar lipids, particularly sphingolipids. These ordered membrane compartments co-exist with the surrounding disordered fluid membranes that are rich in unsaturated lipids [89,90].

Sphingolipids, a prominent lipid in rafts, generates ceramide upon enzymatic hydrolysis by the sphingomyelinase. Ceramide controls the cholesterol content of lipid rafts [91]. Both ceramide and cholesterol are lipids with rather small polar headgroups suggesting that these lipid raft components regulate specific protein interaction by creating a local dehydration with easy accessibility to the lipid interior. Lipid rafts have the characteristics to act as scaffolds that organize the alignment and aggregation of amyloidgenic proteins such as Aβ. Parkinson's disease implicates the filamentous aggregation of the pre-synaptic protein α-synuclein, and lipid rafts may also serve as sites for promoting the oligomerization of this amyloidogenic protein [92].

We propose that lipid rafts, which are supramacromolecular complexes, act as an organizing template for aligning amyloidogenic peptides. They may bring together multiple proteins in close proximity, promoting protein-protein interactions. Lipid rafts are ordered and highly regular structures, and with the potential of Aβ penetrating lipid bilayers, the lipid rafts may provide an opportunity for organizing the repetitive arrangement of these peptides.

Additionally, as described below these floating templates may supply substrates for polymer formation that would support protein aggregation.

Polymeric Underlayment

Functionally different proteins form similar amyloid-like structures. Diverse proteins, which have little biological relationships to link them together conceptually, form similar repetitive arrays. These proteins form polymers that are similar to those seen in silk. These observations have changed our perspective of protein chemistry and have broadened our view of cell dysfunction. Hence, the study of the misfolding of plasma proteins like albumin and transthyretin may prove beneficial in understanding the events associated with Aβ oligomerization and cytotoxicity.

In this context, we propose a novel paradigm in which polymer chemistry, the basis of plastic formation, is a major contributing factor to cell degeneration. We further extend this theme to include that plastic-like polymers may provide a skeletal framework onto which protein aggregation can occur. Various ordered chain assemblies may occur during nonenzymatic polymerization of metabolic byproducts (Figure 10). Polymers [73] may be linear, fully extended and proceeding in one direction, or branched. They may be spiro polymers in which two linear polymers are linked at regular intervals and thus share common points of connection. Ladder polymers are two linear polymers that form rings as their connecting points. Lastly, layer polymers that extend two dimensionally involve multi-ring structures. Below is a discussion on two proposed biologically significant polymeric underlayments that may provide an organizing template for Aβ peptide aggregation or perhaps for aggregation of other proteins in different biological contexts.

Neuromelanin

Neuromelanin comes fundamentally in two forms as eumelanin and pheomelanin. Both appear to be derived from tyrosine precursors with pheomelanin involving the incorporation of cysteine. Melanin is a polymer created largely by nonenzymatic reactions. The production of melanin in the brain appears to be linked to the oxidative stress imposed by the accumulation of catecholamines such as dopamine. The loss of neuromelanin is a feature of Parkinson's disease as the dopaminergic neurons have degenerated creating a dearth of dopamine, which is the precursor to melanin. Neuromelanin is decreased in the AD brain as well [93]. Interestingly, APP has a role in melanin release and deposition in the epidermis [94,95]. The precise function of neuromelanin in brain remains to be elucidated. Neuromelanin is the dark pigment present in substantia nigra, locus ceruleus, dorsal motor nucleus of the vagus nerve and median raphe nucleus of the pons. This pigment develops during maturation and into adulthood [96].

The function of neuromelanin is currently unknown. It is redox active, and is both chemically and photochemically reactive. The duality of being an oxidant and a potential antioxidant suggests a complex nature of this polymer. The loss of pigmented neurons from specific nuclei is seen in neurodegenerative diseases. Loss of dopamine-producing neurons in the substantia nigra occurs in Parkinson's disease. Loss of the norepinephrine-producing neurons of the locus ceruleus occurs in AD. The loss of neurons explains the loss of neuromelanin, but it is unknown whether the neuromelanin played a role in the degeneration of those specific neurons.

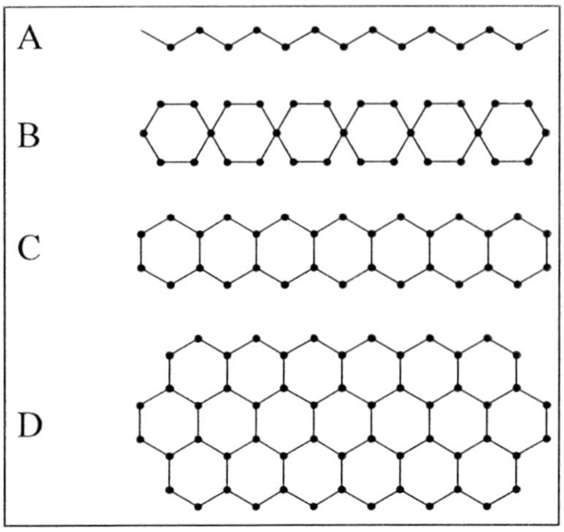

Figure 10. Types of polymeric structures that may act as organizing templates. The dots represent the main atoms of a monomeric compound that can polymerize in diverse ways. Polymers may exist as simple linear arrays (A). Linear organization of cyclic and heterocyclic units may increase the level of complexity (B and C). Additionally, two-dimensional polymerization of cyclic and heterocyclic monomers is also possible creating layered polymers (D) [redrawn from 73].

Eumelanin consists of cross-linked indole derivatives of catecholamines (5,6-dihydroxyindole and 5,6-dihydroxyindole-2-carboxylic acid) that form extensive polymers. The repeating hexameric and pentameric units likely form planar or curvilinear structures that extend two-dimensionally. The electrical properties of eumelanin suggest that the rings are contiguous such that electron flow would generate slow moving current. The precise nature of eumelanin's molecular structure is unknown, though it is likely that the structure resembles a layer polymer (Figure 10D). That eumelanin is found in hair and skin, creating the colors grey, black, yellow, and brown, further indicates the complexity of this molecular entity. The forms that exist in neural systems may suggest new mechanisms of pathogenesis. It appears that the cellular context determines the neurotoxicity of neuromelanin as it does with Aβ [97]. We propose that this two-dimensional redox reactive polymer may provide a molecular framework, or underlayment, onto which protein aggregation can be orchestrated.

Polyacrolein

Polyacrolein is a homopolymer derived from the chain polymerization of the bifunctional acrolein. Prior to our recent publications [65,66], polyacrolein was investigated merely for its commercial applications [98]. Our laboratory was the first to propose a biological role for polyacrolein in pathogenic mechanisms.

Acrolein, a lipid-derived 3-carbon compound, contains a vinyl and a carbonyl group, both of which are reactive. AD brain exhibits high levels of acrolein [99], which is intriguingly produced by Aβ-induced lipid peroxidation. Acrolein is an α, β-unsaturated aldehyde that reacts with histidinyl imidazoles and primary amines. Since Aβ has three histidines and two lysines, adduct formation is possible. Additionally, vinyl groups on acrolein condense via fundamental polymer chemistry. Polymerization also occurs via the carbonyl groups resulting in complicated two-dimensional structures (Figure 11D).

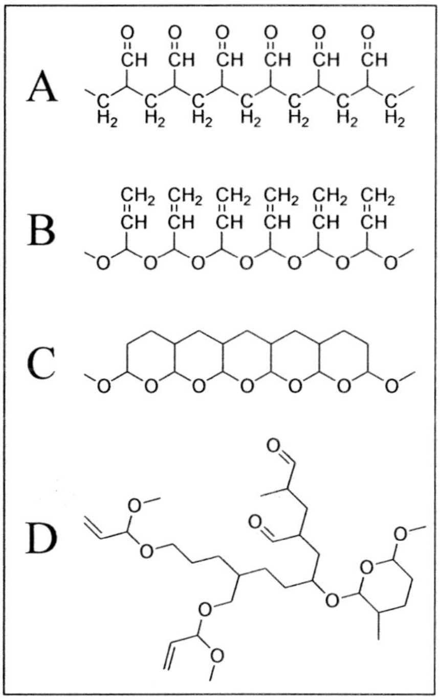

Figure 11. Acrolein reacts to produce various polymeric forms. If only one functional group participates in polymerization whether its the alkene group or the carbonyl group, the resulting linear structure resembles A and B, respectively. The unreacted groups in A and B are available to form covalent linkages with Aβ. Acrolein (form B) may react internally to yield repeating 6-membered rings (C). Lastly, acrolein can react in a more unstructured way that would yield complex branches of polymerized monomers (D).

Polyacrolein may be formed in simple biological systems [65,66]. Aβ's redox and surfactant properties [100,101] contributes to the initiation of acrolein polymerization that consequently forms a composite material. In our model [102], the remaining free carbonyl and vinyl groups on polyacrolein fix the Aβ peptides to the growing polymers. Furthermore, this process appears accelerated at lipid-water interfaces. Aβ-polyacrolein aggregates exist as planar structures that appear polygonal and exhibit an uneven surface. An organized pattern of aligned amylospheroids are embedded in the planar aggregate. Isolated amylospheroids are also observed. Interestingly, atomic force microscopy demonstrates the presence of spherical structures immediately after initiation of Aβ (1-40) fibrillization [103]. The planar aggregates that we observed are derived at least in part from the spherical units likely through a process of polycondensation in which polymer-polymer reactions occur.

Acrolein co-localizes to the Aβ aggregates in extracellular deposits [104] with only light immuno-stain surrounding the core aggregate. The core itself lacks acrolein staining. The lack of acrolein is likely due to its incorporation into nascent polymers though further research needs to substantiate this suggestion. This new perspective of endogenously-derived plastic-like polymers requires tools and technical approaches that are typically associated with material science.

Acrolein-based plastic fragments can form in the absence of industrial processes that typically require harsh conditions [98]. We generate polyacrolein with the simple presence of acrolein and Aβ. Acrolein readily forms covalent bonds with amino acid residues in proteins [105] analogous to glycation reactions, which may provide the chemical environment to initiate polymerization. Aβ's nucleophilic centers may promote free radical reactions that contribute as a catalyst for polymerization of acrolein. Anionic-initiated polymerization may also occur. Endogenously-formed plastic fragments, which are made under simple biological conditions, may contribute to the formation of neurotoxic structures. The intra-bilayer production of two-dimensional films with covalently tagged proteins would alter membrane properties. Nerve cells function by active transmission of electrical signals along the surface membrane, which if altered may dampen depolarization dynamics. Additionally, gas exchange through the membrane may be affected, leading to de-energization of the nerve cell. Polyacrolein may also be involved in the accumulation of mature senile plaques. Lastly, the presence of these polymeric structures as composite material may evoke antigenicity. All of these proposed effects need rigorous *in vivo* validation, but additional chemical identifiers need to be determined prior to effective analysis.

Although the molecular arrangement of the planar aggregates of Aβ-polyacrolein needs further characterization, we propose that plastic may form and persist in biological tissues. In AD, where there is co-localized production of Aβ peptide and acrolein [100,104], unique plastic-like products may be formed via Schiff base attachment or Michael addition of Aβ onto polyacrolein films. The diseased nervous system provides a suitable environment for production of polyacrolein, which when bound to Aβ oligomers may promote cytotoxicity. The high concentrations required for polymerization may be reached by the rapid and focal production of lipid peroxidation products such that the formation rate in the chain reaction of lipid peroxidation exceeds that of diffusion. Additionally, factors that may sequester and concentrate acrolein, such as lipid rafts and inhaled anesthetics [Roberts RD, Fibuch EE, Seidler NW, unpublished data], would create a favorable environment for polymerization reactions. As we get a better understanding of the chemical signatures associated with these proposed structures, we will be able to investigate the presence of these entities in isolated lipid rafts, whole cells, tissues and even autopsy samples.

Acrolein (CH_2=CH-CHO) can polymerize to form linear polymers. This type of polymerization can be done two ways. First, acrolein polymerizes via alkene bonds, creating carbon chain units –CH_2-CH(CHO)– with the side chains being aldehyde groups (Figure 11A). Alternately, acrolein polymerizes via carbon-oxygen double bonds, generating carbon-oxygen units –O-CH(CH=CH_2)– with the side chains being ethylene groups (Figure 11B). If either of these scenarios were the case, the side chains would be available for reaction to Aβ residues. Acrolein can also polymerize to form a ladder-like structure giving six-membered rings in polymer chains (Figure 11C). Acrolein can polymerize to form multiple stacked two-dimensional layers. These polymers would be considered mixed polymers as they would incorporate all of the types of polymer reactions described above. Unreacted side chains would allow for reaction with Aβ, fixing the peptide to the polymeric film. Polycondensation may also occur that involves the reaction of two larger polymeric aggregates to one another, potentially forming multiple layers.

Future Directions

Exhaustive analysis of the innate propensities of the residues in amyloidogenic peptides helps define the rules associated with misfolding. A subcategory of the field of protein folding is protein misfolding. Just as protein folding rules apply to the formation of functional globular enzymes, rules are emerging that dictate the dynamics associated with misfolding as it occurs with Aβ. Misfolding creates structures that contain amyloidogenic potential. Our discussion of Aβ suggests that there are definable rules to which proteins must adhere. As the study of misfolding moves forward, the elaboration of these rules are inevitable and will provide insight to how misfolding leads to diseases such as AD.

Investigation into how interfaces affect conformational transitions in Aβ is pivotal to understanding the essence of misfolding. The mechanism of Aβ propagation as it occurs at interfaces suggests a need to study the chemical composition of surface materials in biological systems. The air-water interface as an experimental model, which is crucial in studying Aβ aggregation, requires a new look in light of our descriptions regarding the effects of shear forces and the role of agitation on mixed samples. Future research in this area would yield valuable information, particularly useful in the discovery of new pharmacological interventions that would work towards preventing protein misfolding.

The deleterious effect of the chemical milieu on the molecular integrity of Aβ suggests that controlling the levels of toxic metabolites may be beneficial in preventing aggregation. For example, therapies such as anti-inflammatory agents that would decrease lipid peroxidation are guided towards this aim. Additionally, glycemic control would moderate glycation reactions, which appear to be associated with AD.

We have identified a novel paradigm, stating how plastic-like polymers may act as templates to direct the oligomerization of amyloidogenic peptides. Polyacrolein represents the prototype for this concept as it orchestrates the alignment of Aβ into structures that may contribute to AD pathology. This allows for new mechanistic models that may spawn more effective interventions.

Acknowledgements

The authors thank Kim Erikson and Deb Mitchell for their excellent clerical assistance in the preparation of this manuscript. Funding support came in part from the Division of Research and the College of Biosciences at Kansas City University of Medicine and Biosciences.

REFERENCES

[1] Kang J, Lemaire HG, Unterbeck A, Salbaum JM, Masters CL, Grzeschik KH, Multhaup G, Beyreuther K, Muller-Hill B. The precursor of Alzheimer's disease amyloid A4 protein resembles a cell-surface receptor. *Nature* 1987;325:733-736.

[2] Kitaguchi N, Takahashi Y, Tokushima Y, Shiojiri S, Ito H. Novel precursor of Alzheimer's disease amyloid protein shows protease inhibitory activity. *Nature* 1988;331:530-532.

[3] Kang J, Muller-Hill B. Differential splicing of Alzheimer's disease amyloid A4 precursor RNA in rat tissues: PreA4(695) mRNA is predominantly produced in rat and human brain. *Biochem Biophys Res Commun* 1990;166:1192-1200.

[4] Lemaire HG, Salbaum JM, Multhaup G, Kang J, Bayney RM, Unterbeck A, Beyreuther K, Muller-Hill B. The PreA4(695) precursor protein of Alzheimer's disease A4 amyloid is encoded by 16 exons. *Nucleic Acids Res* 1989;17:517-522.

[5] Wirths O, Weis J, Szczygielski J, Multhaup G, Bayer TA. Axonopathy in an APP/PS1 transgenic mouse model of Alzheimer's disease. *Acta Neuropathol (Berl)* 2006;111:312-319.

[6] Botelho MG, Gralle M, Oliveira CL, Torriani I, Ferreira ST. Folding and stability of the extracellular domain of the human amyloid precursor protein. *J Biol Chem* 2003;278:34259-34287.

[7] Haass C, Steiner H. Alzheimer disease gamma-secretase: a complex story of GxGD-type presenilin proteases. *Trends Cell Biol* 2002;12:556-562.

[8] Murphy MP, Hickman LJ, Eckman CB, Uljon SN, Wang R, Golde TE. gamma-Secretase, evidence for multiple proteolytic activities and influence of membrane positioning of substrate on generation of amyloid beta peptides of varying length. *J Biol Chem* 1999;274:11914-11923.

[9] Weggen S, Eriksen JL, Das P, Sagi SA, Wang R, Pietrzik CU, Findlay KA, Smith TE, Murphy MP, Bulter T, Kang DE, Marquez-Sterling N, Golde TE, Koo EH. A subset of NSAIDs lower amyloidogenic Abeta42 independently of cyclooxygenase activity. *Nature* 2001;414:212-216.

[10] Berman HM, Westbrook J, Feng Z, Gilliland G, Bhat TN, Weissig H, Shindyalov IN, Bourne PE. The Protein Data Bank. *Nucleic Acids Res* 2000;28:235-242.

[11] Rost B, Sander C. Prediction of protein structure at better than 70% accuracy. *J Mol Biol* 1993;232:584-599.

[12] Rost B, Sander C. Combining evolutionary information and neural networks to predict protein secondary structure. *Proteins* 1994;9:55-72.

[13] Rost B. PHD: predicting one-dimensional protein structure by profile based on neural networks. *Methods Enzymol* 1996;266:525-539.

[14] Karplus K, Barrett C, Hughey R. Hidden Markov models for detecting remote protein homologies. *Bioinformatics* 1998;14:846-856.

[15] Chou PY, Fasman GD. Empirical predictions of protein structure. *Annu Rev Biochem* 1978;47:251-276.

[16] Chou PY, Fasman GD. Prediction of the secondary structure of proteins from their amino acid sequence. *Adv Enzymol* 1978;47:45-148.

[17] Kallberg Y, Gustafsson M, Persson B, Thyberg J, Johansson J. Prediction of amyloid fibril-forming proteins. *J Biol Chem* 2001;276:12945-12950.

[18] Rose GD. Prediction of chain turns in globular proteins on a hydrophathy basis. *Nature* 1978;272:586-590.

[19] Dima RI, Thirumalai D. Exploring the propensities of helices in PrP(C) to form beta sheet using NMR structures and sequence alignments. *Biophys J* 2002;83:1268-1280.

[20] Crescenzi O, Tomaselli S, Guerrini R, Salvadori S, D'ursi AM, Temussi AM, Picone D. Solution structure of the Alzheimer's disease amyloid beta-peptide (1-42). *Eur J Biochem* 2002;269:5642-5648.

[21] Tomaselli S, Esposito V, Vangone P, van Nuland NA, Bonvin AM, Guerrini R, Tancredi T, Temussi PA, Picone D. The alpha-to-beta conformational transition of Alzheimer's A beta-(1-42) peptide in aqueous media is reversible: a step by step conformational analysis suggests the location of beta conformation seeding. *Chembiochem* 2005;7:257-267.

[22] Watson AA, Fairlie DP, Craik DJ. Solution structure of methionine-oxidized amyloid beta-peptide (1-40). Does oxidation affect conformational switching? *Biochemistry* 1998;37:12700-12706.

[23] Coles M, Bicknell W, Watson AA, Fairlie DP, Craik DJ. Solution structure of amyloid beta-peptide(1-40) in a water-micelle environment. Is the membrane-spanning domain where we think it is? *Biochemistry* 1998;37:11064-11077.

[24] Talafous J, Marcinowski KJ, Klopman G, Zagorski MG. Solution structure of residues 1-28 of the amyloid β-peptide. *Biochemistry* 1994;33:7788-7796.

[25] Zirah S, Kozin SA, Mazur AK, Blond A, Cheminant M, Segalas-Milazzo I, Debey P, Rebuffat S. Structural changes of region 1-16 of the Alzheimer disease amyloid beta-peptide upon zinc binding and in vitro aging. *J Biol Chem* 2005;281:2151-2161.

[26] Zhang S, Iwata K, Lachenmann MJ, Peng JW, Li S, Stimson ER, Lu Y, Felix AM, Maggio JE, Lee JP. The Alzheimer's peptide a beta adopts a collapsed coil structure in water. *J Struct Biol* 2000;130:130-141.

[27] Kohno T, Kobayashi K, Maeda T, Sato K, Takashima A. Three-dimensional structures of the amyloid β peptide (25-35) in membrane-mimicking environment. *Biochemistry* 1996;35:16094-16104.

[28] D'Ursi AM, Armenante MR, Guerrini R, Salvadori S, Sorrentino G, Picone D. Solution structure of amyloid beta-peptide (25-35) in different media. *J Med Chem* 2004;47:4231-4238.

[29] Tjernberg LO, Callaway DJ, Tjernberg A, Hahne S, Lilliehook C, Terenius L, Thyberg J, Nordstedt C. A molecular model of Alzheimer amyloid beta-peptide fibril formation. *J Biol Chem* 1999;274:12619-12625.

[30] Tjernberg LO, Naslund J, Lindqvist F, Johansson J, Karlstrom AR, Thyberg J, Terenius L, Nordstedt C. Arrest of beta-amyloid fibril formation by a pentapeptide ligand. *J Biol Chem* 1996;271:8545-8548.

[31] Luhrs T, Ritter C, Adrian M, Riek-Loher D, Bohrmann B, Dobeli H, Schubert D, Riek R. 3D structure of Alzheimer's amyloid-beta(1-42) fibrils. *Proc Natl Acad Sci USA* 2005;102:17342-17347.

[32] Buck M. Trifluoroethanol and colleagues: cosolvents come of age. Recent studies with peptides and proteins. *Q Rev Biophys* 1998;31:297-355.

[33] West MW, Wang W, Patterson J, Mancias JD, Beasley JR, Hecht MH De novo amyloid proteins from designed combinatorial libraries. *Proc Natl Acad Sci USA* 1999;96:11211-11216.

[34] Schwartz R, Istrail S, King J. Frequencies of amino acid strings in globular protein sequences indicate suppression of blocks of consecutive hydrophobic residues. *Prot Sci* 2001;10:1023.

[35] Ma B, Nussinov R. Stabilities and conformations of Alzheimer's β-amyloid peptide oligomers ($A\beta_{16\text{-}22}$, $A\beta_{16\text{-}35}$, and $A\beta_{10\text{-}35}$): Sequence effects. *Proc Natl Acad Sci USA* 2002;99:14126-14131.

[36] Jarrett JT, Berger EP, Lansbury PT Jr. The carboxy terminus of the beta amyloid protein is critical for the seeding of amyloid formation: implications for the pathogenesis of Alzheimer's disease. *Biochemistry* 1993;32:4693-4697.

[37] Thirumalai D, Klimov DK, Dima RI. Emerging ideas on the molecular basis of protein and peptide aggregation. *Curr Opin Struct Biol* 2003;13:146-159.

[38] Eckenhoff RG, Johansson JS, Wei H, Carnini A, Kang B, Wei W, Pidikiti R, Keller JM, Eckenhoff MF. Inhaled anesthetic enhancement of amyloid-beta oligomerization and cytotoxicity. *Anesthesiology* 2004;101:703-709.

[39] Schladitz C, Vieira EP, Hermel H, Mohwald H. Amyloid-beta-sheet formation at the air-water interface. *Biophys J* 1999;77:3305-3310.

[40] Nichols MR, Moss MA, Reed DK, Hoh JH, Rosenberry TL. Amyloid-beta aggregates formed at polar-nonpolar interfaces differ from amyloid-beta protofibrils produced in aqueous buffers. *Microsc Res Tech* 2005;67:164-174.

[41] Nichols MR, Moss MA, Reed DK, Cratic-McDaniel S, Hoh JH, Rosenberry TL. Amyloid-beta protofibrils differ from amyloid-beta aggregates induced in dilute hexafluoroisopropanol in stability and morphology. *J Biol Chem* 2005;280:2471-2480.

[42] James LK, Augenstein LG. Adsorption of enzymes at interfaces: film formation and the effect on activity. *Adv Enzymol* 1966;28:1-40.

[43] Malcolm BR. Molecular structure and deuterium exchange in monolayers of synthetic polypeptides. *Proc R Soc Lond, Ser. A* 1968;305:363-385.

[44] Maltseva E, Kerth A, Blume A, Mohawald H, Brezesinski G. Adsorption of amyloid beta (1-40) peptide at phospholipid monolayers. *Chembiochem* 2005;6:1817-1824.

[45] Kwan AH, Winefield RD, Sunde M, Matthews JM, Haverkamp RG, Templeton MD, Mackay JP. Structural basis for rodlet assembly in fungal hydrophobins. *Proc Natl Acad Sci U S A* 2006;103:3621-3626.

[46] McMasters MJ, Hammer RP, McCarley RL. Surface-induced aggregation of beta amyloid peptide by co-substituted alkanethiol monolayers supported on gold. *Langmuir* 2005;21:4464-4470.

[47] Terzi E, Holzemann G, Seelig J. Interaction of Alzheimer beta-amyloid peptide(1-40) with lipid membranes. *Biochemistry* 1997;36:14845-14852.

[48] Ege C, Lee KY. Insertion of Alzheimer's A beta 40 peptide into lipid monolayers. *Biophys J* 2004;87:1732-1740.

[49] Ji SR, Wu Y, Suo SF. Study of beta-amyloid peptide (Abeta40) insertion into phospholipid membranes using monolayer technique. *Biochemistry (Mosc)* 2002;67:1283-1288.

[50] Blanc EM, Toborek M, Mark RJ, Hennig B, Mattson MP. Amyloid beta-peptide induces cell monolayer albumin permeability, impairs glucose transport, and induces apoptosis in vascular endothelial cells. *J Neurochem* 1997;68:1870-1881.

[51] Rhee SK, Quist AP, Lal R. Amyloid β-protein (1-42) forms calcium-permeable, Zn^{2+}-sensitive channel. *J Biol Chem* 1998;273:13379-13382.

[52] Lambert MP, Barlow AK, Chromy BA, Edwards C, Freed R, Lisoatos M, Morgan TE, Rozovsky I, Trommer B, Biola KL, Wals P, Zhang C, Finch CE, Krafft GA, Klein WL. Diffusible, nonfibrillar ligands derived from Aβ1-42 are potent central nervous system neurotoxins. *Proc Natl Acad Sci U S A* 1998;95:6448-6453.

[53] Hristova K, Dempsey CE, White SH. Structure location, and lipid perturbations of melittin at the membrane interface. *Biophys J* 2001;80:801-811.

[54] Laczko-Hollosi I, Hollosi M, Lee VM, Mantsch HH. Conformational change of a synthetic amyloid analogue des [Ala21,30] A42 upon binding to octyl glucoside micelles. *Eur Biophys J* 1992;21:345-348.

[55] Rangachari V, Reed DK, Moore BD, Rosenberry TL. Secondary structure and interfacial aggregation of amyloid-beta (1-40) on sodium dodecyl sulfate micelles. *Biochemistry* 2006;45:8639-8648.

[56] Crescenzi O, Tomaselli S, Guerrini R, Salvadori S, D'Ursi AM, Temussi PA, Picone D. Solution structure of the Alzheimer amyloid β-peptide (1-42) in an apolar microenvironment. Similarity with a virus fusion domain. *Eur J Biochem* 2002;277:5642-5648.

[57] Reiersen H, Rees AR. Trifluoroethanol may form a solvent matrix for assisted hydrophobic interactions between peptide side chains. *Protein Eng* 2000;13:739-743

[58] Shao H, Jao S, Ma K, Zagorski MG. Solution structures of micelle-bound amyloid beta-(1-40) and beta-(1-42) peptides of Alzheimer's disease. *J Mol Biol* 1999;285:755-773.

[59] Hatters DM, Lawrence LJ, Howlett GJ. Sub-micellar phospholipid accelerates amyloid formation by apolipoprotein C-11. *FEBS Lett* 2001;494:220-224.

[60] Kim J, Lee M. Observation of multi-step conformation switching in beta-amyloid peptide aggregation by fluorescence resonance energy transfer. *Biochem Biophys Res Commun* 2004;316:393-397.

[61] Avdulov NA, Chochina SV, Igbavboa U, Warden CS, Vassiliev AV, Wood WG. Lipid binding to amyloid beta-peptide aggregates: preferential binding of cholesterol as compared with phosphatidylcholine and fatty acids. *Neurochem* 1997;69:1746-1752.

[62] Esposito C, Tedeschi A, Scrima M, D'errico G, Ottaviani MF, Rovero P, D'ursi AM. Exploring interaction of beta-amyloid segment (25-35) with membrane models through paramagnetic probes. *J Pept Sci* 2006;12:766-774.

[63] Chan W, Fornwald J, Brawner M, Wetzel R. Native complex formation between apolipoprotein E isoforms and the Alzheimer's disease peptide A beta. *Biochemistry* 1996;35:7123-7130.

[64] Del Mar Martinez-Senac M, Villalain J, Gomez-Fernandez JC. Structure of the Alzheimer β-amyloid peptide (25-35) and its interaction with negatively charged phospholipid vesicles. *Eur J Biochem* 1999;235:744-753.

[65] Seidler NW, Yeargans GS. Albumin-bound polyacrolein: implications for Alzheimer's disease. *Biochem Biophys Res Commun* 2004;320:213-217.

[66] Seidler NW, Squire TJ. Abeta-polyacrolein aggregates: novel mechanism of plastic formation in senile plaques. *Biochem Biophys Res Commun* 2005;335:501-504.

[67] Li C, Orbulescu J, Sui G, Leblanc RM. Amyloid-like formation by self-assembly of peptidolipids in two dimensions. *Langmuir* 2004;20:8641-8645.

[68] Nichols MR, Moss MA, Reed DK, Lin WL, Mukhopadhyay R, Hoh JH, Rosenberry TL. Growth of beta-amyloid(1-40) protofibrils by monomer elongation and lateral association. Characterization of distinct products by light scattering and atomic force microscopy. *Biochemistry* 2002;41:6115-6127.

[69] Dong J, Apkarian RP, Lynn DG. Imaging amyloid beta peptide oligomeric particles in solution. *Bioorg Med Chem* 2005;13:5213-5217.

[70] Wood SJ, Maleeff B, Hart T, Wetzel R. Physical, morphological and functional differences between ph 5.8 and 7.4 aggregates of the Alzheimer's amyloid peptide Abeta. *J Mol Biol* 1996;256:870-877.

[71] Evans KC, Berger EP, Cho CG, Weisgraber KH, Lansbury PT Jr. Apolipoprotein E is a kinetic but not a thermodynamic inhibitor of amyloid formation: implications for the pathogenesis and treatment of Alzheimer disease. *Proc Natl Acad Sci USA* 1995;92:763-767.

[72] Goldsbury CS, Wirtz S, Muller SA, Sunderji S, Wicki P, Aebi U, Frey P. Studies on the in vitro assembly of a beta 1-40: implications for the search for a beta fibril formation inhibitors. *J Struct Biol* 2000;130:217-231.

[73] Elias H-G. *An Introduction to Plastics*, second edition. Weinheim: Wiley-VCH GmbH & Co., 2003.

[74] Maltseva E, Brezesinski G. Adsorption of amyloid beta (1-40) peptide to phosphatidylethanolamine monolayers. *Chemphyschem* 2004;5:1185-1190.

[75] Esler WP, Stimson ER, Jennings JM, Vinters HV, Ghilardi JR, Lee JP, Mantyh PW, Maggio JE. Alzheimer's disease amyloid propagation by a template-dependent dock-lock mechanism. *Biochemistry* 2000;39:6288-6295.

[76] Guijarro JI, Sunde M, Jones JA, Campbell ID, Dobson CM. Amyloid fibril formation by an SH3 domain. *Proc Natl Acad Sci USA* 1998;95:4224-4228.

[77] Chiti F, Webster P, Taddei N, Clark A, Stefani M, Ramponi G, Dobson CM. Designing conditions for in vitro formation of amyloid protofilaments and fibrils. *Proc Natl Acad Sci USA* 1999;96:3590-3594.

[78] Kolsch H, Heun R, Kerksiek A, Bergmann KV, Maier W, Lutjohann D. Altered levels of plasma 24S- and 27-hydroxycholesterol in demented patients. *Neurosci Lett* 2004;368:303-308.

[79] Kolsch H, Ludwig M, Lutjohann D, Prange W, Rao ML. 7alpha-Hydroperoxycholesterol causes CNS neuronal cell death. *Neurochem Int* 2000;36:507-512.

[80] Chang JY, Liu LZ. Neurotoxicity of cholesterol oxides on cultured cerebellar granule cells. *Neurochem Int* 1998;32:317-323.

[81] Wang K, Bermudez E, Pryor WA. The ozonation of cholesterol: separation and identification of 2,4-dinitrophenylhydrazine derivatization products of 3 beta-hydroxy-5-oxo-5,6-secocholestan-6-al. *Steroids* 1993;58:225-229.

[82] Zhang, O, Powers ET, Nieva J, Huff ME, Dendle MA, Bieschke J, Glabe CG, Eschenmoser A, Wentworth P Jr, Lerner RA, Kelly JW. Metabolite-initiated protein misfolding may trigger Alzheimer's disease. *Proc Natl Acad Sci USA* 2004;101:4752-4757.

[83] Chen K, Maley J, Yu PH. Potential implications of endogenous aldehydes in beta-amyloid misfolding, oligomerization and fibrillogenesis. *J Neurochem* 2006;99:1413-1424.

[84] Yeargans GS, Seidler NW. Carnosine promotes the heat denaturation of glycated protein. *Biochem Biophys Res Commun* 2003;300:75-80.

[85] Seidler NW, Kowalewski C. Methylglyoxal-induced glycation affects protein topography. *Arch Biochem Biophys* 2003;410:149-154.

[86] Yip CM, Darabie AA, McLaurin J. Abeta42-peptide assembly on lipid bilayers. *J Mol Biol* 2002;318:97-107.

[87] Kakio A, Nishimoto S, Yanagisawa K, Kozutsumi Y, Matsuzaki K. Interactions of amyloid beta-protein with various gangliosides in raft-like membranes: importance of GM1 ganglioside-bound form as an endogenous seed for Alzheimer amyloid. *Biochemistry* 2002;41:7385-7390.

[88] Anderson DH, Talaga KC, Rivest AJ, Barron E, Hageman GS, Johnson LV. Characterization of beta amyloid assemblies in drusen: the deposits associated with aging and age-related macular degeneration. *Exp Eye Res* 2004;78:243-256.

[89] Brown DA, London E. Structure and origin of ordered lipid domains in biological membranes. *J Memb Biol* 1998;164:103-114.

[90] Rietveld A, Simons K. The differential miscibility of lipids as the basis for the formation of functional membrane rafts. *Biochim Biophys Acta* 1998;1376:467-479.

[91] Megha, London E. Ceramide selectively displaces cholesterol from ordered lipid domains (rafts): implications for lipid raft structure and function. *J Biol Chem* 2004;279:9997-10004.

[92] Kubo S, Nemani VM, Chalkley RJ, Anthony MD, Hattori N, Mizuno Y, Edwards RH, Fortin DL. A combinatorial code for the interaction of alpha-synuclein with membranes. *J Biol Chem* 2005;280:31664-31672.

[93] Reyes MG, Faraldi F Rydman R, Wang CC. Decreased nigral neuromelanin in Alzheimer's disease. *Neurol Res* 2003;25:179-182.

[94] Quast T, Wehner S, Kirfel G, Jaeger K, De Luca M, Herzog V. sAPP as a regulator of dendrite motility and melanin release in epidermal melanocytes and melanoma cells. *FASEB J* 2003;17:1739-1741.

[95] Herzog V, Kirfel G, Siemes C, Schmitz A. Biological roles of APP in the epidermis. Eur *J Cell Biol* 2004 ;83:613-624.

[96] Prota G, D'Ischia M, Napolitano A. The chemistry of melanins and related metabolites. In: Nordlund JJ, Boissy RE, Hearing VJ, King RA, Ortonne J-P, editors. *The Pigmentary System*. Oxford University Press; 1988.

[97] Rao KS, Hegde ML, Anitha S, Musicco M, Zucca FA, Turro NJ, Zecca L. Amyloid beta and neuromelanin--toxic or protective molecules? The cellular context makes the difference. *Prog Neurobiol* 2006;78:364-373.

[98] Chang M, Richards G, Rembaum A. Polyacrolein microspheres: preparation and characteristics. *Methods Enzymol* 1985;112:150-164.

[99] Lovell MA, Xie C, Markesbery WR. Acrolein is increased in Alzheimer's disease brain and is toxic to primary hippocampal cultures. *Neurobiol Aging* 2001;22:187-194.

[100] Butterfield DA, Castegna A, Lauderback CM, Drake J. Evidence that amyloid beta-peptide-induced lipid peroxidation and its sequelae in Alzheimer's disease brain contribute to neuronal death. *Neurobiol Aging* 2002;23:655-664.

[101] Soreghan B, Kosmoski J, Glabe C. Surfactant properties of Alzheimer's A beta peptides and the mechanism of amyloid aggregation. *J Biol Chem* 1994;269:28551-28554.

[102] Seidler NW, Craig HD, Squire TJ. Endogenous plastic composite material in the Alzheimer's brain. *Med Hypotheses* 2006;67:467-470.

[103] Blackley HK, Patel N, Davies MC, Roberts CJ, Tendler SJ, Wilkinson MJ, Williams PM. Morphological development of beta (1-40) amyloid fibrils. *Exp Neurol* 1999;158:437-443.

[104] Calingasan NY, Uchida K, Gibson GE. Protein-bound acrolein: a novel marker of oxidative stress in Alzheimer's disease. *J Neurochem* 1999;72:751-756.

[105] Uchida K, Kanematsu M, Sakai K, Matsuda T, Hattori N, Mizuno Y, Suzuki D, Miyata T, Noguchi N, Niki E, Osawa T. Protein-bound acrolein: potential markers for oxidative stress. *Proc Natl Acad Sci USA* 1998;95:4882-4887.

In: Alzheimer's Disease Research Trends
Editor: A.P. Chan, pp. 57-89

ISBN 978-1-60021-712-8

Chapter IV

DUAL INHIBITORS OF ACETYLCHOLINESTERASE AND SEROTONIN TRANSPORTER TARGETING POTENTIAL AGENTS FOR ALZHEIMER'S DISEASE

Narihiro Toda[1,3], Tsugio Kaneko[2,4] and Hiroshi Kogen[1,5,*]

[1]Exploratory Chemistry Research Laboratories, [2]Neuroscience and Immunology Research Laboratories, Sankyo Co., Ltd., Tokyo, Japan;

[3]Present address: Lead Discovery Research Laboratories, Sankyo Co., Ltd., Tokyo, Japan;

[4]Present address: Pharmacodynamics Research Laboratories, Sankyo Co., Ltd., Tokyo, Japan;

[5]Present address: R&D Strategy Department, Sankyo Co., Ltd., Tokyo, Japan.

ABSTRACT

To date, acetylcholinesterase (AChE) inhibitors are clinically effective drugs for a palliative treatment of Alzheimer's disease, but their clinical efficacy is limited mainly due to their adverse effects on peripheral organs. Since patients of Alzheimer's disease often exhibit depression as well as memory impairment, dual inhibitors of AChE and serotonin transporter (SERT) would be a better therapeutic method. Anti-depressive effects based on SERT inhibition would reduce dose-related side effects of AChE inhibitors.

Such dual inhibitors were designed by the hybridization of rivastigmine and fluoxetine based on a hypothetical model of the AChE active site. Various derivatives were synthesized and evaluated for their *in vitro* inhibition, and then (*S*)-**2j** (RS-1259),

* Correspondence concerning this article should be addressed to Dr. Hiroshi Kogen R&D Strategy Department, Sankyo Co., Ltd., 1-2-58 Hiromachi, Shinagawa-ku, Tokyo 140-8710, Japan; e-mail: hkogen@sankyo.co.jp.

which possessed balanced inhibitory activities of AChE (IC_{50} = 101 nM) and SERT (IC_{50} = 42 nM), was successfully obtained.

Molecular modeling studies of several compounds were performed to analyze their inhibitory activities against AChE. The results corresponded well with their potencies and provided some useful information about enzyme–inhibitor interaction.

An *ex vivo* experiment in mice indicated that (*S*)-2j (RS-1259) simultaneously inhibited AChE and SERT in the brain following an oral administration. The simultaneous elevation of extracellular levels of acetylcholine and serotonin in the rat hippocampus was actually confirmed by microdialysis. Both the cholinergic and serotonergic activation in the brain were confirmed by pharmacological tests such as the water maze test, and the merits of SERT inhibition were demonstrated.

Keywords: Alzheimer's disease, acetylcholinesterase, serotonin transporter, dual inhibitors.

1. Introduction

1-1. What is Dementia

Dementia, a condition where parts of the brain stop working, occurs more frequently as people age. As a result, in societies where the expectancy of life has been extended, dementia is one of the most severe health problems of the aging population. Approximately 15 percent of those who live to the age of 65 will show some symptoms of dementia. Currently, there are about 18 million people with dementia in the world. The number of people with dementia is expected to increase globally to about 34 million by 2025 [1]. People with dementia are unable to take care of themselves and need help in their daily life, since symptoms of dementia include breakdown of memory, judgment, reasoning and emotion.

The most common cause of dementia is Alzheimer's disease (AD), which accounts for 55% of all origins in the world. The second cause of dementia is vascular dementia (VD), which makes up 20% of all cases [2]. Consequently, it is important to introduce new therapeutic agents for AD in order to alleviate dementia.

1-2. About Alzheimer's Disease

AD, a neurodegenerative disorder discovered by Alois Alzheimer in 1907, is characterized by a progressive deterioration of memory and cognition [3]. Neuropathologically, AD is identified by three major signs: amyloid-β plaques (Aβ), neurofibrillary tangles (NFT) and synaptic loss [4]. In particularly, the degeneration of cholinergic neurons in the cortex and hippocampus and a loss of acetylcholine (ACh), a neurotransmitter for cholinergic neurotransmission, in the brain are characteristically observed in AD patients [5].

So far, no single factor of AD has been identified. It is likely that a combination of several factors, such as age and genetic makeup, and environmental factors are involved [6].

1-3. Treatment of Alzheimer's Disease

A deficiency in cholinergic neurotransmission is considered to play an important role in the learning and memory impairments of AD patients. Therefore, cholinergic enhancement is believed to be an effective therapeutic method to treat AD [7].

In the course of neurotransmission at cholinergic synapses (Figure 1), ACh is released from the presynapse into the synaptic cleft and binds to muscarinic and nicotinic receptors on the postsynapse. This nerve impulse transmission at cholinergic synapses is terminated by acetylcholinesterase (AChE), which catalyzes the hydrolysis of ACh.

To date, several strategies have been explored on the basis of the above neurotransmission mechanism in order to enhance cholinergic functions.

These are:

(1) AChE inhibitors, which increase the level of ACh in the synaptic cleft [8]
(2) ACh precursors, such as choline [9]
(3) ACh releasers, which advance the release of ACh from presynapses [10]
(4) muscarinic agonists, which activate muscarinic receptors on postsynapses [11]
(5) nicotinic agonists, which activate nicotinic receptors on postsynapses [12].

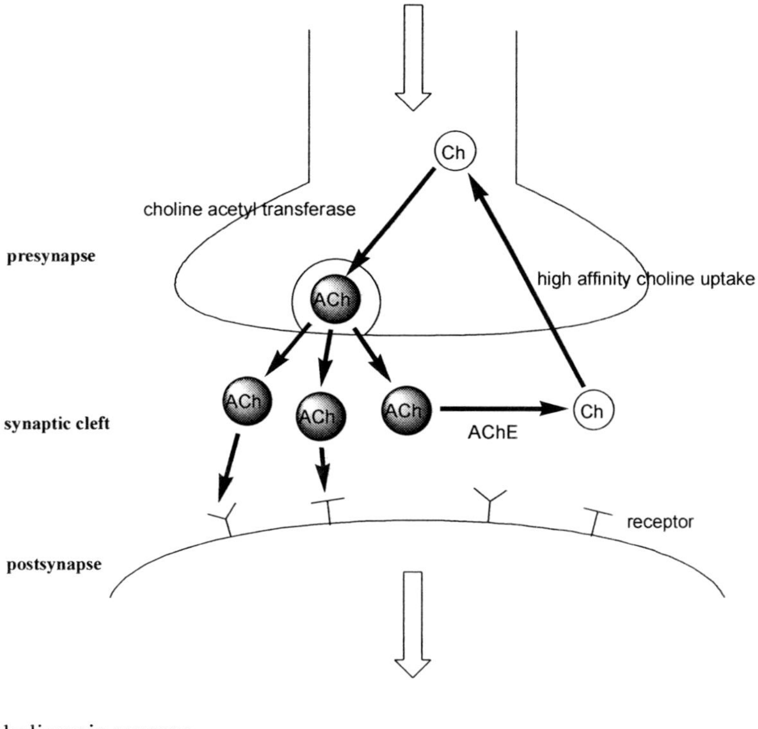

Figure 1. The cholinergic synapse.

Among these strategies, it is known that the only clinically effective strategy for a palliative treatment of AD is to inhibit AChE [13]. At present, several AChE inhibitors have successfully reached the market, such as tacrine (Cognex®), donepezil (Aricept®), rivastigmine (Exelon®) and galanthamine (Reminyl®) (Figure 2) [14,15,16,17].

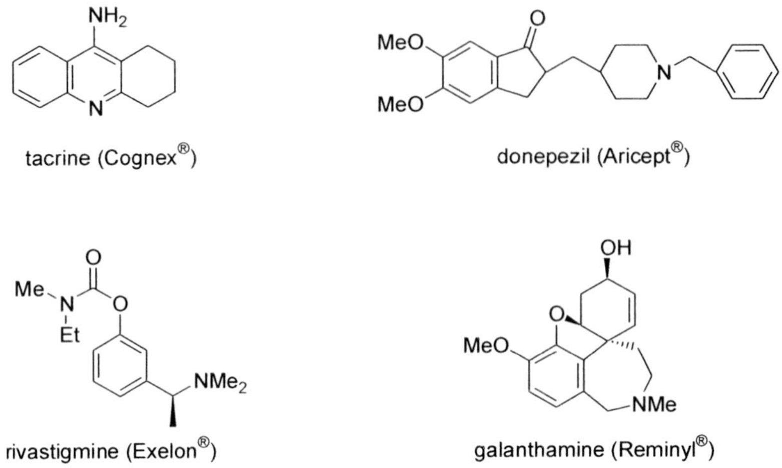

Figure 2. Structure of marketed AChE inhibitors.

Tacrine (Cognex®), a reversible AChE inhibitor, was the first approved drug for AD from Warner–Lambert. It can improve some symptoms of AD patients. However, it also causes a potentially serious side effect, liver damage.

Donepezil (Aricept®), a reversible AChE inhibitor, was produced by Eisai. It has now replaced tacrine because of its convenient once a day dosing regimen (tacrine, four times daily). In addition, it does not cause hepatotoxic effects.

Rivastigmine (Exelon®) was produced by Novartis Pharmaceuticals. From a structural viewpoint, it has a carbamate moiety which is considered to interact with the AChE active center. Recently, Bar-on *et al.* reported that rivastigmine was a pseudo-irreversible inhibitor of AChE based on structure interaction studies [18].

Galanthamine (Reminyl®), a tertiary alkaloid isolated from several plants, was co-developed by Shire Pharmaceuticals and the Janssen Research Foundation. It works as not only an AChE inhibitor but also as a nicotinic agonist.

These drugs do not provide complete cures, but stabilize some of the symptoms of AD patients for a limited time. However, the usefulness of these AChE inhibitors in the clinical setting is limited mainly due to their adverse effects on peripheral organs, since ACh works as the primary neurotransmitter in the whole body as well as in the brain [19].

1-4. Structure of Acetylcholinesterase

Sussman *et al.* reported on the determination of the crystal structure of AChE from *Torpedo californica* by X-ray analysis to 2.8 angstrom resolution (Figure 3) [20]. The AChE enzyme is an α/β protein that contains 537 amino acids forming 12 β-sheets surrounded by 14 α helices. The catalytic triad consisting of Ser200, His400 and Glu327, is located at the bottom of a deep and narrow gorge. The gorge is lined with the side chain rings of 14 aromatic residues.

With respect to donepezil, complex structure models and their binding interactions were simulated by molecular modeling methods [21]. Recently, Susmman *et al.* solved the complex crystal structure of donepezil with *Torpedo californica* AChE and reported three major binding interactions: the benzyl moiety to Trp84 at the bottom of the gorge; the charged nitrogen of the piperidine ring to Phe330 in the middle of the gorge; and the indanone ring to Trp279 at the top of the gorge (Figure 4) [22]. These studies provide useful information, for example, on inhibitor–enzyme interactions and possible binding sites, for the design of potent AChE inhibitors.

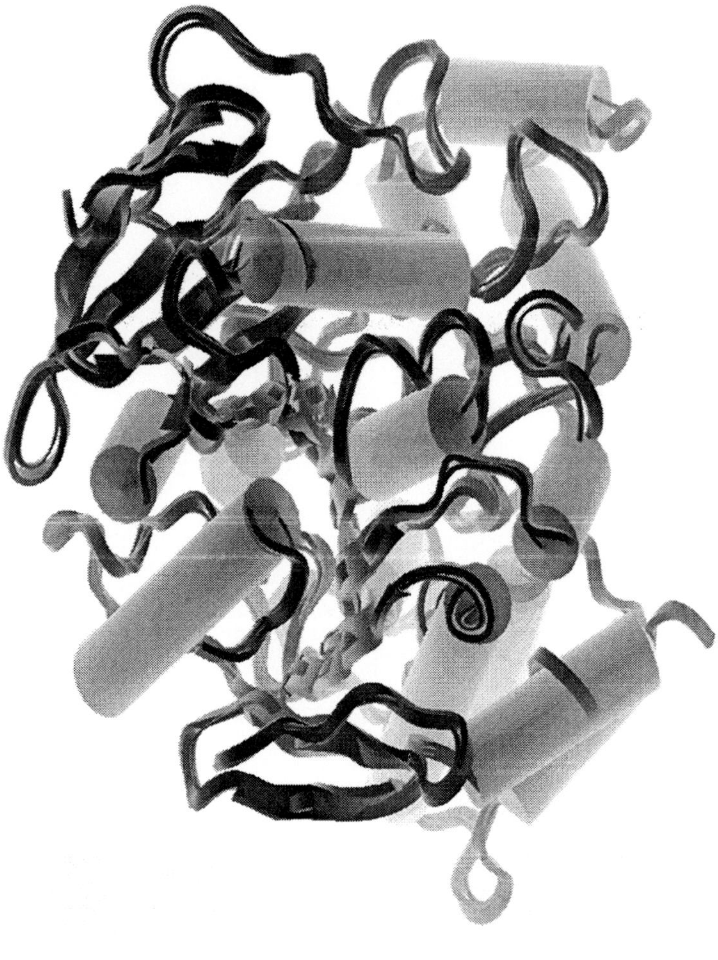

Figure 3. Crystal structure of AChE.

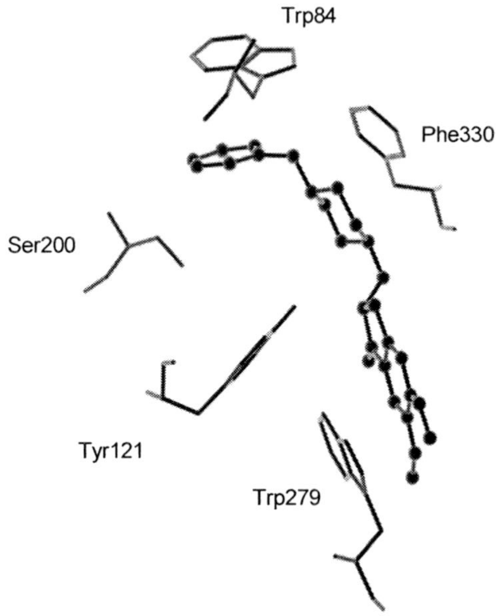

Figure 4. Major binding interactions of donepezil and *Torpedo californica* AChE.

1-5. Depression in Alzheimer's Disease

Recent studies suggest that cholinergic dysfunction does not completely explain the age-related cognitive deficits [23]. The hypofunction of several other neuronal systems such as the glutamatergic, GABAergic and monoaminergic systems in the brain of AD patients may be partly responsible for the cognitive decline [24]. There are many experimental reports suggesting that several neurotransmitters, including serotonin, norepinephrine, dopamine and GABA, appear to play a role in cognitive processes and interact with the cholinergic systems [25].

Moreover, AD patients often exhibit several behavioral abnormalities such as irritability, anxiety and depression, as well as cognitive impairment [26]. These psychiatric symptoms are sometimes controlled by psychotropic agents [27]. Among these symptoms, it is most often reported that depression is present in about 40% of patients with dementia [28]. Currently, depression in AD patients has been successfully treated with serotonin transporter (SERT) inhibitors [29], a type of antidepressant which has no anticholinergic side effect, since serotonin is known to be a neurotransmitter associated with many psychiatric symptoms including depression. At serotonergic synapses, serotonin is released in the brain synaptic cleft and binds to a receptor. Upon its reuptake into the presynaptic neuron by SERT, which terminates the action of serotonin, it is recycled into the neurotransmitter pool (Figure 5). Therefore, inhibition of SERT results in an increased concentration of serotonin in the brain synaptic cleft, i.e. an enhanced serotonergic neurotransmission.

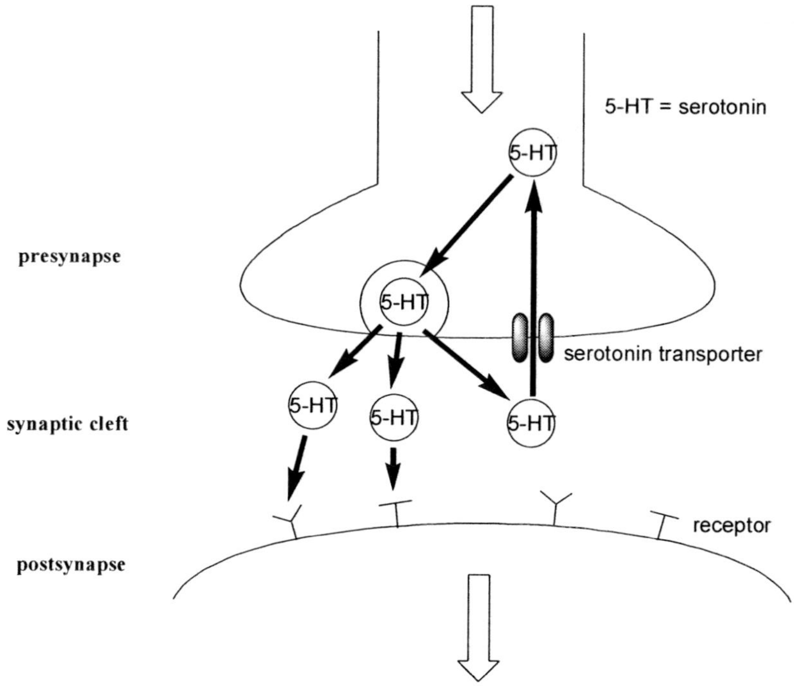

Figure 5. Serotonin reuptake process in the serotonergic synapse.

1-6. Concept of Dual Inhibitors of AChE and SERT as Therapeutic Agents for Alzheimer's Disease

To date, AChE inhibitors are able to enhance memory in AD patients, but their clinical efficacy is limited mainly due to their adverse peripheral effects [19]. SERT inhibitors which have no anticholinergic side effect are also useful for controlling depression in AD patients [29]. However, co-administration of SERT and AChE inhibitors is considered undesirable due to the difficulty in managing their different pharmacodynamics and pharmacokinetics properties. Moreover, it may cause harmful drug–drug interactions [30].

In order to overcome these disadvantages, a drug inhibiting both SERT and AChE but in a balanced manner is considered to be a promising method. This combined SERT and AChE inhibition would bring about greater therapeutic benefits than AChE inhibition alone, since further improvement of cognitive deficits could be achieved without the dose-related adverse effects caused by excessive AChE inhibition. Thus, AChE–SERT dual inhibitors would make a novel class of anti-AD drugs that is more effective in alleviating the symptoms of AD than known AChE inhibitors (Figure 6).

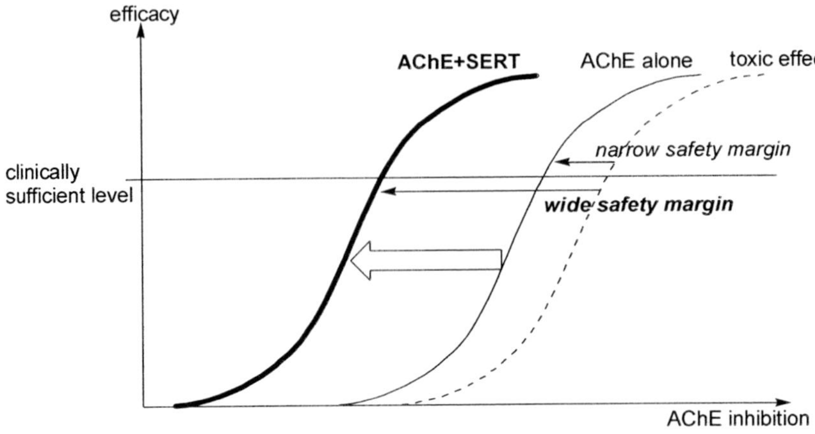

Figure 6. Wider safety margin of AChE–SERT dual inhibitors.

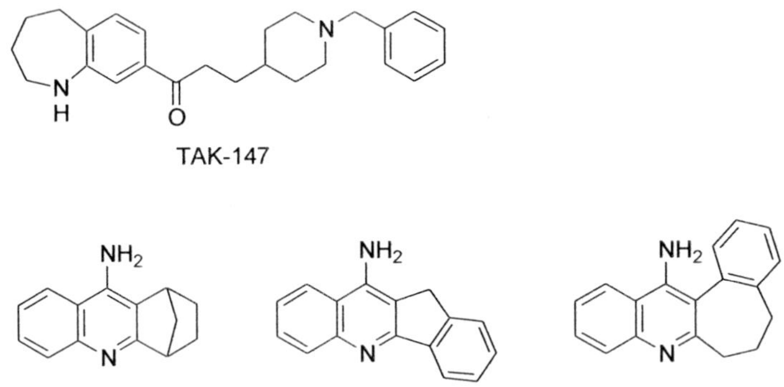

Figure 7. Reported AChE–SERT dual inhibitors: Hirai's TAK-147 and McKenna's tacrine analogues.

So far, only two groups have studied AChE inhibitors that also possess SERT inhibitory activity. Hirai *et al.* reported that TAK-147 showed potent AChE inhibition (IC_{50} = 51 nM) (Figure 7). Furthermore, it weakly inhibited norepinephrine transporter and SERT (IC_{50} = 4020 and 1350 nM, respectively) [31]. McKenna *et al.* reported that several analogues of tacrine could be useful templates for further investigation of dual AChE and SERT inhibitors (Figure 7) [32]. The compounds described from these two groups showed potent AChE inhibitory activities and moderate SERT inhibitory activities *in vitro*. However, the extent of inhibition against each was imbalanced when it came to *in vivo* dual inhibition. Consequently, the antidepressive effect resulting from SERT inhibition was not observed due to the dominating effect of increased cholinergic transmission. It is clear that the balance between AChE and SERT inhibition is crucial for the simultaneous activation of the cholinergic and serotonergic transmissions in the brain *in vivo*. Therefore, the creation of a balanced dual inhibitor of AChE and SERT, that can achieve the same pharmacological effects as those observed *in vivo*, would be challenging but important.

2. Design of Dual Inhibitors of AChE and SERT

A deficiency in the cholinergic neurotransmission is considered to play an important role in the learning and memory impairments of AD patients. Enhancement of the cholinergic function by inhibiting AChE, which terminates nerve impulse transmission at cholinergic synapses by catalyzing the hydrolysis of ACh, is the only clinically effective method for a palliative treatment of AD [13]. However, the usefulness of AChE inhibitors in the clinical setting is limited mainly due to their adverse effects on peripheral organs [19].

Furthermore, AD patients often suffer from psychiatric disorder-related symptoms, such as irritability, anxiety and depression [26]. Among these symptoms, it is especially known that depression is seen in almost 40% of patients with dementia [28]. Currently, the most commonly used treatments for depression in AD patients are SERT inhibitors such as fluoxetine and paroxetine which have no anticholinergic side effects (Figure 8) [29,33,34].

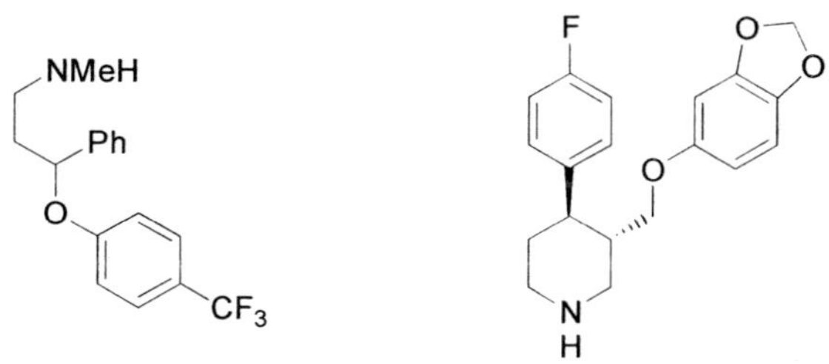

fluoxetine (Prozac®)   paroxetine (Paxil®)

Figure 8. Examples of SERT inhibitors.

Thus, combined SERT and AChE inhibition is considered to bring about greater therapeutic benefits than AChE inhibition alone since further improvement of cognitive deficits could be achieved and dose-related adverse effects caused by excessive AChE inhibition could be avoided (Figure 6).

There is no information about three-dimensional structure of SERT since it has yet to be elucidated. Meanwhile, the crystal structure of AChE from *Torpedo californica* has been revealed. Moreover, the complex crystal structure of donepezil with *Torpedo californica* AChE was recently solved [22]. It revealed three major binding interactions: a hydrophobic interaction at the bottom of the gorge; a cation–π interaction in the middle of the gorge; a hydrophobic interaction at the top of the gorge. Knowledge of the three-dimensional structure of AChE and ligand binding interactions is highly useful for rational drug design.

Thus, in an attempt to design novel AChE–SERT dual inhibitors as a new class of anti-AD drugs, we proposed a hypothetical model of the AChE active site on the basis of the crystal structure of AChE with donepezil and molecular modeling studies (Scheme 1) [21,35]. Our hypothetical model consists of four enzyme-binding sites and corresponding binding elements. We selected rivastigmine, one of the marketed AChE inhibitors, as a lead compound because rivastigmine possesses three binding elements: a carbamate moiety at the catalytic triad site; an aromatic ring at the hydrophobic site A; and an amine moiety at the ionic site. Focusing on the fourth binding site of our model, we selected fluoxetine as a pharmacophoric element corresponding to the hydrophobic site B. Fluoxetine has potent

SERT inhibitory activity and possesses an ethylamine moiety that could be overlapped with that of rivastigmine. Therefore, we designed a type A compound by the hybridization of these two compounds at the common ethylamine moiety. Our designed type A compound was anticipated to be a dual inhibitor of AChE and SERT.

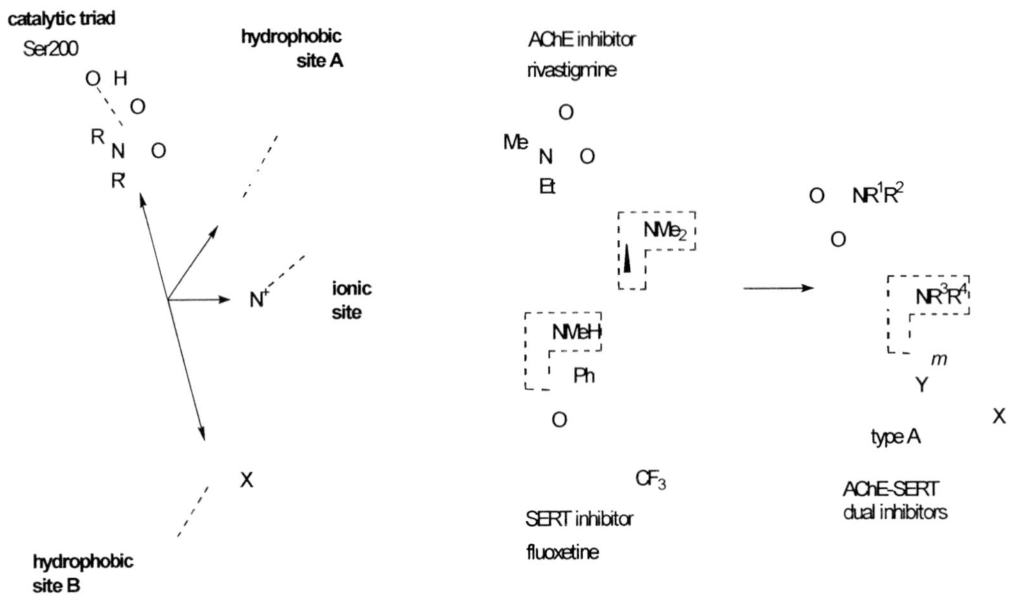

Scheme 1. Design of AChE–SERT dual inhibitors based on a hypothetical model of an AChE active site with a proposed pharmacophore.

3. Synthesis and Structure–Activity Relationships of AChE–SERT Dual Inhibitors

Various type A compounds were synthesized and evaluated for their inhibitory potencies of AChE and SERT [36].

Table 1 summarizes the inhibitory activities of compounds 1a–f (m = 1, Y = O, $R^1 = R^2 = R^3$ = Me, R^4 = H) which possess the dimethylcarbamate at the *meta* position similarly to rivastigmine. For comparison, the assay data of rivastigmine, donepezil and fluoxetine are also included. The effect of the electron-donating (1a,b) and electron-withdrawing (1c–f) substituents X at the 4-position of the phenyl ether moiety was examined. Nearly all of the 4-substituted derivatives 1a–e exhibited potent inhibitory activity against SERT (IC_{50} = <50 nM) but much lower activity against AChE (IC_{50} = >1000 nM). However, only the 4-nitro-substituted derivative 1f was found to be a potential dual inhibitor of AChE (IC_{50} = 221 nM) and SERT (IC_{50} = 52 nM).

Table 1. *In vitro* AChE and SERT inhibitory activity of *meta*-carbamate derivatives

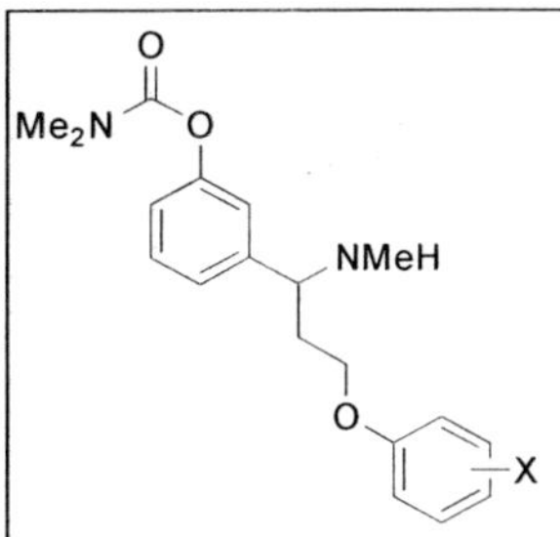

Compound[a]	X	IC_{50} (nM)	
		AChE[b]	SERT[c]
rivastigmine		11000	>1000
donepezil		10	>1000
fluoxetine		>10000	180
1a	4-OMe	>1000	38
1b	4-Me	>1000	49
1c	4-Cl	870	81
1d	4-F	870	16
1e	4-CF_3	>1000	13
1f	4-NO_2	221	52

[a]Compounds were tested as their hydrochloride salts.
[b]From mouse brain. [c]From rat synaptosome.

Table 2. *In vitro* AChE and SERT inhibitory activity of *para*-carbamate derivatives

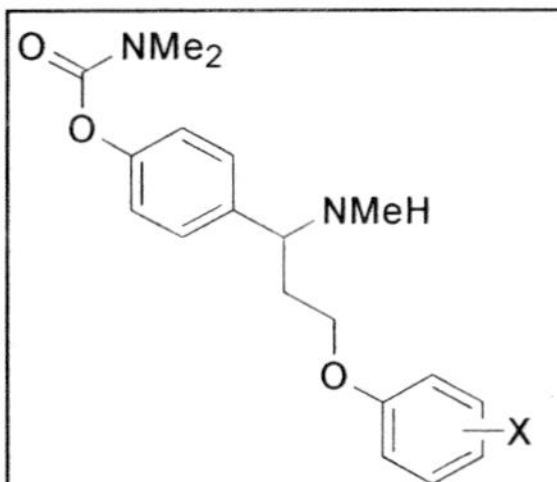

Compound[a]	X	IC_{50} (nM)	
		AChE[b]	SERT[c]
2a	4-OMe	220	310
2b	4-Me	726	230
2c	H	341	>1000
2d	4-Cl	493	210
2e	4-F	594	790
2f	4-CF_3	572	130
2g	4-CN	330	500
2h	2-NO_2	52	>1000
2i	3-NO_2	14	175
2j	4-NO_2	125	44

[a]Compounds were tested as their hydrochloride salts.
[b]From mouse brain. [c]From rat synaptosome.

Changing the location of the dimethylcarbamate from the *meta* position to the *para* position mostly increased the potency against AChE (Table 2). The potency against SERT was modestly maintained. *p*-Carbamate derivatives were potential AChE–SERT dual inhibitors as expected. Among the compounds 2a–j, the 4-nitro-substituted derivative 2j was revealed to possess good potencies against both AChE (IC_{50} = 125 nM) and SERT (IC_{50} = 44 nM), inhibiting them both to a suitable extent.

The effect of the carbamate moiety in 2j was examined (Table 3). The carbamate derivatives 3a,b had good anti-SERT activity but moderate anti-AChE activity. The dimethylamide derivative 3d no longer exhibited an inhibitory effect against AChE, whereas its anti-SERT activity was maintained. The removal of the dimetylcarbamate moiety from 2j led to a loss of the inhibitory activities against both AChE and SERT (3c). These results suggest that the dimethylcarbamate moiety is essential for anti-AChE activity.

Table 3. *In vitro* AChE and SERT inhibitory activity of derivatives with different carbamates

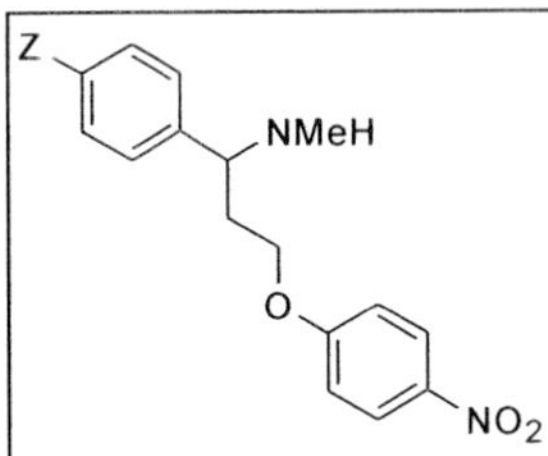

Compound[a]	Z	IC_{50} (nM) AChE[b]	SERT[c]
2j	$-OCONMe_2$	125	44
3a	-OCONMeH	497	32
3b	-OCONEtH	>1000	46
3d	$-CH_2CONMe_2$	>1000	60
3c	-OH	>1000	>1000

[a]Compounds were tested as their hydrochloride salts.
[b]From mouse brain. [c]From rat synaptosome.

Table 4. *In vitro* AChE and SERT inhibitory activity of derivatives with various amines

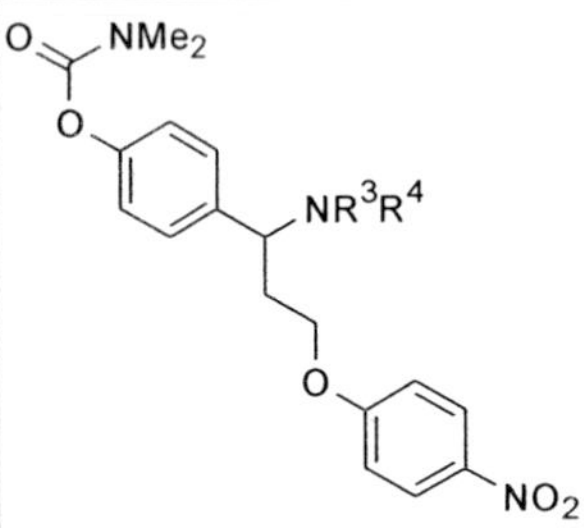

Compound[a]	NR^3R^4	IC_{50} (nM) AChE[b]	SERT[c]
2j	NMeH	125	44
4a	NMe_2	319	87
4b	N^+Me_3	>1000	44
4c	NEtH	326	>1000
4d	NMeEt	378	980
4e	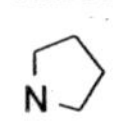	852	>1000
4f	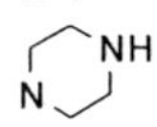	>1000	500
4g	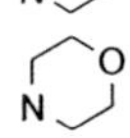	>1000	>1000

[a]Compounds were tested as their hydrochloride salts.
[b]From mouse brain. [c]From rat synaptosome.

The optimization of the methylamine moiety in 2j is shown in Table 4. The dimethylamine derivative 4a was found to be less potent than 2j. Increasing the size of the amine (4c–g) resulted in a sharp decline of inhibitory potencies against both AChE and SERT. Ammonium derivative 4b was found to have lost its inhibitory activities against AChE (IC_{50} = >1000 nM), whereas the potency against SERT was maintained (IC_{50} = 44 nM). In general, it seems that a small amine group like methylamine is particularly favorable for dual inhibition of AChE and SERT. However, the primary amine derivative (R^3 = R^4 = H) no longer displayed anti-SERT activity.

Table 5. *In vitro* AChE and SERT inhibitory activity of derivatives with different tethers and substituted heteroatoms

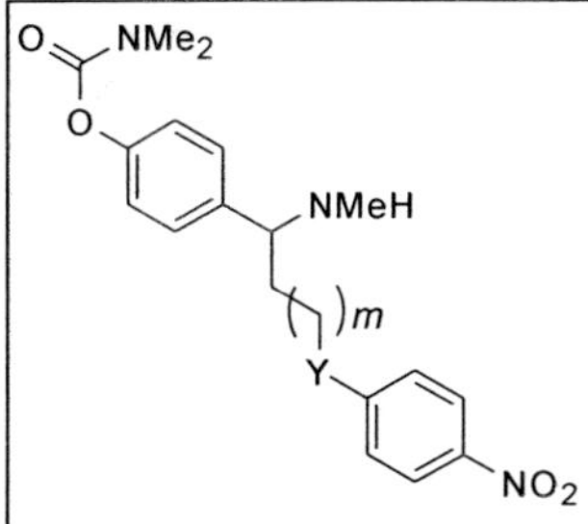

Compound[a]	m	Y	IC_{50} (nM) AChE[b]	IC_{50} (nM) SERT[c]
5	0	O	>1000	>1000
2j	1	O	125	44
6	2	O	77	>1000
7	1	NH	36	>1000
8	1	NAc	>1000	>1000
9	1	S	61	680
10	1	none	524	670

[a]Compounds were tested as their hydrochloride salts.
[b]From mouse brain. [c]From rat synaptosome.

As shown in Table 5, the effects of the tether length and the replacement of the hetero atom were examined. Compound 5 (m = 0, Y = O) possessing a shorter tether length exhibited much less activity toward both AChE and SERT than 2j (m = 1, Y = O). However, compound 6 possessing a longer tether length (m = 2, Y = O) displayed stronger activity against AChE (IC_{50} = 77 nM) than 2j (IC_{50} = 125 nM) but lower potency against SERT (IC_{50} = >1000 nM). It seems that the nitrophenoxy moiety of compound 6 interacted more efficiently with the hydrophobic site B in our hypothetical model of the AChE active site than compounds 2j and 5. The replacement of oxygen by nitrogen (7 and 8, Y = NH and NAc, respectively) or sulfur (9, Y = S) resulted in a reduction of inhibitory potency particularly against SERT. Compound 10 in which the ethereal oxygen was removed from 2j, was found to be a moderate dual inhibitor of AChE (IC_{50} = 524 nM) and SERT (IC_{50} = 670 nM). These replacement studies revealed that the ethereal oxygen was crucial for the inhibition of both AChE and SERT.

Since we described that racemic 2j was the best dual inhibitor of AChE and SERT, both enantiomers of 2j were synthesized from known chiral amines (*S*)-11 and (*R*)-11 as shown in Scheme 2 [36].

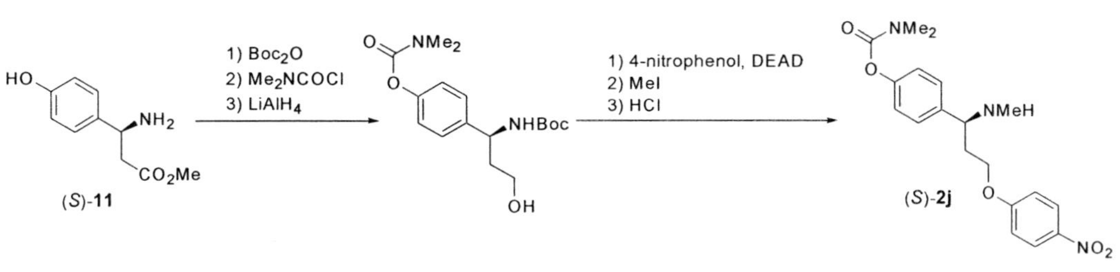

Scheme 2. Synthesis of an enantiomer of 2j, an AChE and SERT dual inhibitor

The inhibitory activities of both enantiomers were evaluated (Table 6). Compound (*S*)-2j showed potent inhibitory potencies against both AChE (IC_{50} = 101 nM) and SERT (IC_{50} = 42 nM). There was little difference in AChE inhibitory activity between the stereoisomers of 2j. However, SERT inhibition of (*S*)-2j was threefold more potent than that of (*R*)-5j. This difference in inhibitory activity due to stereochemistry was also observed in the enantiomers of 2d which possess a chlorine instead of a nitro group. Both enantiomers of 2d showed similar anti-AChE activities, and (*S*)-2d exhibited a threefold higher inhibitory activity than (*R*)-2d. These results showed that the (*S*)-configuration in type A compounds was desirable to obtain a strong SERT inhibitory activity. In addition, compound (*S*)-2j showed little inhibitory activity against various transporters including norepinephrine and dopamine transporters, butylcholinesterase and choline acetyltransferase.

Table 6. *In vitro* AChE and SERT inhibitory activity of 2j and 2d enantiomers

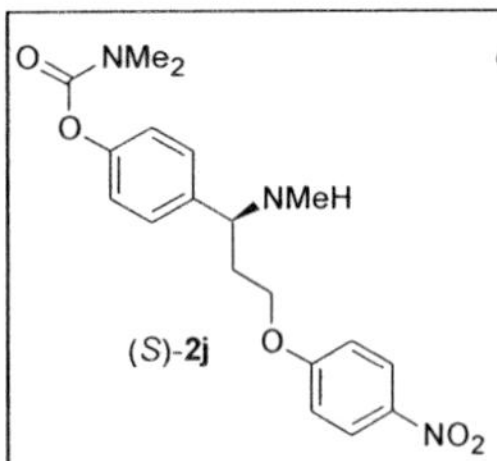

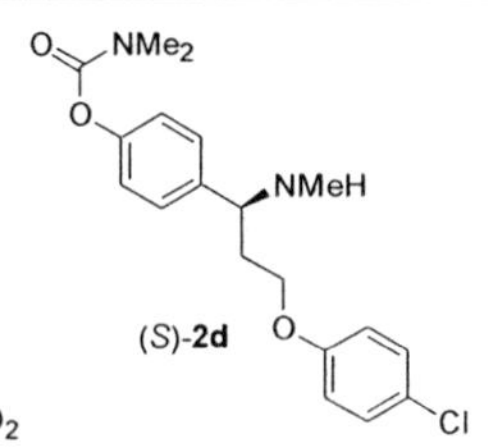

Compound[a]	IC_{50} (nM)	
	AChE[b]	SERT[c]
rac-**2j**	125	44
(*R*)-**2j**	143	135
(*S*)-**2j**	101	42
rac-**2d**	493	210
(*R*)-**2d**	343	270
(*S*)-**2d**	377	83

[a]Compounds were tested as their hydrochloride salts.
[b]From mouse brain. [c]From rat synaptosome.

4. A Conformational Restriction Approach to the Development of AChE–SERT Dual Inhibitors

For further development of dual inhibitory activities of AChE and SERT, conformationally restricted type B derivatives were designed by linking the methylamine moiety and *ortho*-carbon atom of the phenyl ring of (*S*)-2j with a carbon chain of appropriate length (Figure 9) [37].

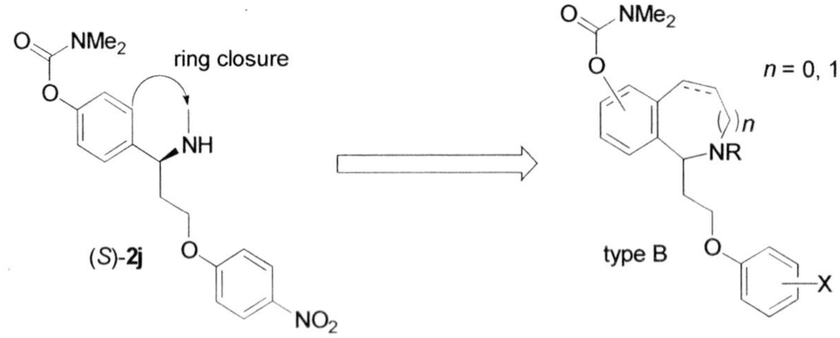

Figure 9. Development of AChE–SERT dual inhibitors using a conformational restriction approach.

Table 7 summarizes the inhibitory activities against AChE and SERT of the conformationally restricted derivatives containing a 1,2,3,4-tetrahydroisoquinoline skeleton (12a,b, 13a,b, 14a–g, 15 and 16a,b). As shown in the preceding section, it was revealed that a nitro group for substituent X on the phenyl ether moiety and *para*-carbamate substitution were crucial for potent dual inhibitory activities. However, 1,2,3,4-tetrahydroisoquinoline derivatives were reinvestigated with respect to substituent X using, in particular, an electron-withdrawing group, and ideal carbamate position. A series of 1,2,3,4-tetrahydroisoquinoline derivatives dramatically enhanced the inhibitory activity toward AChE, but their inhibitory activity toward SERT almost disappeared. We supposed that the conformational restriction of the flexible amine moiety resulted in the appropriate binding to AChE. The reason for the disappearance of anti-SERT activity could not be determined because we had no information on the structure of SERT. Among the compounds with 1,2,3,4-tetrahydroisoquinoline structure, 12a (R = H, X = 4-NO_2) showed the most potent inhibitory activity against AChE (IC_{50} = 8 nM). In comparison with compound (*S*)-2j (IC_{50} = 101 nM against AChE), 12a was about 13 times more active against AChE. Similarly to type A derivatives, compound 12a possessed a 4-NO_2 group as substituent X and 6-substituted carbamate moiety on the 1,2,3,4-tetrahydroisoquinoline skeleton.

Table 7. *In vitro* AChE and SERT inhibition activity of 1,2,3,4-tetrahydroisoquinoline derivatives

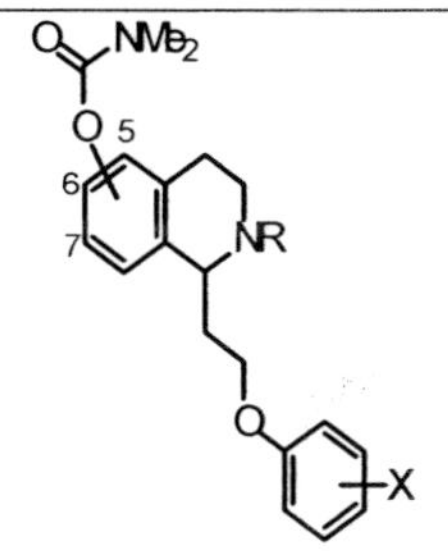

Compound[a]	carbamate position	R	X	IC_{50} (nM) AChE[b]	IC_{50} (nM) SERT[c]
12a	6-	H	4-NO_2	8	>1000
12b	6-	H	4-Cl	17	>1000
13a	7-	H	4-NO_2	101	>1000
13b	7-	H	4-Cl	219	>1000
14a	6-	Me	4-NO_2	11	940
14c	6-	Me	3-Me-4-NO_2	16	170
14d	6-	Me	3-NO_2	11	125
14b	6-	Me	4-Cl	33	660
14e	6-	Me	4-F	49	>1000
14f	6-	Me	4-Br	34	>1000
14g	6-	Me	4-OMe	20	>1000
15	5-	Me	4-NO_2	56	750
16a	7-	Me	4-NO_2	161	>1000
16b	7-	Me	4-Cl	265	520

[a]Compound were tested as their hydrochloride salts. [b]From mouse brain. [c]From rat synaptosome

Table 8. ***In vitro*** **AChE and SERT inhibition activity of derivatives with a seven-membered ring**

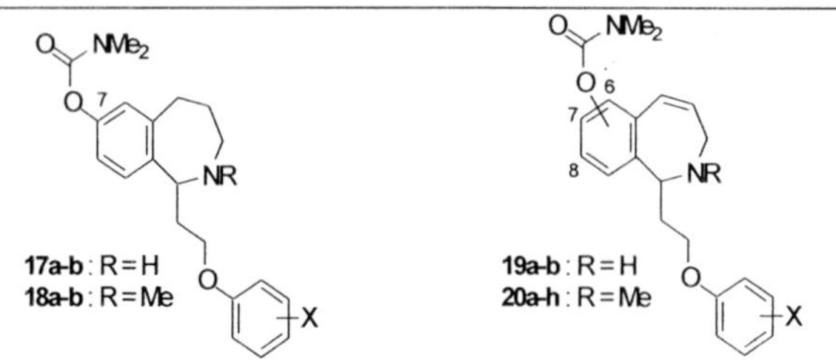

Compound[a]	carbamate position	R	X	IC_{50} (nM) AChE[b]	IC_{50} (nM) SERT[c]
17a	7-	H	4-NO_2	55	>1000
17b	7-	H	4-Cl	215	>1000
18a	7-	Me	4-NO_2	61	>1000
18b	7-	Me	4-Cl	116	>1000
19a	7-	H	4-NO_2	92	>1000
19b	7-	H	3-Me-4-Cl	153	>1000
20a	7-	Me	4-NO_2	66	63
20b	7-	Me	3-Me-4-Cl	103	61
20c	7-	Me	4-Cl	139	71
20d	7-	Me	4-F	135	850
20e	7-	Me	4-CF_3	285	62
20f	6-	Me	3-Me-4-Cl	146	900
20g	8-	Me	4-NO_2	>1000	>1000
20h	8-	Me	4-Cl	>1000	>1000

[a]Compound were tested as their hydrochloride salts. [b]From mouse brain. [c]From rat synaptosome

Next, we examined the rigid derivatives 17a,b, 18a,b containing a saturated seven-membered ring and 19a,b, 20a–h containing an unsaturated seven-membered ring (Table 8). Compounds 17a,b (R = H) and 18a,b (R = Me) showed higher inhibitory potencies against AChE but much lower potencies against SERT similarly to 1,2,3,4- tetrahydroquinoline derivatives. Compounds 19a,b (R = H) which possessed a double bond on the seven-membered ring also exhibited good inhibitory activities but only against AChE, whereas compounds 20a–e (R = Me) surprisingly showed potent inhibitory activities against not only AChE but also SERT. We have not determined the reason for this striking improvement in anti-SERT activities obtained by changing the secondary amine (R = H) to a tertiary amine (R = Me) on the seven-membered ring. However, it is clear that the olefin moiety on the seven-membered ring is essential for the inhibitory potency of SERT as can be seen by comparing derivatives 20a–e with 18a,b. Compound 20a was the most potent dual inhibitor of AChE (IC_{50} = 66 nM) and SERT (IC_{50} = 63 nM). Changing the substitution position of the dimethylcarbamate from 7- to 6- (20f) and 8- (20g,h) resulted in the loss of inhibitory potency for SERT.

Table 9 shows the effects of changing the substituent on the olefin moiety of compound 20a. Derivatives 21a,b, which have small substituents (R' = Me, vinyl) maintained their inhibitory activities against AChE (IC_{50} = 60 and 43 nM, respectively), but lost their inhibitory activities against SERT (both IC_{50} = >1000 nM). Derivative 21d, which has a large substituent (R' = *p*-chlorophenyl), had little inhibitory activity against both AChE (IC_{50} = >1000 nM) and SERT (IC_{50} = >1000 nM). Exo olefin derivative 22 also had little inhibitory activity against SERT (IC_{50} = >1000 nM). These results revealed that a 7-membered internal olefin without substituents at the double bond was essential for SERT inhibition.

Table 9. Effect of various substituents on the inhibitory activity of 20a

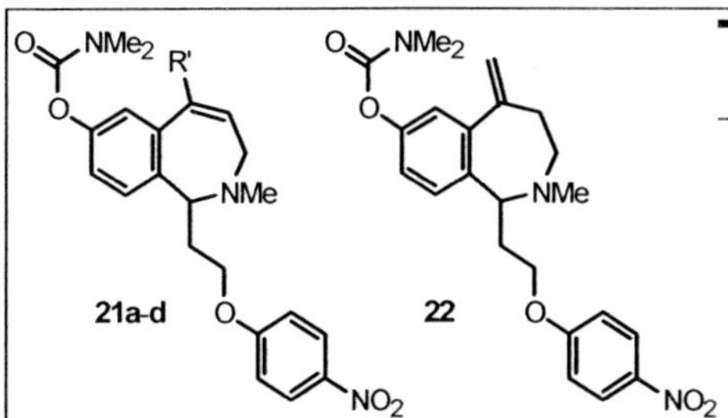

Compound[a]	R'	IC_{50} (nM) AChE[b]	IC_{50} (nM) SERT[c]
20a	H	66	63
21a	Me	60	>1000
21b	Vinyl	43	>1000
21c	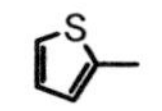	150	>1000
21d	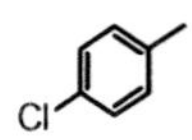	>1000	>1000
22		27	>1000

[a]Compound were tested as their hydrochloride salts.
[b]From mouse brain. [c]From rat synaptosome

Consequently, compound 20a was the most potent type B dual inhibitor, and both enantiomers of 20a were synthesized as shown in Scheme 3 [37]. Ester 24 derived from phenol 23 was subjected to a chiral amination reaction with (*S*)-25, which was reported by Davies, followed by deprotection and Boc-protection to yield (*R*)-26 (99% ee). Styrene (*R*)-27, a precursor for ring-closing olefin metathesis, was synthesized from compound (*R*)-26 in several steps. Ring-closing olefin metathesis of (*R*)-27 with 10 mol% of Grubbs catalyst 28 gave the desired seven-membered ring product in high yield. The resulting cyclic product led to (*R*)-20a in two steps.

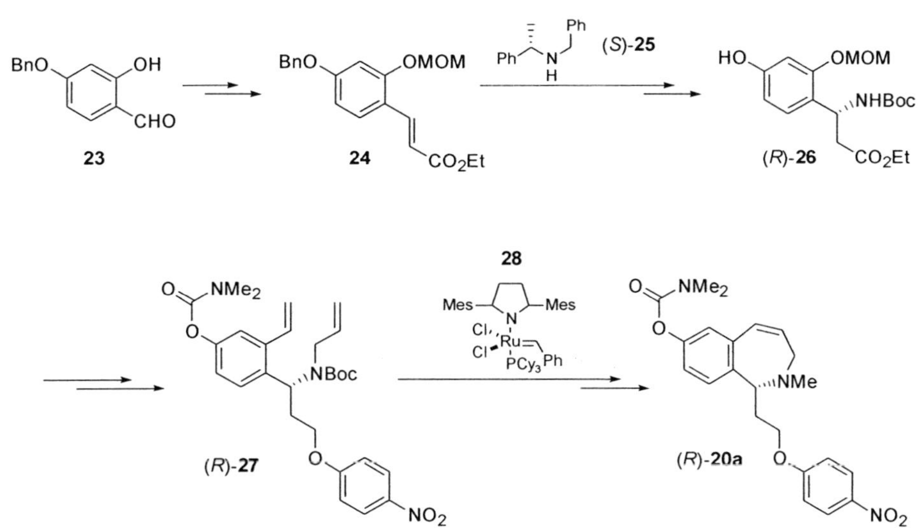

Scheme 3. Synthesis of an enantiomer of **20a**, an AChE and SERT dual inhibitor.

The inhibitory activity of both enantiomers of 20a was evaluated as shown in Table 10. Surprisingly, the enantiomer (*R*)-20a showed extremely potent inhibitory activities against both AChE (IC_{50} = 14 nM) and SERT (IC_{50} = 6 nM) as compared to type A dual inhibitors (*S*)-2j. Although both enantiomers of 2j showed similar levels of AChE inhibition, (*R*)-20a showed a 44 times stronger inhibitory activity against AChE than (*S*)-20a. This difference in AChE inhibition would result from the conformational rigidity of 20a. Similarly (*R*)-20a exhibited a 155 times stronger inhibitory activity against SERT than (*S*)-20a. Compound (*R*)-20a showed extremely weak inhibitory activities against butylcholinesterase, choline acetyltransferase, norepinephrine and dopamine transporters.

Table 10. *In vitro* AChE and SERT inhibition activity of 20a enantiomers

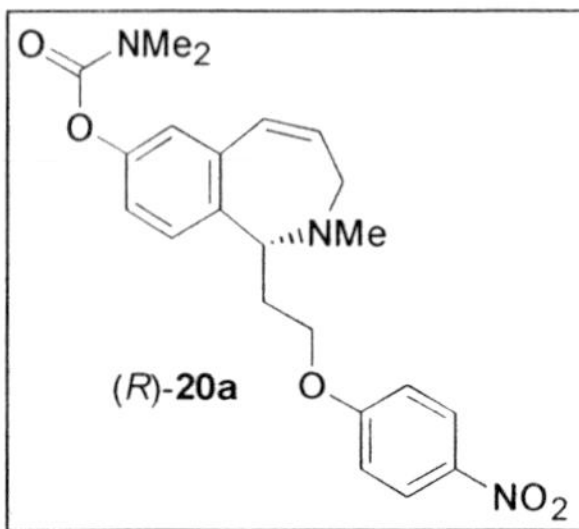

(*R*)-**20a**

Compound[a]	IC_{50} (nM)	
	AChE[b]	SERT[c]
rac-**20a**	66	63
(*R*)-**20a**	14	6
(*S*)-**20a**	609	930

[a]Compound were tested as their hydrochloride salts.
[b]From mouse brain. [c]From rat synaptosome

5. Docking Study of Dual AChE–SERT Inhibitors

A conformational analysis and a docking study of derivatives 2j, 5, 6 and 20a with AChE were performed in order to analyze their AChE inhibitory potencies (Figure 10) [38].

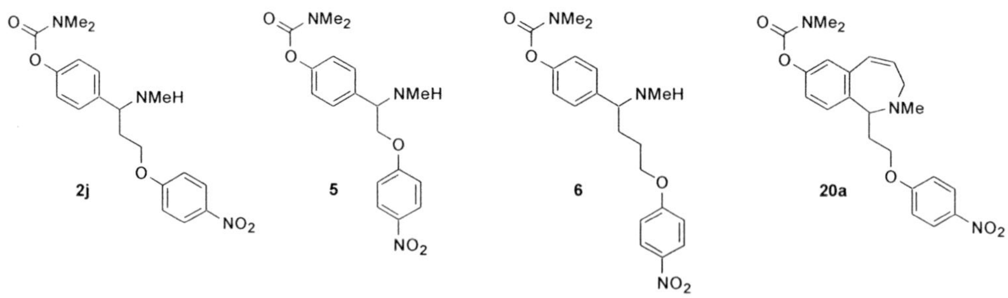

Figure 10. Chemical structures of AChE–SERT dual inhibitors 2j, 5, 6 and 20a.

Each compound was model-built using the QUANTA system in the protonated form with respect to the basic amine. A conformational analysis using molecular dynamics and molecular mechanics was performed using the CHARMm force field [39,40]. The docking study of the inhibitors was carried out with the QUANTA/CHARMm system based on several low energy conformations obtained by the conformational analysis. A series of initial positions and conformations of the inhibitors were manually set and stable complex structures were obtained by energy minimization with the enzyme structure being fixed.

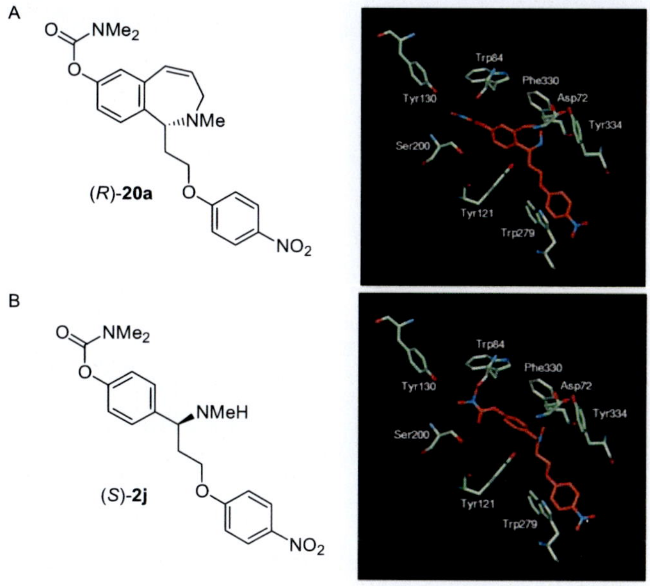

Figure 11. Complex structure models of AChE and (*R*)-20a (A) or (*S*)-2j (B).

From the results, comparable interaction energies were obtained for (*R*)-2j and (*S*)-2j. This is consistent with the fact that only a slight difference was observed for the IC_{50} values of the isomers of 2j. On the other hand, the interaction energy of the most stable model of (*R*)-20a was about 6 kcal/mol more stable than that of (*S*)-20a, which is consistent with the observed potencies of the isomers of 20a, i.e., (*R*)-20a is around 40 times more potent than (*S*)-20a.

The most stable complex structure models of (*R*)-20a and (*S*)-2j are shown in Figure 11. As it can be seen for both cases, the carbamate moiety was located near catalytic Ser200 and the phenyl ring was located in the hydrophobic pocket near Phe330, which is located deep in the gorge. The proton of the tertiary ammonium group did not interact directly with the carboxyl group of Asp72. The positive charge is considered to be stabilized by the aromatic ring of Tyr334 through an aromatic–ammonium interaction [41]. This kind of interaction is observed in several complex crystal structures such as those of donepezil [42]. The 4-nitrophenoxy moiety was located near the indole ring of Trp279 at the top of the gorge.

In the case of compounds 2j, 5 and 6, the length of the methylene chain between the benzylamine and nitrophenoxy moieties is an important factor affecting the potency. Compound 5 with a shorter tether group showed very weak inhibitory activity (IC_{50} = >1000 nM). In contrast, compound 5 showed a slightly higher potency (IC_{50} = 77 nM) than compound 2j (IC_{50} = ~100 nM). In order to explain the difference among 2j, 5 and 6, we focused on the position of the nitrophenoxy group at the binding site (Figure 12). The nitrophenoxy group of 2j was involved in the hydrophobic interaction with the indole group of Trp279 as mentioned above. In the case of 5, the distance between the nitrophenoxy group and indole rings became 0.2 Å longer than that of (*S*)-2j. The shorter tether for 5 would prevent both phenyl and nitrophenoxy groups to simultaneously interact with the hydrophobic pocket at the bottom and top of the gorge, respectively. On the other hand, the distance between the nitrophenoxy group of 6 and the indole ring of Trp279 was 0.4 Å shorter than that of (*S*)-2j, leading to an enlarged ring overlap. Moreover, the interaction at the peripheral hydrophobic site seemed to be more favorable due to the additional hydrophobic methylene group of 6, even though its larger number of rotatable bonds was more disadvantageous with respect to entropy compared to 2j. This resulted in a slight improvement of the inhibitory activity of 6.

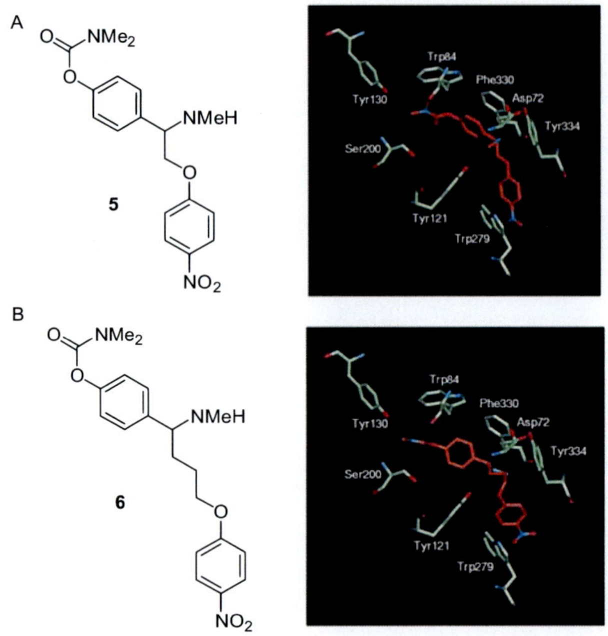

Figure 12. Complex structure models of AChE and 5 (A) or 6 (B).

6. Pharmacological Effects of Dual AChE–SERT Inhibitors

Pharmacological properties of (*S*)-2j, the most potent type A compound, and (*R*)-20a, the most potent type B compound, were evaluated in order to show efficacy as a drug for AD [43]. In the experiments, (*S*)-2j was used as a (fumaric acid)$_{1/2}$ salt (RS-1259) for solidification and (*R*)-20a was used as a hydrochloride salt (Figure 13).

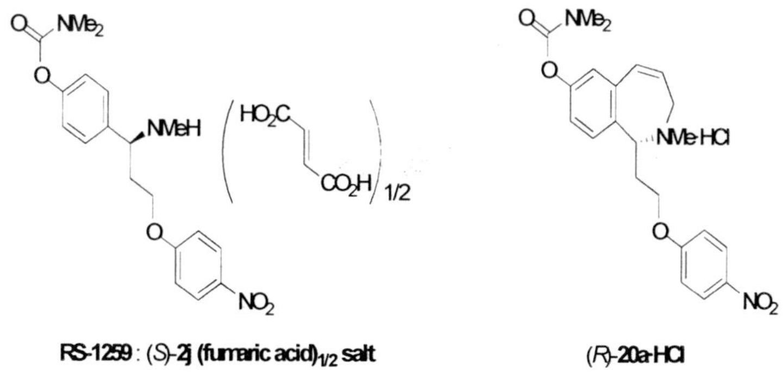

Figure 13. Chemical structures of AChE–SERT dual inhibitors RS-1259 and (*R*)-20a.

Ex Vivo Inhibition of AChE and SERT

The result of the ex vivo inhibitory effects on AChE and SERT of RS-1259 in the mouse brain is shown in Figure 14A. Table 11 summarizes the inhibition of AChE and SERT in mice and rats. The inhibition results of donepezil and fluoxetine are also included for comparison. After oral administration, compound RS-1259 inhibited both AChE and SERT in the mice brain with a potency several fold weaker than donepezil and equivalent to fluoxetine, respectively. Compound (*R*)-20a, the most potent type B dual inhibitor, was not used in further experiments because a low penetration into the brain was predicted based on the ex vivo experiment of AChE inhibition in mice. The doses necessary for 50% efficacy (ED_{50}) of RS-1259, donepezil and rivastigmine were larger in rats than those in mice, although the potency order of compounds was the same in each species. RS-1259 was as potent as fluoxetine and more potent than fluvoxamine for SERT inhibition ex vivo in mice.

Table 11. Inhibition of AChE and SERT in the brain 60 min after oral administration of RS-1259, donepezil and rivastigmine in mice and rats

	ED_{50} values (mg/kg, p.o.)	
AChE	mice	rats
RS-1259	13 (11-15, *n*=5)	43 (31-75, *n*=5)
donepezil	5.1 (4.6-5.6, *n*=10)	16 (12-21, *n*=10)
rivastigmine	0.70 (0.64-0.77, *n*=10)	4.1 (2.7-7.5, *n*=10)
SERT	mice	rats
RS-1259	2.4 (1.9-2.9, *n*=5)	<8 (66%inh. at 8mg/kg, *n*=5)
fluoxetine	2.2 (2.0-2.5, *n*=10)	not determined
fluvoxamine	4.6 (4.2-4.9, *n*=10)	not determined

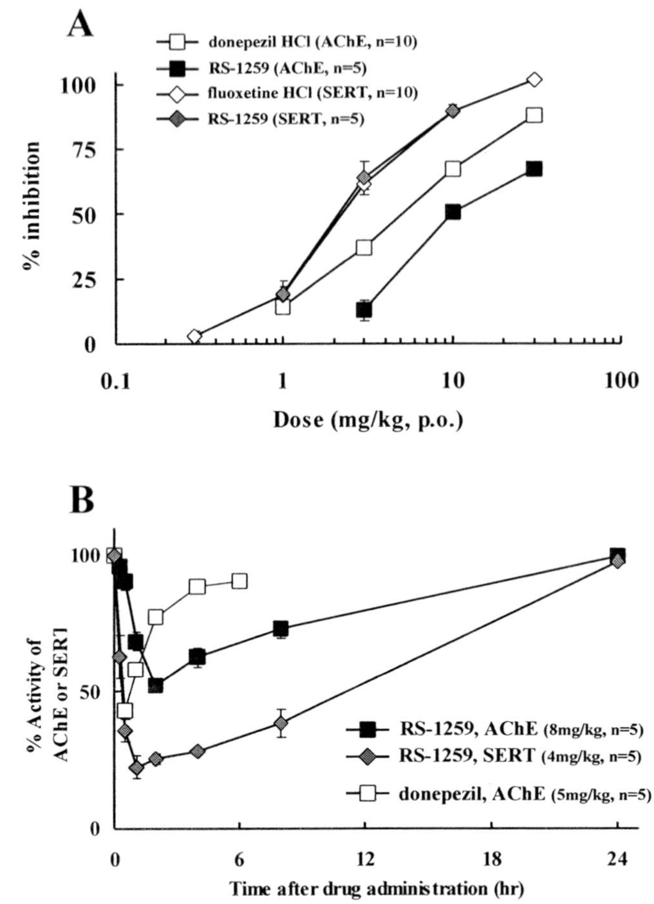

Figure 14. Dose-dependency (A) and time course (B) of inhibition of AChE and SERT in the mouse brain following oral administration of RS-1259, donepezil and fluoxetine. *Ex vivo* inhibition was measured at 60 min (A) and at other time points (B) after administration. Symbols represent the mean and S.E.M. of 5 animals.

RS-1259 is the first compound that can facilitate both cholinergic and serotonergic transmission in the brain following oral administration. The balanced inhibition of AChE and SERT by RS-1259 demonstrated the unique property of this compound and its potentially high efficacy *in vivo*. A single oral administration of RS-1259 inhibited AChE and SERT in the central nervous system in a similar time frame, as expected.

After oral administration, RS-1259 inhibited AChE and SERT in the mouse brain in a similar manner over time. The inhibition of AChE and SERT which reached a maximum at 1–2 hr, was still observed at 8 hr and fully disappeared at 24 hr after administration. The time to reach maximum AChE inhibition and the duration of the inhibitory effect by donepezil were much shorter than that of RS-1259 in mice (Figure 14B).

Microdialysis in the rat Hippocampus

An actual simultaneous elevation of extracellular levels of serotonin and ACh in the rat hippocampus due to the inhibition of both AChE and SERT was confirmed by microdialysis (Figure 15). RS-1259 simultaneously elevated extracellular levels of ACh and 5-HT in the hippocampus of freely moving rats. Donepezil and fluoxetine only increased ACh and 5-HT levels, respectively. ACh was increased to a similar extent by RS-1259 and donepezil at doses of 64 and 16 mg/kg, respectively. At such high doses, all rats showed cholinergic symptoms such as muscle fasciculation, salivation and lacrimation. The rate of 5-HT increase induced by fluoxetine at a dose of 32 mg/kg was slower and the overall 5-HT values were lower than those by RS-1259 at 64 mg/kg. The flat body posture elicited by fluoxetine could not be distinguished from the abnormal posture resulting from the cholinergic symptom which was observed when rats were treated with RS-1259.

Both the ex vivo measurements of AChE and SERT inhibition and the microdialysis experiment indicated that RS-1259 was 3–4 times weaker than donepezil and almost equipotent to fluoxetine in exerting central cholinergic and serotonergic effects, respectively.

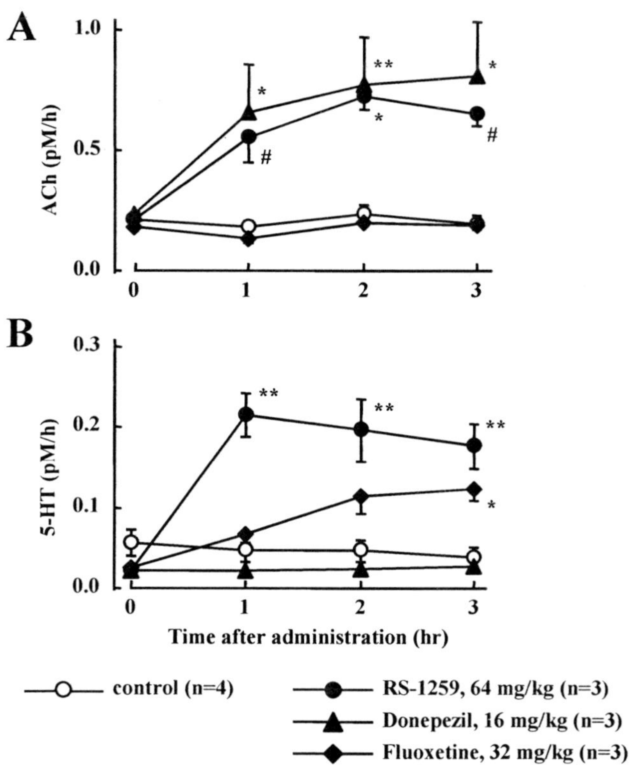

Figure 15. Extracellular concentrations of ACh and 5-HT in the rat hippocampus increased by RS-1259, donepezil and fluoxetine. Compounds or the vehicle was orally administered just after the first sampling (–60–0 h). Each symbol represents the mean of 3–4 animals, with the S.E.M. indicated by a bar. The values indicated by #, * and ** are statistically different ($p<0.1$, 0.05 and 0.01, respectively).

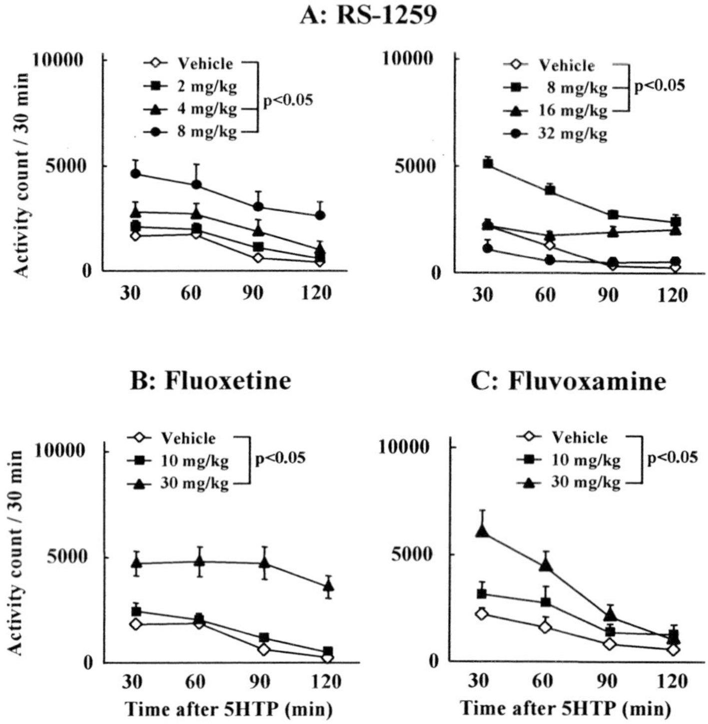

Figure 16. 5HTP-enhancing effect of RS-1259 (A), fluoxetine (B) and fluvoxamine (C) in mice. Each symbol represents the mean of 8 mice, with S.E.M. indicated by a bar. ANOVA of repeated measures and a post-hoc analysis, Fisher's PLSD, indicated that oral doses at 4, 8 and 16 mg/kg of RS-1259, and at 30 mg/kg of fluoxetine and fluvoxamine enhanced 5HTP-induced locomotor activity ($p<0.05$).

5-HTP-Enhancement in Mice

RS-1259 enhanced 5-HTP-induced locomotor activity in a bell-shaped dose-response relationship with maximum enhancement at 8 mg/kg (Figure 16A). The locomotor activity in mice treated with doses larger than 8 mg/kg was reduced as the cholinergic symptoms appeared. Fluoxetine (Figure 16B) and fluvoxamine (Figure 16C) were effective in the test with a longer duration of action for fluoxetine than for fluvoxamine.

RS-1259 was as effective as the serotonin-selective re-uptake inhibitors in the 5-HTP enhancement test in mice, suggesting an anti-depressant effect could be expected with the compound. It was somewhat surprising that RS-1259 was effective at doses lower than the effective dose of fluoxetine, since the potencies of both compounds were similar in the ex vivo measurement of SERT inhibition in the brain. Such low doses of RS-1259 alone did not increase the locomotor activity in mice and fluoxetine-induced 5-HTP enhancement was not affected by a co-administration of donepezil at doses that do not induce cholinergic symptoms. The above inconsistency may be due to the difference in the pharmacokinetic properties between RS-1259 and fluoxetine. The doses of RS-1259 and donepezil eliciting similar increases of ACh in the hippocampus correlated well with their ED_{50} for the ex vivo inhibition of brain AChE. An oral dose four times higher than donepezil was necessary for RS-1259 to achieve a similar inhibition level of the brain AChE in mice and rats. Thus, it was concluded that the potency of RS-1259 following oral administration was approximately a quarter of that of donepezil with respect to AChE inhibition whereas it was equipotent to fluoxetine with respect to SERT inhibition in the central nervous system in vivo.

Amelioration of Memory Deficits of Aged Rat

It has been reported that not only cholinergic but also serotonergic impairments in the brain are involved in causing cognitive deficits in aged animals and in human [44,45]. The effectiveness of RS-1259 in improving these deficits related to the central nervous system was compared to that of donepezil by evaluating two models, i.e., memory deficits in aged rats and the daytime consciousness level of rats with nocturnal habits [46].

Short-term memory is severely affected early on the course of Alzheimer's disease as well as in the normal aging process [47], and it is reported that short-term memory is preferentially impaired in aged animals [48]. To examine whether RS-1259 could improve age-related cognitive decline, the spatial short-term memory was evaluated by using the two-platform task (TPT) using a water maze in aged rats. Briefly, two visible platforms of identical appearance (diameter: 12 cm), one fixed and the other floating, were simultaneously placed at the center of two non-neighboring quadrants (e.g., north and south) in the same pool as that in the pretraining. The surfaces of the platforms were set 0.5 cm above the water surface. A trial began by releasing a rat into the water facing the wall of the pool from one of the remaining two quadrants. The various patterns of platform locations and start positions are shown in Figure. 17A. One session consisting of 6 trials was given each day. Rats were released from the two start positions, alternately the trial ended when the rat reached either platform. At 24–25 months of age, 11 rats showing a significant decline in the TPT performance were orally administered AChE inhibitors or the vehicle 60 min before each test. In the first test, both donepezil (0.5 mg/kg) and RS-1259 (1 mg/kg, but not 0.5 mg/kg) significantly ameliorated the aged-related short-term memory impairment (Figure 16B). In the second test, at half the dose, donepezil (0.25 mg/kg) also improved the memory impairment, although at twice the dose (1 mg/kg) it did not (Figure 17C). A higher dose of RS-1259 (2 mg/kg) was also effective in recovering the memory deficit (Figure 17C). The parameters to evaluate sensorimotor acitivities, i.e., the swimming distance, the swimming speed, the floating time, and the swimming time of rats, were not affected by the drug treatments (data not shown).

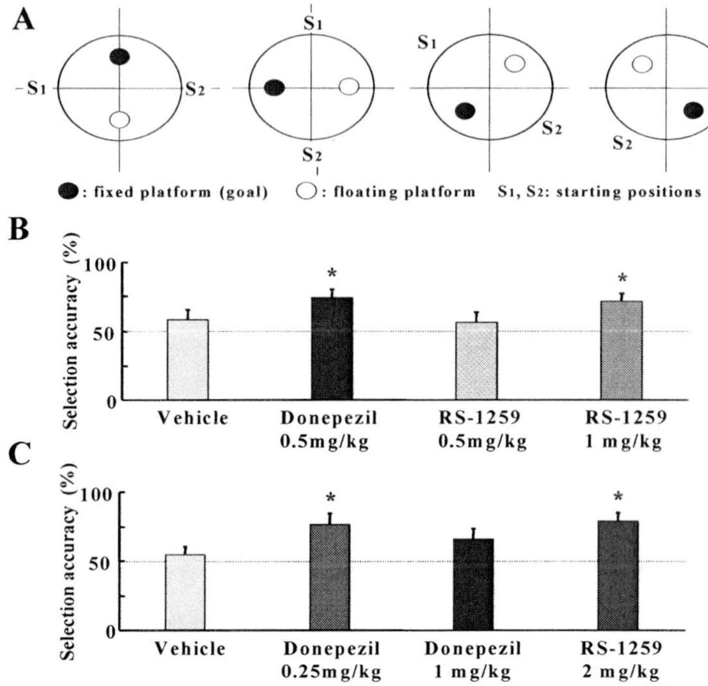

Figure 17. Amelioration of memory deficits in aged rats by RS-1259 and donepezil. (A) Four representative patterns of the platform locations and start positions are shown. Locations of the fixed platform and floating platform were randomly changed at each session. Closed circles, fixed platform; open circles, floating platform; S_1 and S_2, start positions. (B) and (C) represent the results of two separate drug tests. Animals were orally treated with AChE inhibitors or distilled water 60 min before a test session. Each column represents the mean accuracy of 11 rats, with the S.E.M. indicated by a bar. As determined by Wilcoxon's analysis, an amelioration of the reduced accuracy by RS-1259 and donepezil at doses of 1 and 2, and 0.25 and 0.5 mg/kg, respectively, was detected ($p<0.05$).

Both RS-1259 and donepezil ameliorated the low TPT performance of aged rats, but the effective dose of RS-1259 was approximately four times higher than that of donepezil, suggesting that no advantage was obtained by a dual activation of cholinergic and serotonergic transmissions over a solely cholinergic activation in the brain with respect to memory enhancement. TPT is reported to be highly sensitive to cholinergic deficits. We failed to observe any increase in extracellular levels of ACh and 5-HT in the rat hippocampus by fluoxetine and donepezil, respectively, even at high doses. A positive interaction between cholinergic and serotonergic transmissions in the central nervous system may not exist, at least not in the hippocampus. A higher TPT score by RS-1259 was probably obtained solely by improvements in the cholinergic transmission and not the serotonergic one. The simultaneous serotonergic activation by RS-1259 seemed not to affect the cholinergic transmission involved in the memory system.

Elevation of Daytime Consciousness Level in Rats

The daytime consciousness level of rats in a familiar cage was low. The total awake (10–20 min), slow wave sleep (35–45 min) and paradoxical sleep (about 5 min) episodes for every 60 min were stable during the recording period except for the initial 1 hr when the awake episode increased and the other episodes decreased due to the handling necessary for oral administration. RS-1259 and donepezil, at all doses tested, increased the awake episode and decreased slow wave sleep as well as paradoxical sleep episodes in the initial 1 hr following oral administration (Figure 18). The consciousness level remained elevated up to 3 hr after the highest dose of RS-1259 was administered whereas it returned to control levels after 2–3 hr in rats given the highest dose of donepezil. RS-1259 was also effective for the elevation of the daytime consciousness level in rats where the serotonergic neurons in the brain had been degenerated by an intracerebroventricular injection of 5,7-dihydroxytriptamine except the minimum effective dose of 4 mg/kg (Table 12) [49]. No abnormal behavior was observed throughout the recording period at any dose tested.

The consciousness level is associated with several neurotransmitter systems in the brain including cholinergic and serotonergic systems. Dringenberg and Diavolitsis reported that a co-activation of the cortical cholinergic and serotonergic transmissions restored the electrocephalogram (EEG) activation abolished by a monoaminergic-cholinergic blockade [50]. The authors used a complicated pharmacological procedure to induce the blockade and a co-activation of cholinergic and serotonergic transmissions in the cortex, without considering any possible drug-drug interaction between the compounds used. Using the dual inhibitor of AChE and SERT, we were able to evaluate the pharmacological effects of a simultaneous activation of both cholinergic and serotonergic transmissions in the brain without having to take into account any drug-drug interaction. We compared the effect of RS-1259 with that of donepezil on the daytime consciousness level of rats, which is low when they are in a familiar surrounding. Both compounds increased the consciousness level at similar doses. Considering the fact that RS-1259 inhibited brain AChE with a potency four times weaker than that of donepezil, this result clearly indicates that a simultaneous activation of the central serotonergic system could reduce the dose of AChE inhibitor needed to maintain an active consciousness level. This notion was confirmed by the observation that a larger dose of RS-1259 was required for the elevation of consciousness level in rats subjected to serotonergic denervation than that in normal rats.

It was confirmed that the degree of cholinergic activation required in maintaining the brain active could be reduced by a simultaneous activation of the central serotonergic transmission, using the dual AChE–SERT inhibitor.

Currently, BTG International Ltd is clinically developing the dual AChE–SERT inhibitor, RS-1259, as “BGC20-1259” in AD patients.

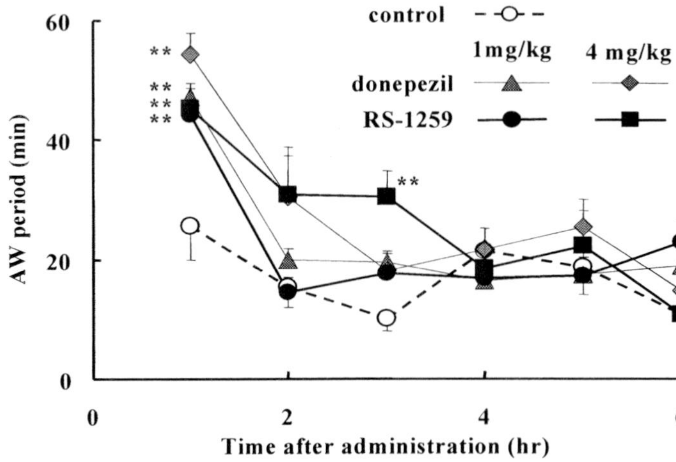

Figure 18. Effects of RS-1259 and donepezil on the daytime consciousness level of rats. The total time of awake episodes was calculated every 60 min after a single oral administration of AChE inhibitors or the vehicle. Each symbol represents the mean awake episode of 5 rats during 60 min, with the S.E.M. indicated by a bar. ** p<0.01 vs. vehicle control (ANOVA).

Table 12. Effects of RS-1259 on the daytime consciousness level in the intact rats and serotonergic denervated rats with 5,7-DHT

		Awake episode (min)	
	Dose (mg/kg)	Intact rats (*n*=5)	5,7-DHT treated ratsw (*n*=5)
Vehicle	-	51.0 ± 5.4	101.0 ± 7.4
RS-1259	1	76.2 ± 6.0	Not tested
	2	82.4 ± 9.3 *	131.2 ± 13.0
	4	106.6 ± 9.8 **	155.4 ± 7.3 ***

Numbers represent the mean of total time of awake episodes in the period of 180 min after a single oral administration of RS-1259, with the S.E.M.

* p<0.05, ** p<0.01, vs. vehicle control in the intact rats.

*** p<0.01, vs. vehicle control in 5,7-DHT treated rats.

The statistical differences were calculated in each group of intact and 5,7-DHT treated rats independently with Dunnett's t-test.

7. Conclusion

Dual AChE and SERT inhibition is considered to be a highly effective method for treating AD because further enhancement of cognitive decline could be achieved and dose-related adverse effects caused by excessive AChE inhibition could be avoided.

To create dual AChE–SERT inhibitors, the hypothetical model of the AChE active center was conceived from the complex crystal structure of AChE and donepezil. Subsequently, a hybrid compound of rivastigmine and fluoxetine was designed as a novel dual AChE–SERT inhibitor.

As a result of structure-activity relationship studies, compound (*S*)-2j which possessed balanced inhibitory activities of AChE and SERT, was successfully obtained.

Moreover, conformationally restricted compounds of (*S*)-2j were designed for further improvement of inhibition potency. Among them, (*R*)-20a, which was successfully synthesized using the ring-closing olefin metathesis reaction, showed the strongest inhibition of both AChE and SERT as anticipated.

Molecular modeling studies of several compounds including 2j and 20a were performed to analyze their inhibitory activities against AChE. The results corresponded with their potencies well and provided some useful information about enzyme-inhibitor interaction.

We confirmed that the degree of cholinergic activation required in maintaining the brain active could be reduced by a concurrent activation of the central serotonergic transmission, using the dual inhibitor RS-1259, an (*S*)-2j (fumaric acid)$_{1/2}$ salt. Thus, it was anticipated that cognitive disorders such as Alzheimer's disease would be effectively and safely treated with dual inhibitors of AChE and SERT.

Currently BTG International Ltd is conducting a clinical trial of RS-1259 as BGC20-1259, the most promising inhibitor of AChE and SERT.

REFERENCES

[1] Alzheimer's Society; http://www.alzheimers.org.uk/

[2] Shibayama, H; Kobayashi, H; Nakagawa, M; Marui, Y; Miyachi, T; Kayukawa, Y; Yamada, K; Iwata, H; Takeuchi, T; Iwai, K; Kogawa, S; Kagawa, N; Imai, M; Mizuno, Y; Hashimoto, N; Ibuki, Y; Ogasawara, S; Tadano, F; Nakagawa, T; Ohta, T. Prevalence of dementia among the elderly in a Japanese community population–comparative study on the 1983 and 1996 survey: The Aichi study. *Psychogeriatrics* 2001, 1, 309-317.

[3] (a)Wurtman, RJ. Alzheimer's disease. *Scientific American* 1985, 252, 62-74. (b) Altman, HJ, Ed. *Alzheimer's diseases problems, prospects and perspectives*; Plenum Press: New York, 1987.

[4] Roberson, MR; Harrell, LE. Cholinergic activity and amyloid precursor protein metabolism. *Brain Res. Rev.* 1997, 25, 50-59.

[5] (a)Davies, P; Maloney, AJ. Selective loss of central cholinergic neurons in Alzheimer's disease. Lancet 1976, 2, 1403-1404. (b) Terry, RD; Masliah, E; Salmon, DP. Physical basis of cognitive alterations in Alzheimer's disease: Synaptic loss is the major correlate of cognitive impairment. *Ann. Neurol.* 1991, 572-580.

[6] Selkoe, DJ. Alzheimer's disease--genotypes, phenotype, and treatments. *Science* 1997, 275, 630-631.

[7] (a)Bartus, RT; Dean, RL; Beer, B; Lippa, AS. The cholinergic hypothesis of geriatric memory dysfunction. *Science* 1982, 217, 408-414. (b) Dunnnett, SB; Fibiger, HC. Role of forebrain cholinergic systems in learning and memory: relevance to the cognitive deficits of aging and Alzheimer's dementia. *Prog. Brain. Res.* 1993, 98,

413-420. (c) Weinstock, M. Possible role of the cholinergic system and disease models. *J. Neural. Transm.* 1997, 49, 93-102.

[8] McGleenon, BM; Dynan, KB; Passmore, AP. Acetylcholinesterase inhibitors in Alzheimer's disease. *Br. J. pharmacol.* 1999, 48, 471-480.

[9] Dolmella, A; Bandoli, G; Nicolini, M. Alzheimer's disease: a pharmacological challenge. *Adv. Drug Res.* 1994, 25, 207-294.

[10] Wesseling, A; Agoston, S. Effects of 4-aminopyridine in elderly patients with Alzheimer's disease. *N. Engl. J. Med.* 1984, 310, 988-989.

[11] Greenlee, W; Clader, J; Asberom, T; McCombie, S; Ford, J; Guzik, H; Kozlowski, J; Li, S; Liu, C; Lowe, D; Vice, S; Zhao, H; Zhou, G; Billard, W; Binch, H; Crosby, R; Duffy, R; Lachowicz, J; Coffin, V; Watkins, R; Ruperto, V; Strader, C; Taylor, L; Cox, K. Muscarinic agonists and antagonists in the treatment of Alzheimer's disease. *Farmaco* 2001, 56, 247-250.

[12] Maelicke, A; Albuquerque, EX. New approach to drug therapy in Alzheimer's dementia. Drug Discovery Today 1996, 1, 53-59.

[13] (a)Enz, A; Amstutz, R; Boddeke, H; Gmelin, G; Malanowski, J. Brain selective inhibition of acetylcholinesterase: a novel approach to therapy for Alzheimer's disease. *Prog. Brain Res.* 1993, 98, 431-438. (b) Millard, CB; Broomfield, CA. Anticholinesterases: Medical applications of neurochemical principles. *J. Neurochem.* 1995, 64, 1909-1918.

[14] Summers, WK; Majovski, LV; Marsh, GM; Tachiki, K; Kling, A. Oral tetrahydroaminoacridine in long-term treatment of senile dementia, Alzheimer type. *N. Engl. J. Med.* 1983, 315, 1241-1245.

[15] Rogers, SL; Farlow, MR; Doody, RS; Mohs, R; Friedhoff, LT. A 24-week, double-blind, placebo-controlled trial of donepezil in patients with Alzheimer's disease. *Neurology* 1998, 50, 136-145.

[16] Forette, F; Anand, R; Gharabawi, G. A phase II study in patients with Alzheimer's disease to assess the preliminary efficacy and maximum tolerated dose of rivastigmine (Exelon). *Eur. J. Neurol.* 1999, 6, 423-429.

[17] Coyle, J; Kershaw, P. Galantamine, a cholinesterase inhibitor that allosterically modulates nicotinic receptors: effects on the course of Alzheimer's disease. *Biol. Psych.* 2001, 49, 289-299.

[18] Bal-On, P; Millard, CB; Harel, M; Dvir, H; Enz, A; Sussman, JL; Silman, I. Kinetic and structural studies on the interaction of cholinesterases with the anti-Alzheimer drug rivastigmine. *Biochemistry* 2002, 41, 3555-3564.

[19] (a)Benzi, G; Moretti, A. Is there a rationale for the use of acetylcholinesterase inhibitors in the therapy of Alzheimer's disease? *Eur. J. Pharmacol.* 1998, 346, 1-13. (b) Giacobini, E. From Molecular Structure to Alzheimer Therapy. *Jpn. J. Pharmacol.* 1997, 74, 225-241.

[20] Sussman, JL; Harel, M; Frolow, F; Oefner, C; Goldman, A; Toker, L; Silman, I. Atomic structure of acetylcholinesterase from Torpedo californica: a prototypic acetylcholine–binding protein. *Science* 1991, 253, 872-879.

[21] Sugimoto, H; Yamanishi, Y; Iimura, Y; Kawakami, Y. Donepezil hydrochloride (E2020) and other acetylcholinesterase inhibitors. *Curr. Med. Chem.* 2000, 7, 303-339.

[22] Kryger, G; Silman, I; Sussman, JL. Structure of acetylcholinesterase complexed with E2020 (Aricept®): implications for the design of new anti-Alzheimer drugs. *Structure* 1999, 7, 297-307.

[23] (a)Wenk, GL; Pierce, DJ; Struble, RG; Price, DL; Cork, LC. Age-related changes in multiple neurotransmitter systems in the monkey brain. *Neurobiol Aging* 1989, 10, 11-19. (b) Palmer, AM; DeKosky, ST. Monoamine neurons in aging and Alzheimer's disease. *J. Neural. Transm.* 1993, 91, 135-159.

[24] Rossor, M; Iversen, LL. Non-cholinergic neurotransmitter abnormalities in Alzheimer's disease. *Br. Med. Bull.* 1986, 42, 70-74.

[25] Decker, MW; McGaugh, JL. The role of interactions between the cholinergic system and other neuromodulatory systems in learning and memory. *Synapse* 1991, 7, 151-168.

[26] (a)Berger, AK.; Fratiglioni, L; Forsell, Y; Winblad, B; Backman, L. The occurrence of depressive symptoms in the preclinical phase of ad: a population-based study. *Neurology* 1999, 53, 1998-2002. (b) Harwood, DG; Sultzer, DL; Wheatley, MV. Impaired insight in Alzheimer disease: association with cognitive deficits, psychiatric symptoms, and behavioral disturbances. *Neuropsychiatry Neuropsychol. Behav. Neurol.* 2000, 13, 83-88. (c) Sweet, RA; Nimgaonkar, VL; Devlin, B; Lopez, OL; DeKosky, ST. Increased familial risk of the psychotic phenotype of Alzheimer disease. *Neurology* 2002, 58, 907-911.

[27] Nyth, AL; Gottfries, CG. The clinical efficacy of citalopram in treatment of emotional disturbances in dementia disorders. *Br. J. Psychiatry* 1990, 157, 894-901. (b) Burke, WJ; Dewan, V; Wengel, SP; Roccaforte, WH; Nadolny, GC; Folks, DG. The use of selective serotonin reuptake inhibitors for depression and psychosis complicating dementia. *Int. J. Ger. Psych.* 1997, 12, 519. (c) Street, JS; Clark, WS; Gannon, KS. Olanzapine treatment of psychotic and behavioral symptoms in patients with Alzheimer disease in nursing care facilities: a double-blind, randomized, placebo-controlled trial. *Arch. Gen. Psych.* 2000, 57, 968-976.

[28] Mendez, MF; Martin, RJ; Smyth, KA; Whitehouse, PJ. Psychiatric symptoms associated with Alzheimer's disease. *J. Neuropsych. Clin. Neurosci.* 1990, 2, 28-33.

[29] Lyketsos, CG; Sheooard, JM; Steele, CD; Kopunek, S; Steinberg, M; Baker, AS; Brandt, J; Rabins, PV. Randomized, placebo-controlled, double-blind clinical trial of sertraline in the treatment of depression complicating Alzheimer's disease: initial results from the depression in Alzheimer's disease study. *Am. J. Psychiatry* 2000, 157, 1686-1689.

[30] (a)Hemeryck, A; Belpaire, FM. Selective serotonin reuptake inhibitors and cytochrome P-450 mediated drug-drug interactions: an update. *Curr Drug Met.* 2002, 3, 13-37. (b) Jann, MW; Shirley, KL; Small, GW. Clinical pharmacokinetics and pharmacodynamics of cholinesterase inhibitors. *Clin. Pharmacokinet.* 2002, 41, 719-739.

[31] Hirai, K; Kato, K; Nakayama, T; Hayako, H; Ishihara, Y; Goto, G; Miyamoto, M. Neurochemical effects of 3-[1-(phenylmethyl)-4-piperidinyl]-1-(2,3,4,5-tetrahydro-1H-1-benzazepin-8-yl)-1-propanone fumarate (TAK-147), a novel acetylcholinesterase inhibitor, in rats. *J. Pharmocol. Exp. Ther.* 1997, 280, 1261-1269.

[32] Mackenna, MT; Proctor, GR; Young, LC; Harvey, AL. Novel tacrine analogues for potential use against Alzheimer's disease: Potent and selective acetylcholinesterase inhibitors and 5-HT uptake inhibitors. *J. Med. Chem.* 1997, 40, 3516-3523.

[33] Golstein, J; Schreiber, S; Velkeniers, B; Vanhaelst, L. Effect of fluoxetine, a serotonin reuptake inhibitor, on the pituitary-thyroid axis in rat. *Eur. J. Pharmacol.* 1983, 91, 239-243.

[34] Dechant, KL; Clissold, SP. Paroxetine: a review of its pharmacodynamic and pharmacokinetic properties, and therapeutic potential in depressive illness. *Drugs* 1991, 41, 225-253.

[35] Kogen, H; Toda, N; Tago, K; Marumoto, S; Takami, K; Ori, M; Yamada, N; Koyama, K; Naruto, S; Abe, K; Yamazaki, R; Hara, T; Aoyagi, A; Abe, Y; Kaneko, T. Design and synthesis of dual inhibitors of acetylcholinesterase and serotonin transporter targeting potential agents for Alzheimer's disease. *Org. Lett.* 2002, 4, 3359-3362.

[36] Toda, N; Tago, K; Marumoto, S; Takami, K; Ori, M; Yamada, N; Koyama, K; Naruto, S; Abe, K; Yamazaki, R; Hara, T; Aoyagi, A; Abe, Y; Kaneko, T; Kogen, H. Design, synthesis and structure–activity relationships of dual inhibitors of acetylcholinesterase and serotonin transporter as potential agents for Alzheimer's disease. *Bioorg. Med. Chem.* 2003, 11, 1935-1955.

[37] Toda, N; Tago, K; Marumoto, S; Takami, K; Ori, M; Yamada, N; Koyama, K; Naruto, S; Abe, K; Yamazaki, R; Hara, T; Aoyagi, A; Abe, Y; Kaneko, T; Kogen, H. A conformational restriction Approach to the development of dual inhibitors of acetylcholinesterase and serotonin transporter as potential agents for Alzheimer's disease. *Bioorg. Med. Chem.* 2003, 11, 4389-4415.

[38] Toda, N; Iwata, Y; Tago, K; Kogen, H; Kaneko, T; Miyamoto, S. Conformational analysis and docking study of potent acetylcholinesterase inhibitors having a benzylamine moiety. *Chem-Bio Informatics Journal* 2003, 3, 46-57; http://www.jstage.jst.go.jp/browse/cbij/.

[39] QUANTA, Version 98. Accelerys, Inc., San Diego, Calif.; http://www. accelerys.com.

[40] CHARMm, Version 23. Accelerys, Inc., San Diego, Calif.; http://www. accelerys.com.

[41] (a)Levitt, M; Perutz, M. F. Aromatic rings act as hydrogen bond acceptors. J. Mol. Biol.1998, 201, 751-754. (b) Dougherty, DA; Stauffer, DA. Acetylcholine binding by a synthetic receptor: implications for biological recognition. *Science* 1990, 250, 1558-1560.

[42] Berman, HM; Westbrook, J; Feng, Z; Gilliland, G; Bhat, TN; Weissig, H; Shindyalov, IN; Bourne, PE. The protein data bank. *Nucleic Acids Res.* 2000, 28, 235-242.

[43] Abe, Y; Aoyagi, A; Hara, T; Abe, K; Yamazaki, R; Kumagae, Y; Naruto, S; Koyama, K; Marumoto, S; Tago, K; Toda, N; Takami, K; Yamada, N; Ori, M; Kogen, H; Kaneko, T. Pharmacological characterization of RS-1259, an orally active dual inhibitor of acetylcholinesterase and serotonin transporter in rodents: possible treatment of Alzheimer's disease. *J. Pharmacol. Sci.* 2003, 93, 95-105.

[44] Richter-Levin, G; Segal, M. Serotonin, aging, and cognitive functions of the hippocampus. *Rev. Neurosci.* 1996, 7, 103-113.

[45] Porter, RJ; Lunn, BS; Walker, LL; Gray, JM; Ballard, CG; O'Brien, JT. Cognitive deficit induced by acute tryptophan depletion in patients with Alzheimer's disease. *Am. J. Psychiatry* 2000, 157, 638-640.

[46] Iwata, N; Kozuka, M; Hara, T; Kaneko, T; Tonohiro, T; Sugimoto, M; Niitsu, Y; Kondo, Y; Yamamoto, T; Sakai, J; Nagano, M. Activation of cerebral function by CS-932, a functionally selective M_1 partial agonist: neurochemical characterization and pharmacological studies. *Jpn. J. Pharmacol.* 2000, 84, 266-280.

[47] Mitrushina, M; Drebing, C; Uchiyama, C; Satz, P; Van Gorp, W; Chervinsky, A. The pattern of deficit in different memory components in normal aging and dementia of Alzheimer's type. *J. Clin. Psychol.* 1994, 50, 591-596.

[48] Markowska, AL; Price, D; Koliatsos, VE. Selective effects of nerve growth factor on spatial recent memory as assessed by a delayed nonmatching-to-position task in the water maze. *J. Neurosci.* 1996, 16, 3541-3548.

[49] Björklund, A; Baumgarten, HG; Rensch, A. 5,7-Dihydroxytryptamine: improvement of its selectivity for serotonin neurons in the CNS by pretreatment with desipramine. *J. Neurochem.* 1975, 24, 833-835.

[50] Dringenberg, AC; Diavolitsis, P. Electroencephalographic activation by fluoxetine in rats: role of 5-HT_{1A} receptors and enhancement of concurrent acetylcholinesterase inhibitor treatment. *Neuropharmacol.* 2002, 42, 154-161.

In: Alzheimer's Disease Research Trends
Editor: A.P. Chan, pp. 91-116

ISBN 978-1-60021-712-8

Chapter V

EARLY ONSET DEMENTIA WITH ABUNDANT NON-NEURITIC Aβ PLAQUES AND WITHOUT SIGNIFICANT NEURONAL LOSS: REPORT OF TWO JAPANESE AUTOPSY CASES

***Osamu Yokota*[1,2,*,Δ], *Kuniaki Tsuchiya*[1,3,4], *Shigetoshi Kuroda*[2]**

[1]Department of Neuropathology, Tokyo Institute of Psychiatry, 2-1-8 Kamikitazawa, Setagaya-ku, Tokyo 156-8585, Japan;

[2]Department of Neuropsychiatry, Okayama University Graduate School of Medicine, Dentistry and Pharmaceutical Sciences, 2-5-1 Shikata-cho, Okayama 700-8558, Japan;

[3]Department of Laboratory Medicine and Pathology, Tokyo Metropolitan Matsuzawa Hospital, Tokyo, Japan;

[4]Department of Neurology, Tokyo Metropolitan Matsuzawa Hospital, Tokyo, Japan.

ABSTRACT

The presence of Aβ-positive neuritic plaques with dense cores is considered an essential pathological marker of Alzheimer's disease (AD). However, there are atypical cases that have abundant non-cored plaques with surrounding minor dystrophic neurites. The atypical plaques are called 'cotton wool plaques', and AD with cotton wool plaques is thought to be one of the variants of AD. Cotton wool plaques are usually large, round, and eosinophilic, and appear to displace surrounding normal structures. Inflammatory glial response is mild. We here describe two autopsy cases of early-onset dementia with abundant eosinophilic non-cored Aβ plaques, the histopathological features of which are

* Correspondence concerning this article should be addressed to Dr. Osamu Yokota, Department of Neuropsychiatry, Okayama University Graduate School of Medicine, Dentistry and Pharmaceutical Sciences, 2-5-1 Shikata-cho, Okayama 700-8558, Japan. TEL: +81-86-235-7242, FAX: +81-86-235-7246, e-mail: oyokota1@yahoo.co.jp.

Δ This work was supported by a grant-in-aid for scientific research from the Ministry of Education, Culture, Sports, Science and Technology (14570957) and a research grant from the Zikei Institute of Psychiatry.

different. Patient 1 was a 44-year-old man at the time of death, with a clinical course of 8 years. Nine relatives in three generations had died in their thirties to forties, and some of them were verified to have had dementia. The proband presented clinically with spastic paraparesis at age 36 prior to the development of dementia. The brain weight was 1330 g. Macroscopically, only mild atrophy was found in the frontal, temporal, and parietal cortices. Histopathological examination revealed abundant, large, eosinophilic, non-cored plaques having the typical appearance of cotton wool plaques. The plaques were more strongly immunopositive for Aβ42 than Aβ40. A moderate number of neurofibrillary changes were found in the hippocampus and parahippocampal gyrus, but only a few in other anatomical regions, including the neocortex. The pyramidal tract was degenerated. Although moderate neuronal loss was found in the insular and entorhinal cortices, the other cerebral cortices were relatively spared. Genetic analysis demonstrated the G384A presenilin-1 gene mutation. Patient 2 was a 46-year-old man at the time of death, with a clinical course of 8 years. His family had no history of neurological diseases in the previous three generations. He presented with memory impairment at the age of 39. Subsequently, he showed disinhibition, impulsiveness, and paranoid ideation, but no neurological abnormality. The brain weight was 1700 g. Macroscopically, neither brain atrophy nor edema was observed. Histopathological examination disclosed abundant eosinophilic non-cored plaques in all cerebral cortices. The diameters were 40-100 μm, including plaques smaller than those in patient 1. The plaques showed little tendency to displace normal structures, but did not contain neurons. Intriguingly, the plaques in this case were were more strongly immunoreactive for Aβ40 than for Aβ42. In the cerebral cortex including the hippocampus, neurons were well preserved, and glial response was slight. In the pyramidal tract, glial proliferation was evident, although loss of myelin was not noted. No tau-positive lesions were found in any region. No mutations in presenilin-1, presenilin-2, or amyloid precursor genes were revealed by genetic analysis using formalin-fixed paraffin-embedded tissue. These findings suggest that factors besides neuritic plaques, neurofibrillary tangles, and severe neuronal loss play a pivotal role in the occurrence of cognitive decline in AD patients.

INTRODUCTION

The presence of Aβ-positive senile plaques is considered to be an essential pathological marker of Alzheimer's disease (AD). Senile plaques are classified into several morphological subtypes. The most representative subtype is a classic mature plaque with a dense amyloid core and surrounding dystrophic neurites with reactive glial cells. They are often called neuritic plaques, and the presence of neuritic plaques is an essential criterion for pathological diagnosis of AD [1,2]. Another pivotal subtype is the diffuse plaque, which is visualized with Aβ immunostaining but not hematoxylin-eosin (H&E) staining. Diffuse plaques are ill-defined and lack inflammatory glial response. In addition to the formation of senile plaques, variable degrees of neurofibrillary changes usually develop in AD cases. The severity of neurofibrillary changes rather than that of senile plaques correlates with the severity of AD [3]. However, because the presence of senile plaques rather than that of neurofibrillary changes is more specific for AD, the formation of senile plaques is considered to be more closely related to the pathogenesis of AD.

In 1998, Crook et al. [4] reported an unusual variant AD bearing deletion of exon 9 of the presenilin-1 (PS1) gene. This variant was clinically characterized by dementia with spastic paraparesis, and pathologically, by the occurrence of large non-cored plaques with minor neuritic changes. Thereafter, familial cases with different PS1 gene mutations or deletions, as well as a few sporadic cases, were also reported. The atypical plaques in this variant were large, round, well-defined, and eosinophilic, and were called cotton wool plaques (CWPs). They had few dystrophic neurites and little surrounding glial response, and appeared to displace surrounding normal structures. This variant AD with CWPs (CWP-AD) raised the question of how the atypical plaques resulted in the neurodegeneration of CWP-AD, and whether the presence of mature plaques with dystrophic neurites is really necessary in the development of dementia in AD.

We here describe two autopsy cases of early-onset dementia with abundant eosinophilic non-cored Aβ plaques. Case 1 had abundant large Aβ plaques having morphological features consistent with those of CWPs reported previously. This case also had neurofibrillary changes corresponding to Braak stage V. Neurons in the superficial layer in the cerebral cortex were slightly reduced in number. Case 2 also had abundant eosinophilic Aβ-positive plaques. These plaques varied in size from 40-100 μm, including plaques of rather small size. They were often ill-defined and lacked the tendency to displace surrounding normal structures. In contrast to the remarkable Aβ deposition, neither amyloid angiopathy nor glial response was observed in the cerebral cortex. Furthermore, intriguingly, no tau-positive lesions were noted in any anatomical region. Neurons and the laminar structure of the cerebral cortex were well preserved despite the presence of dementia.

MATERIALS AND METHODS

Brains tissue samples from both subjects were fixed post mortem with 10% formaldehyde and embedded in paraffin. Ten-μm-thick sections from the frontal, temporal, parietal, occipital, insular, and cingulate cortices, hippocampus, amygdala, basal ganglia, midbrain, pons, medulla oblongata, cerebellum, and spinal cord were prepared. These sections were stained by the hematoxylin-eosin (H&E), Klüver-Barrera (KB), Holzer, periodic acid-Schiff stain (PAS), methenamine silver, Bodian, modified Bielschowsky silver, and Gallyas-Braak silver methods.

Sections from the various regions in the cerebrum, brainstem, and spinal cord were examined immunohistochemically using anti-Aβ42 antibody (rabbit, polyclonal, 1:750, FCA3542, courtesy of Dr. F. Checler [5]), anti-Aβ40 antibody (rabbit, polyclonal, 1:750, FCA3340, kindly provided by Dr. F. Checler [5]), anti-Aβ antibody (against Aβ a.a.17-24, mouse, monoclonal, 1:2000, 4G8, Senetek), anti-Aβ antibody (against Aβ a.a.1-17, mouse, monoclonal, 1:2000, 6E10, Senetek), phosphorylated tau (AT8, mouse, monoclonal, 1:3,000, Innogenetics), phosphorylated α-synuclein (pSyn#64, mouse, monoclonal, 1:1,000, Wako), prion protein (3F4, mouse, monoclonal, 1:1000, Dako), and glial fibrillary acidic protein (GFAP, rabbit, polyclonal, 1:5,000, Dako). Deparaffinized sections were incubated with 1% H_2O_2 in methanol for 20 min to eliminate endogenous peroxidase activity in the tissue. Sections were treated with 0.2% TritonX-100 for 5 min and washed in phosphate-buffered saline (PBS, pH 7.4). Sections were pretreated with formic acid (99%, 5 min; Sigma) for antigen retrieval when using anti-Aβ, anti-α-synuclein, and anti-prion protein antibodies. After blocking with 10% normal serum, sections were incubated 72 hours at 4°C with one of the primary antibodies in 0.05 M Tris-HCl buffer, pH 7.2, containing 0.1% Tween and 15 mM NaN_3. After three 10-min washes in PBS, sections were incubated in biotinylated anti-rabbit or anti-mouse secondary antibody for 1 h, and then in avidin-biotinylated horseradish peroxidase complex (ABC Elite kit, Vector) for 1 h. The peroxidase labeling was visualized with 0.2% 3,3'-diaminobenzidine (DAB) or diaminobenzidine-nickel as the chromogen.

Neuronal loss and gliosis in representative regions were semiquantitatively evaluated. In the cerebral cortex, the degree of degeneration was assessed on H&E, KB-, and GFAP-stained sections according to the grading system employed in our previous studies [6-11]: -, no histopathological alteration is observed; +, slight neuronal loss and gliosis are observed only in the superficial layers; ++, obvious neuronal loss and gliosis are found in cortical layers II and III, often accompanied by status spongiosis and relative preservation of neurons in layers V and VI; +++, pronounced neuronal loss with gliosis is found in all cortical layers with prominent fibrous gliosis exhibited in adjacent subcortical white matter. In the basal ganglia and brainstem nuclei, the degree of neuronal loss and gliosis was assessed on H&E, KB-, and GFAP-stained sections according to the following grading system: -, neither neuronal loss nor gliosis is observed; ±, mild gliosis is observed on H&E-stained sections or GFAP-immunostained sections, but neurons are not reduced in number; +, mild gliosis and mild neuronal loss are present; ++, neuronal loss and gliosis are moderate, but tissue rarefaction is absent; +++, severe neuronal loss, severe fibrous gliosis, and tissue rarefaction are observed. The degeneration of the corticospinal tract was assessed based on the loss of myelin, glial proliferation, and appearance of macrophages at the level of the medulla oblongata and spinal cord, and indicated as + or –.

Genomic DNA was extracted from paraffin-embedded brain sections. The regions encoding exons 3-12 of PS1, exons 3-12 of PS2, exons 16 and 17 of APP, and the regions including codons 112 and 158 of the apo E gene were amplified by PCR using unique primer sets according to previously described procedures [12,13]. Designation of the number of each exon of the PS1 follows Hutton's nomenclature [12]. PCR products of PS1 were directly sequenced. The apo E genotype was determined by restriction fragment length polymorphism analysis using *Cfo*I.

CASE REPORTS

Case 1

Clinical Course

This man was 44 years old at the time of death. Figure 1 shows the pedigree of this case (IV.6). At least nine relatives in three generations suffered from dementia. The age at onset in all affected members was in the 30s, and the age at death was in the 40s [14]. A part of the clinical information and the pathological findings of this case have been reported in Japanese

[15,16]. This patient had a history of polyneuropathy at the age of 33, but without aftereffect. At the age of 36, in 1979, he initially complained of numbness in the legs. In 1981, his stance became wide-based, and he walked in a forward-bent posture. In addition, his dysarthria and forgetfulness were first noticed by his wife. Reduction of spontaneity, dysarthria, and gait instability developed subsequently. In 1983, neurological examination disclosed dysarthria, pyramidal signs, cerebellar signs, and memory impairment. Deep tendon reflexes were exaggerated in all four extremities, and Babinski signs were bilaterally positive. Swallowing function was not disturbed. Mild dysmetria in the left arm and left side-predominant bilateral adiadochokinesis were noted. His score on the Hasegawa Dementia Scale (HDS), which is most frequently employed to assess cognitive function of people with dementia in Japan and correlates well with the score of the Mini Mental State examination, was 28.5 points (full score 32.5 points), indicating normal cognitive function. He obtained a verbal IQ score of 100, a performance IQ score of 86, and a full scale IQ of 99 on the Wechsler Adult Intelligence Scale-revised (WAIS-R). Cerebrospinal fluid examination demonstrated a mild increase in protein concentration. One year later, at age 40, neurological reexamination revealed progression of memory impairment, dysarthria, ataxia, and gait disturbance. Both verbal IQ and performance IQ were under 60 on the WAIS-R. Ocular movement was not restricted but saccadic. Rigidity was found in the upper extremities, and rigospasticity in the lower extremities. Deep tendon reflexes were apparently increased. Babinski signs, palmomental reflexes, and snout reflex were positive. Clonus was not found. Diadochokinesis was bilaterally impaired. Cerebellar ataxia was also noted. Muscle atrophy, weakness, or involuntary movements were not noted. Bladder and erectile functions were impaired. Blood and urine examinations were within normal limits. Cerebrospinal fluid examination again demonstrated a mild elevation of protein concentration. He was clinically suspected of having Gerstmann-Sträussler-Scheinker syndrome. He was admitted to a psychiatric hospital at age 41. On admission, he presented with dementia, severe memory impairment, dysarthria, and gait disturbance. His score on the Hasegawa Dementia Scale Revised (HDS-R: full score 30 points, cutoff 19/20) was 10 points, indicating moderate dementia. Baseline examinations of blood, urine, and cerebrospinal fluid were within normal limits. Electroencephalography registered much diffuse slow wave activity. Head computed tomography (CT) showed mild dilation of the Sylvian fissures and lateral ventricles. Cortical atrophy in the cerebrum was not evident. The cerebellum was unremarkable. One year later, CT revealed mild atrophy in the frontal and temporal cortices, and ventricular enlargement and atrophy in the brainstem were evident. At age 43, he walked dragging his legs while extending his knees. His gait was wide-based but not ataxic. He could not comprehend simple neurological examination instructions such as the finger-nose test and eye-tracking test. Pyramidal signs, pseudobulbar sign, and slight cerebellar ataxia were observed. Parkinsonism or primitive reflexes were not found. CT revealed moderate cerebral atrophy; however, the severity was far milder than expected from severe dementia. The atrophy in the brainstem progressed. At age 44, he could not walk without support. Spontaneity was increasingly reduced, and emaciation became evident. He finally became bedridden, and he died of pneumonia at age 44 in 1988, 8 years after the disease onset. No respiratory support was given throughout the clinical course. The final neurological diagnosis was unclassified presenile dementia.

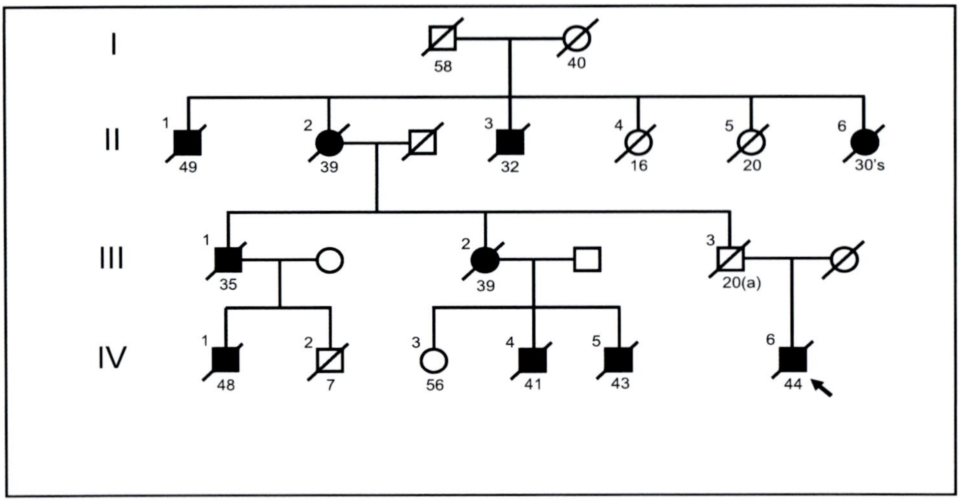

Figure 1. Family tree of case 1 (arrow). Squares = males; circles = females; filled symbols = affected; slashes = deceased. G384A presenilin-1 mutation was found in cases IV.1 and IV.6. (a) Killed in the World War II.

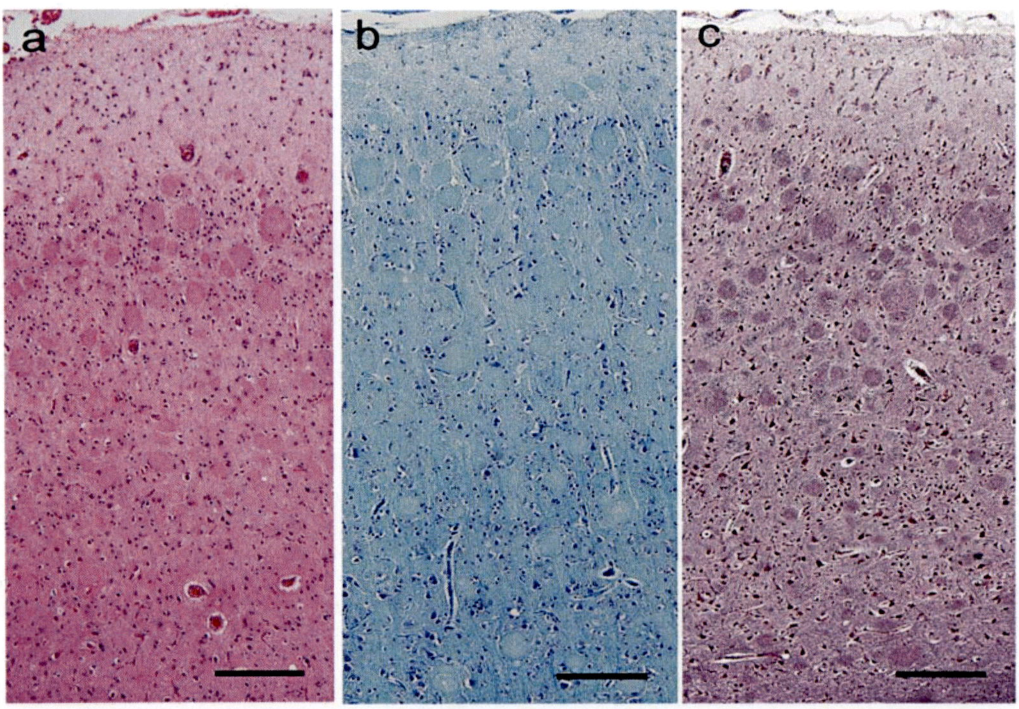

Figure 2. The temporal cortex in case 1. (a) Hematoxylin-eosin stain. Many large round eosinophilic cotton wool plaques are easily detected in the cortical layers II and III and layers V and VI. (b) Klüver-Barrera stain also reveals cotton wool plaques. In the deep cortical layers, the neuropil is more intensely stained rather than the cotton wool plaques. (c) Bodian stain. Many cotton wool plaques are easily detected. The plaques are mainly distributed in the deep and upper layers. All scale bars = 200 μm.

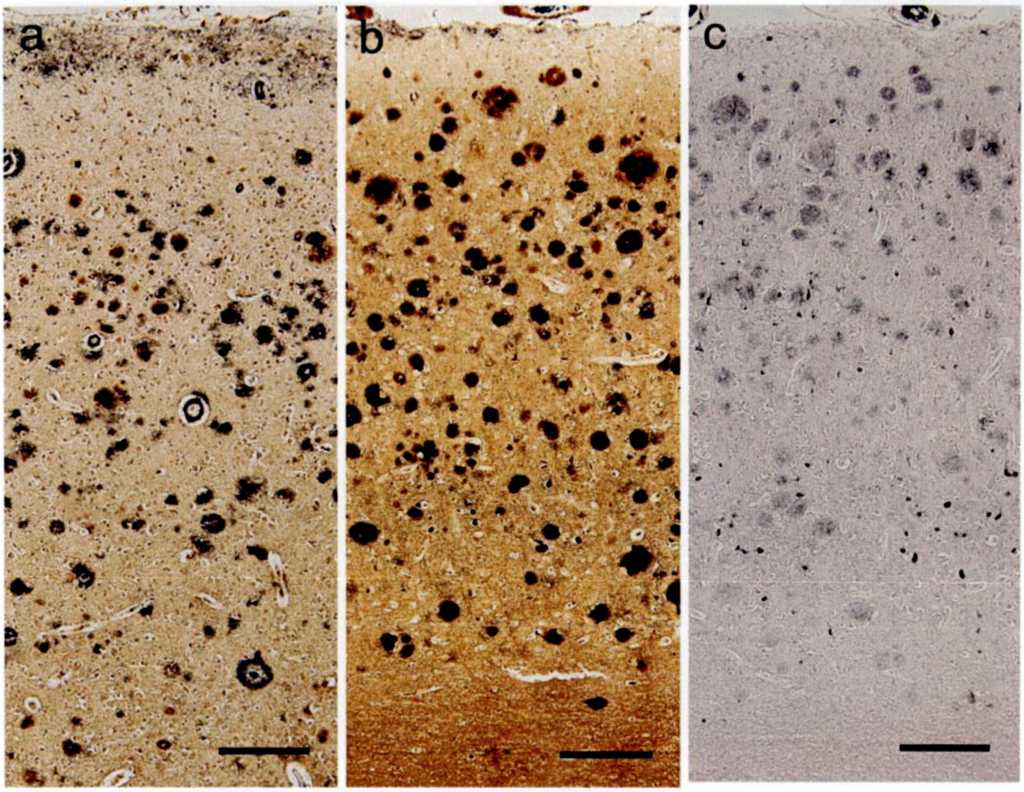

Figure 3. The temporal cortex in case 1. (a) Methenamine silver stain. Many cotton wool plaques and a small number of cored plaques are seen. (b) Modified Bielschowsky silver stain also reveals cotton wool plaques. (c) Gallyas-Braak silver stain. Cotton wool plaques are faintly argyrophilic. Neurofibrillary changes are found in the deep cortical layers. All scale bars = 200 μm.

Pathological Findings

The brain weight was 1330 g after fixation. Macroscopically, mild cerebral atrophy in the frontal, temporal, and parietal lobes was found. The bilateral anterior horns of the lateral ventricles were dilated. The substantia nigra and locus coeruleus showed mild depigmentation.

Microscopically, the most striking feature was the occurrence of numerous atypical senile plaques. They were large, round, and eosinophilic, and distributed throughout the cerebral cortex (Figure 2a) and limbic system. Almost all of the plaques lacked cores, and surrounding neuritic changes were scarce. These morphological features were consistent with those of CWPs [4]. The non-cored plaques were most frequently encountered in cortical layers II and III, but they were also found in the deep layers, although in rather small numbers. The plaques in the upper cortical layers were larger than those in the deep layers. The plaques were easily detected on H&E-stained sections (Figures 2a, 4a, 4b). On KB-stained sections also, the plaques were visible, but the intensity of the staining was weak compared with that of myelin (Figures 2b, 4c, 4d). The plaques were stained with Bodian stain (Figures 2c, 5a). The plaques showed argyrophilia on methenamine and Bielschowsky silver stains (Figures 3a, 3b, 5b). On Gallyas-Braak silver-stained sections, the plaques were weakly argyrophilic (Figures 3c, 5c). The diameters of the plaques were often over 100 µm, and some of the plaques had a glial nucleus in the central portion (Figures 4b, 5a, 5b, 5c). Silver stains revealed minor neuritic changes surrounding the plaques (Figure 5c). On the other hand, only a few mature plaques with amyloid cores and surrounding neuritic changes were seen. Glial response surrounding non-cored plaques was almost totally lacking, in contrast to the evident proliferation of reactive astrocytes associated with classic cored plaques (Figure 5d). In the cerebellum, H&E stain revealed a few cored plaques in the molecular layer. Moderate numbers of neurofibrillary tangles (NFTs) were observed in the hippocampus and parahippocampal gyrus. NFTs were encountered in the middle and deep cortical layers in the temporal and frontal cortices (Figure 3c). NFTs were also found in the nucleus basalis of Meynert, caudate nucleus, putamen, and hippocampal dentate gyrus. Although the number of NFTs was small, the distribution fits Braak stage V.

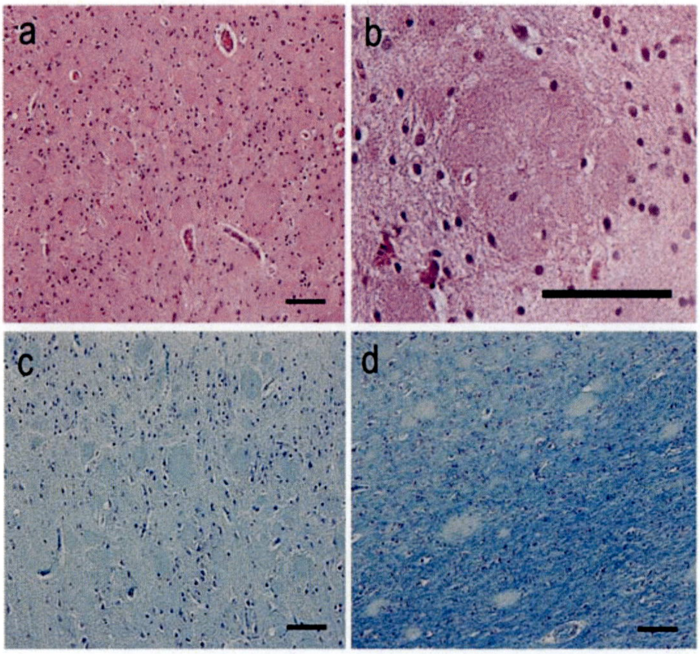

Figure 4. Cotton wool plaques in the temporal cortex in case 1 at higher magnification. (a) Hematoxylin-eosin stain. Many round plaques appear to displace surrounding normal structures. Inflammatory response is not evident. (b) Hematoxylin-eosin stain. A large cotton wool plaque of over 100 µm in diameter. A glial nucleus, but not an amyloid core, is present in the central portion. Surrounding glial response is not evident. (c) Klüver-Barrera stain. Neurons are displaced by many cotton wool plaques, but relatively preserved. (d) Cotton wool plaques in the white matter of the temporal lobe. Klüver-Barrera stain. All scale bars = 100 µm.

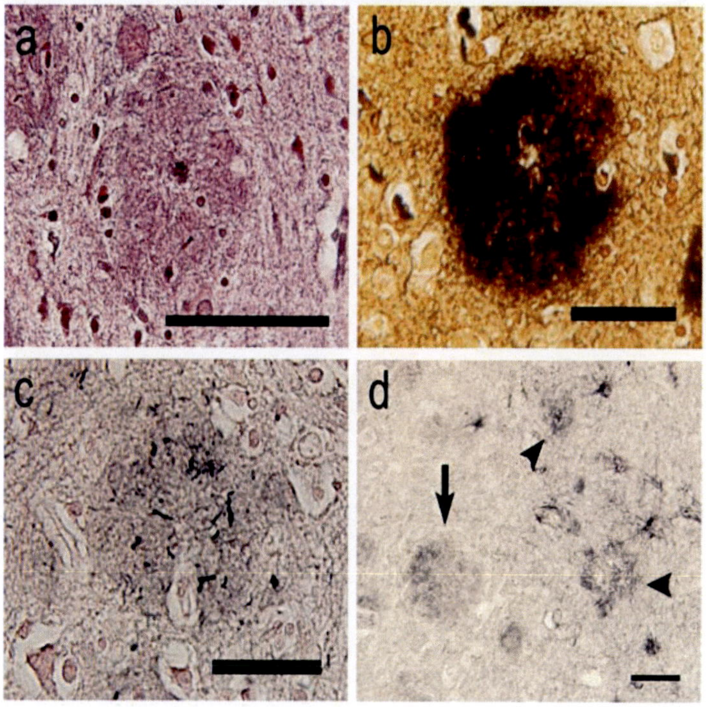

Figure 5. Cotton wool plaques in case 1. (a) Bodian stain. A plaque without neuritic changes in the temporal cortex. A glial nucleus is seen in the central portion. There is no amyloid core. (b) Modified Bielschowsky stain. A plaque without neuritic changes in the temporal cortex. (c) Gallyas-Braak silver stain. A plaque with a few neuritic changes in the temporal cortex. (d) GFAP immunohistochemistry. Reactive astrocytes are found around classic cored plaques (arrowheads). By contrast, a cotton wool plaque (arrow) lacks them. Scale bars = (a) 100 μm, (b) 50 μm, (c) 50 μm, (d) 50 μm.

In contrast to the abundant CWPs, the degree of neuronal loss in the cerebral cortex was generally mild (Table). Severe neuronal loss involving all cortical layers was not found in any region. Moderate neuronal loss with preservation of the cortical layers V and VI was found only in the entorhinal cortex and the ventral portion of the insular cortex. Slight neuronal loss involving the superficial cortical layer alone was noted in the cingulate, frontal, and temporal cortices, prarahippocampal gyrus, and ambient gyrus. In the primary motor cortex, mild neuronal loss involving the upper cortical layers alone were found; however, loss of Betz cells, with small groupings of lipofuscin-laden macrophages in the holes from which the Betz cells had presumably disappeared, was found in this site. Neurons in the hippocampus and subiculum were not reduced in number. The number of neurons in the nucleus basalis of Meynert and locus coeruleus was also reduced. The pyramidal tract was involved at the levels of the midbrain and medulla oblongata (Figures 6a, 6b). The lower motor neurons in the hypoglossal nuclei were preserved in number.

Table. Distribution of neuronal loss and astrocytosis in the present cases

	Case 1	Case 1
Superior frontal gyrus	+	+
Medial frontal gyrus	+	-
Inferior frontal gyrus	+	-
Orbital gyrus	+	-
Primary motor cortex	+	+
Superior temporal gyrus	+	+
Medial temporal gyrus	+	+
Inferior temporal gyrus	+	+
Insular cortex	++	+
Cingulate gyrus	+	+
Amygdala	±	n.a.
Ambient gyrus	+	n.a.
CA1 in hippocampus	-	-
Hippocampal dentate gyrus	-	-
Subiculum	-	-
Entorhinal cortex	++	n.a.
Parahippocampal gyrus	+	+
Caudate nucleus	-	-
Putamen	-	-
Globus pallidus	-	-
Thalamus	±	-
Subthalamic nucleus	-	-
Nucleus basalis of Meynert	++	±
Dentate nucleus of cerebellum	-	±
Trochlear nucleus	n.a.	-
Oculomotor nucleus	±	n.a.
Substantia nigra	±	-
Red nucleus	-	n.a.
Locus coeruleus	+	n.a.
Pontine nucleus	-	-
Dorsal vagal nucleus	±	-
Hypoglossal nucleus	±	-
Inferior olivary nucleus	±	±
Corticospinal tract	+	+ (a)
Anterior horn	n.a.	n.a.

The severity of degeneration in the cerebral cortex: -, no histopathological alteration; +, slight neuronal loss and gliosis only in the superficial layers; ++, obvious neuronal loss and gliosis in cortical layers II and III, often accompanied by status spongiosis and relative preservation of neurons in layers V and VI; +++, pronounced neuronal loss with gliosis in all cortical layers with prominent fibrous gliosis in adjacent subcortical white matter. The severity of neuronal loss and gliosis in the basal ganglia and brainstem nuclei: -, neither neuronal loss nor gliosis; ±, mild gliosis on H&E- and GFAP-immunostained sections, but neurons e preserved; +, mild gliosis and mild neuronal loss; ++, neuronal loss and gliosis, but tissue rarefaction absent; +++, severe neuronal loss, severe gliosis, and tissue rarefaction. The degeneration of the corticospinal tract was assessed at the level of the medulla oblongata or spinal cord, and the existence of degeneration was indicated as + or - . n.a., not available. (a) Although loss of myelin was not evident, glial proliferation was observed.

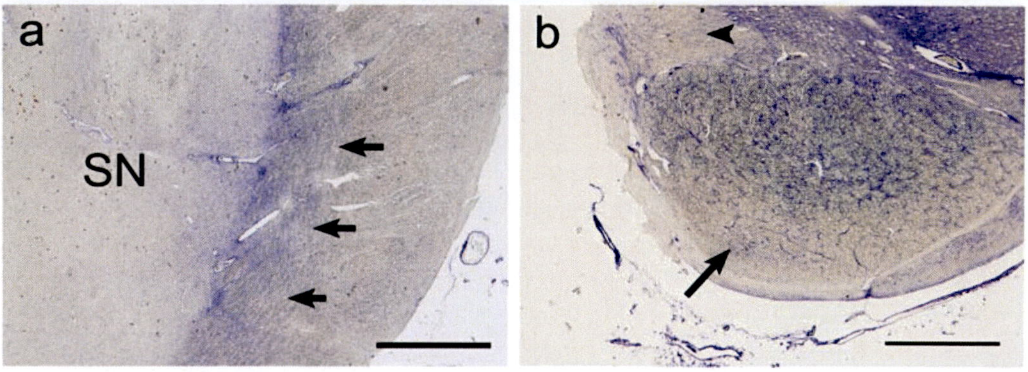

Figure 6. Pyramidal tract involvement in case 1. (a) Evident gliosis in the pyramidal tract at the level of the midbrain (arrows). SN indicates the substantia nigra. (b) Gliosis in the pyramidal tract at the level of the medulla oblongata (arrow) is also evident in comparison with the medial lemniscus (arrowhead). Holzer stain. All scale bars = 1 mm.

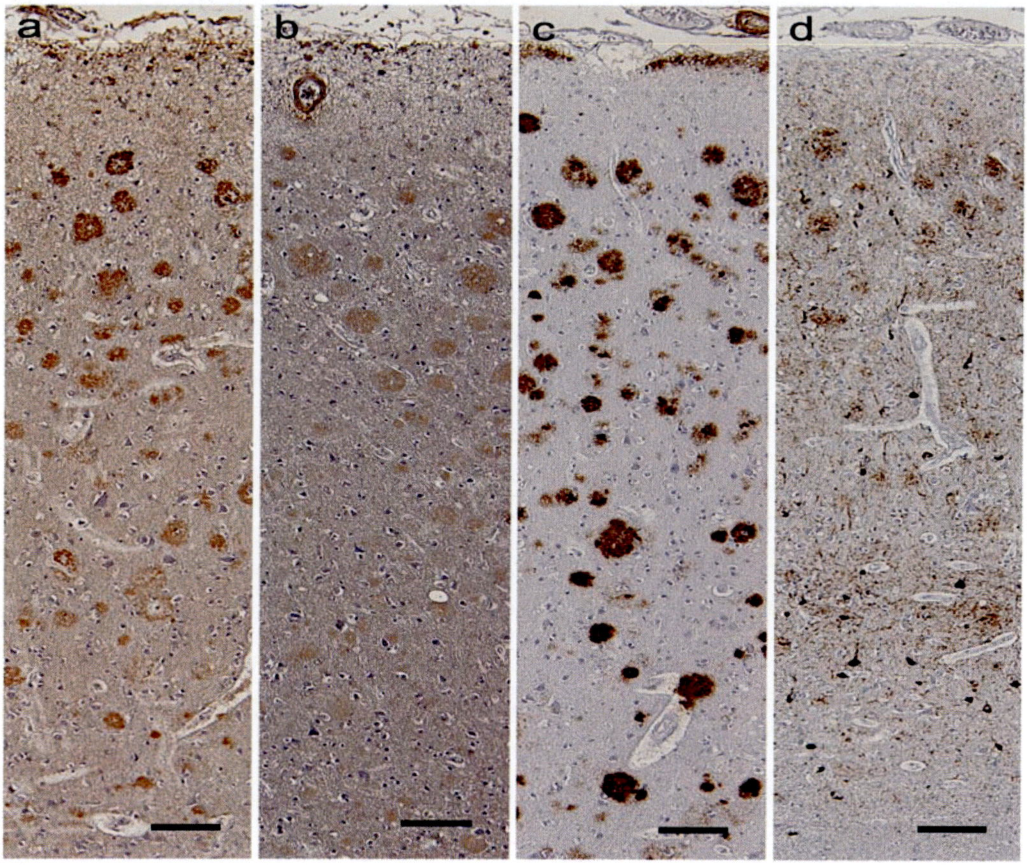

Figure 7. Aβ and tau immunohistochemistry in case 1. (a) Aβ42-positive cotton wool plaques. (b) Aβ40-positive plaques. Aβ42 rather than Aβ40 is predominantly deposited in the cerebellum. Amyloid angiopathy is also found. (c) Cotton wool plaques are intensely labeled with 4G8. (d) Some of the plaques are faintly tau positive. However, few tau-positive dystrophic neurites are noted in the cotton wool plaques. (a) FCA3542 (Aβ42) immunostain, (b) FCA3340 (Aβ40) immunostain, (c) 4G8 immunostain, (d) AT-8 immunostain. All scale bars = 200 μm.

Cotton wool plaques were immunostained with anti-Aβ antibodies (Figures 7a, 7b, 7c). They were immunolabeled with anti-Aβ42 more strongly than Aβ40 antibodies. The plaques were found in all cortical layers, but mainly distributed in the upper and deep layers. Aβ deposits in the subpial region were often observed (Figure 7c). Cerebral amyloid angiopathy was labeled with anti-Aβ40 antibody (Figure 7b). Some CWPs were slightly tau-positive; however, there were few tau-positive neuritic changes in CWPs. Tau-positive NFTs were scattered mainly in the deep cortical layers (Figure 7d). Neither α-synuclein-positive nor prion protein-positive lesions were present in any region.

Genetic analysis using paraffin-embedded brain sections revealed a G384A mutation in the PS1 gene. The Apo E genotype was not examined.

Case 2

Clinical Course

This was a 46-year-old man at the time of death with a clinical course of 8 years. The detailed clinical course and conventional pathological findings of this case were first described by Hayashi et al. in Japanese in 1967 [17], and a clinical summary and additional immunohistochemical findings were reported recently [18]. This patient was initially aware of forgetfulness and a reduction of spontaneity at the age of 39 in 1958. The first neurological examination at a university hospital in 1960 revealed memory impairment, but no other neurological abnormalities. He had no family history of neurological disorders in the previous three generations. He was clinically diagnosed as having Alzheimer's disease. Subsequently, disinhibition, disorientation in time and place, restlessness, and indifference occurred, and he admitted to a psychiatric hospital in 1963. His restlessness, irritability, anxiety, and a tendency to exaggerate things were remarkable. Recent memory, but not remote memory, was severely impaired. He often lost his way in the ward. Calculation ability was impaired. He obtained an IQ score of 58 on the Wechsler-Bellevue Intelligence Scale. Parkinsonism was not found. Baseline examinations of blood and urine were within normal limits. Electroencephalogram showed a basic activity of 9-11 Hz and a high voltage slow wave in the frontal and parietal regions. His appetite gradually declined, and seizures and prolonged coma developed. He died of an unknown cause in 1965. Repeated neurological examinations during the clinical course did not disclose parkinsonism, pyramidal signs, or cerebellar signs. Genetic analysis using paraffin-embedded brain sections did not reveal any mutation in exons 3 to 12 of the PS1 gene, exons 3-12 of the PS2 gene, or exons 16 and 17 of the APP gene, which included all coding regions. The Apo E genotype was ε3/ε4.

Pathological Findings

Brain weight was 1700 g. Macroscopically, neither brain atrophy nor edema was found. Arteriosclerosis was not noted in the basilar artery. The bilateral mamillary bodies were atrophic. The cerebellum and brainstem were unremarkable. Coronal sections showed only slight dilation of the third ventricle and bilateral lateral ventricles, but not cortical atrophy (Figures 8a, 8b).

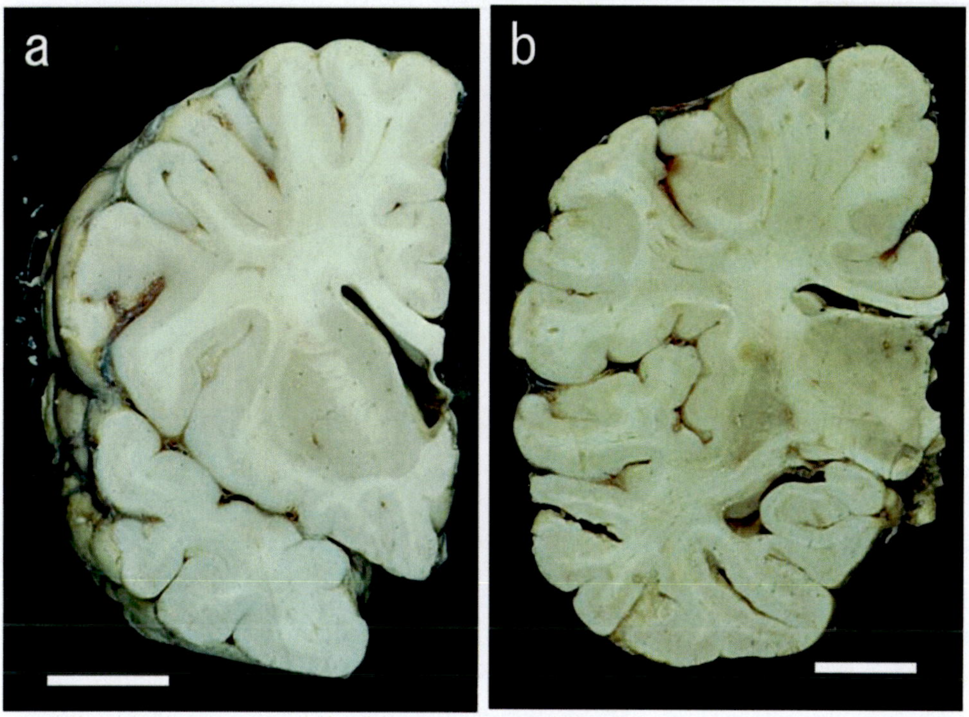

Figure 8. Coronal sections of case 2. (a) The frontal and temporal lobes and basal ganglia are unremarkable. (b) The hippocampal region is not atrophic. All scale bars = 2 cm.

Microscopically, the most remarkable finding was the occurrence of abundant atypical plaques, easily visible on H&E-stained sections (Figures 9a, 11a). The eosinophilic plaques were distributed in all cortical layers. The sizes of the plaques were variable, with diameters of 40-100 μm. These plaques often showed ill-defined boundaries. These plaques lacked cores, and no typical senile plaque with an amyloid core was found. The plaques did not appear to displace surrounding normal structures. The plaques were hardly stained with KB stain (Figure 9b), but easily visible with Bodian (Figures 9c, 11b), Gallyas-Braak silver (Figures 10b, 11d), and PAS stains (Figure 10c). The plaques showed no argyrophilia on methenamine silver-stained sections, and slight argyrophilia on modified Bielschowsky silver-stained sections (Figures 10a, 11c). No dystrophic neurites were revealed by any silver stain (Figures 12a, 12b, 12c). In contrast to the existence of numerous plaques, neurons and laminar structure in the cerebral cortex were well spared (Figure 9b). In the cerebellum, large eosinophilic plaques associated with the blood vessels were frequently encountered (Figure 15a).

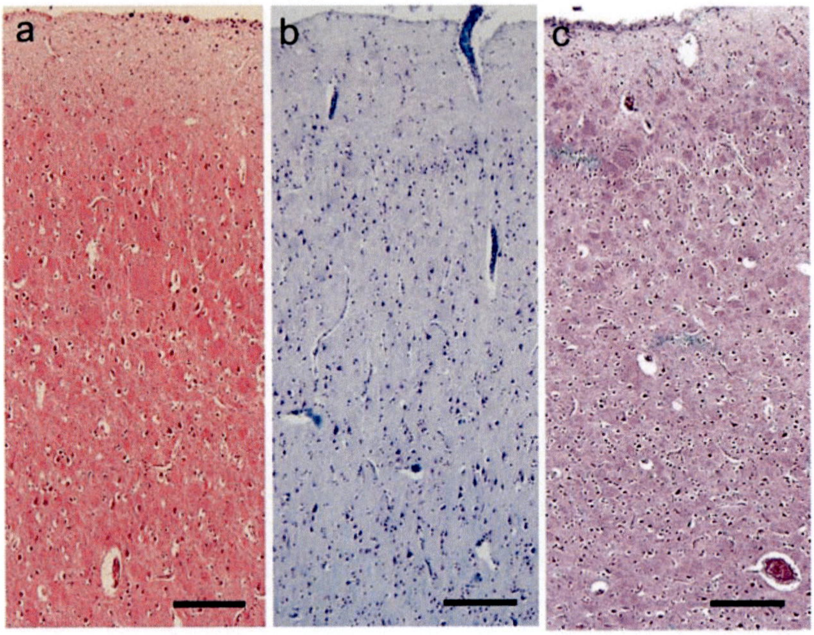

Figure 9. The temporal cortex in case 2. (a) Hematoxylin-eosin stain shows abundant irregularly shaped plaques in all cortical layers. (b) Klüver-Barrera stain. The cortical laminar structure is relatively well preserved, although neurons in the superficial layer are reduced in number. (c) Bodian stain also shows many slight argyrophilic plaques in all cortical layers. All scale bars = 200 μm.

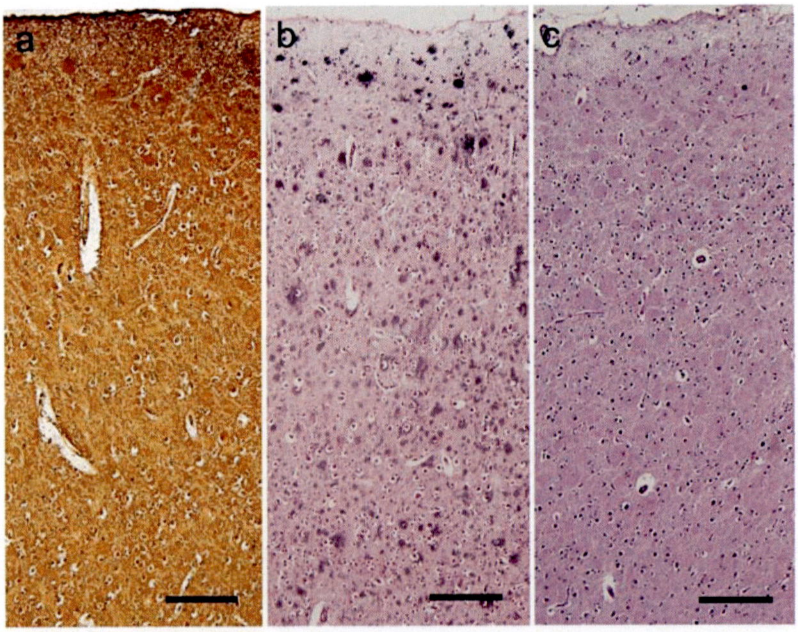

Figure 10. The temporal cortex in case 2. (a) Bielschowsky silver stain. Plaques are faintly argyrophilic. (b) Gallyas-Braak silver stain reveals many small plaques, but no neuritic changes are found. (c) PAS stain. Many plaques are found in all cortical layers. All scale bars = 200 μm.

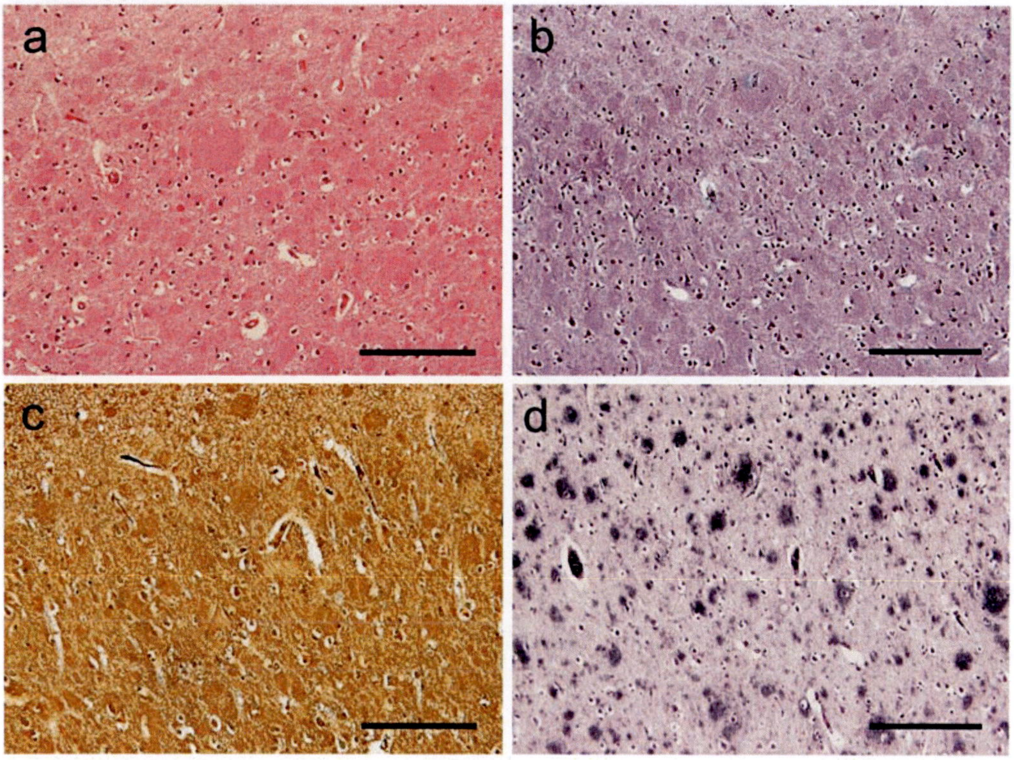

Figure 11. The temporal cortex in case 2 at higher magnification. (a) Many irregularly shaped plaques with ill-defined boundaries are found on hematoxylin-eosin stained sections. Variable sizes of plaques are also found on (b) Bodian, (c) Bielschowsky, and (d) Gallyas-Braak silver stains. All scale bars = 200 μm.

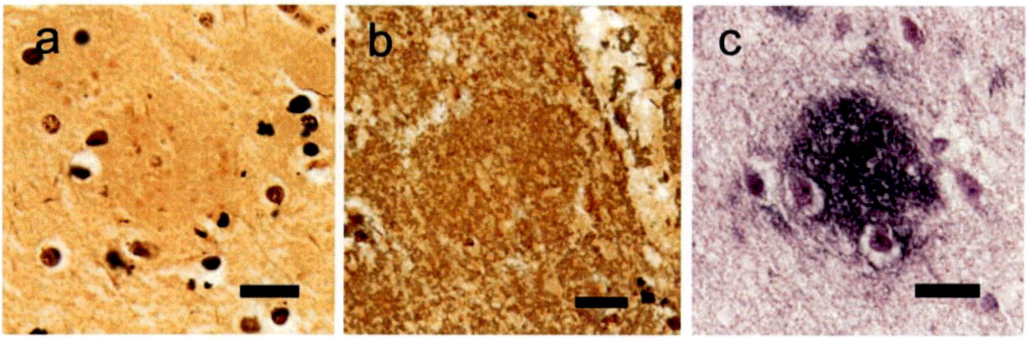

Figure 12. Plaques in the temporal cortex in case 2. Core and dystrophic neurites are not revealed with (a) methenamine, (b) Bielschowsky, or (c) Gallyas-Braak stains. All scale bars = 20 μm.

Neurons in the cerebral cortex, basal ganglia, and brainstem nuclei were surprisingly well preserved in number despite the occurrence of abundant plaques (Table). In the cerebral cortex, slight loss of neurons in the superficial layers was noted in a part of the frontal and temporal cortices. In the basal ganglia, neurons in the nucleus basalis of Meynert were spared in number, although glial proliferation was evident. The other sites in the basal ganglia and brainstem nuclei were not affected by neuronal loss. In the pyramidal tract, although loss of myelin was not noted, glial proliferation was evident. Lower motor neurons in the hypoglossal nuclei were not reduced in number.

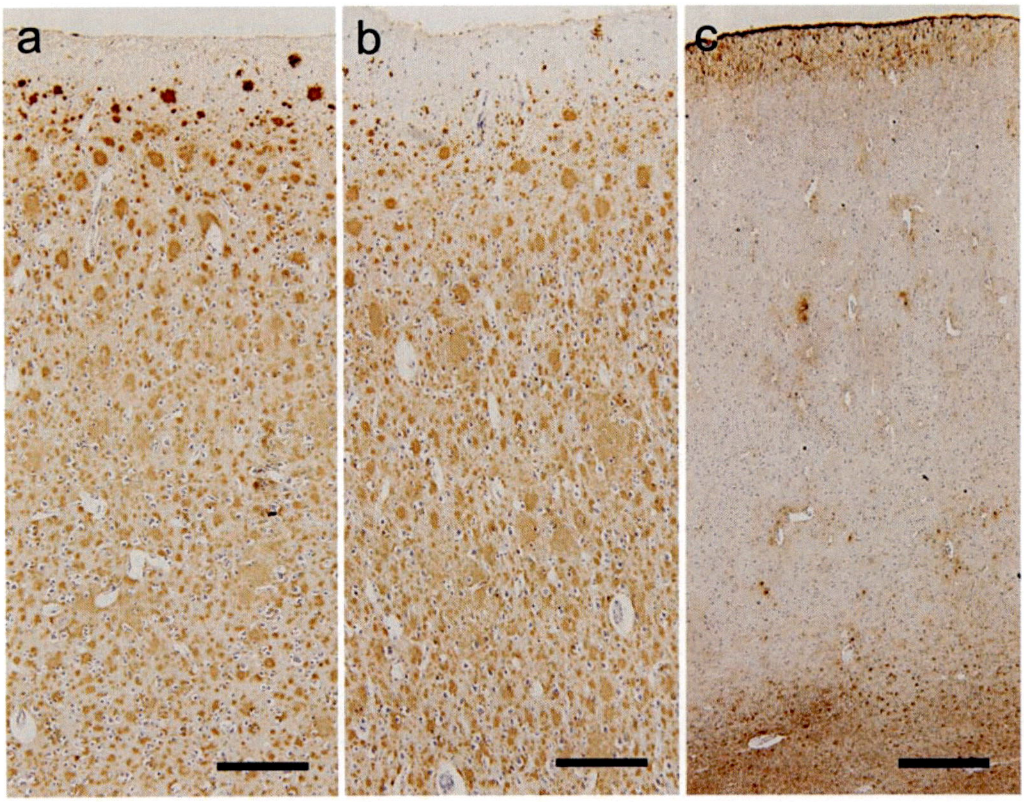

Figure 13. Aβ and GFAP immunohistochemistry in the temporal cortex in case 2. Abundant plaques with variable size are visualized with (a) 6E10 and (b) 4G8. Aβ deposits are not found in the subpial region. (c) GFAP immunohistochemistry reveals a few reactive astrocytes in the cortex, in contrast to the evident gliosis in the subpial region and subcortical white matter. Scale bars = (a, b) 200 μm, (c) 500 μm.

Aβ immunohistochemistry demonstrated abundant Aβ deposits in the entire cerebral cortex (Figures 13a, 13b). The Aβ deposits were distributed in all cortical layers; however, they were not noted in the subpial region. Most of the plaques were irregularly round or oval, and the boundary was often ill-defined. The plaques in the cerebral cortex were not associated with blood vessels. The diameter of the plaques was 40-100 μm. Most of the plaques were smaller than those in case 1; however, they often conglomerated and formed large plaques. Unusually, Aβ40 rather than Aβ42 was predominantly deposited in these plaques (Figures 14a, 14b). In addition, no amyloid angiopathy was encountered in any region in the cerebral cortex. In the cerebellum, Aβ was severely deposited in the molecular layer, and to a lesser degree, in the Purkinje cell layer and granular cell layer. As in the cerebral cortex, Aβ40 rather than Aβ42 was predominantly accumulated in these plaques (Figures 15b, 15c). In contrast to the plaques in the cerebral cortex, Aβ deposits in the molecular layer in the cerebellum frequently surrounded the blood vessels. Neither α-synuclein-positive nor prion protein-positive lesions were noted in any regions.

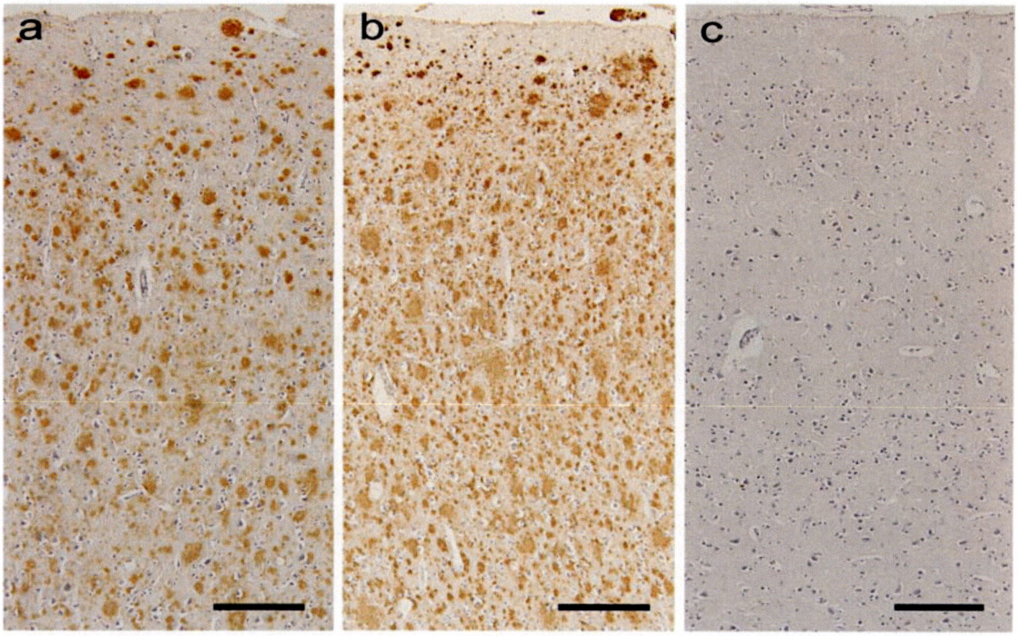

Figure 14. Aβ40 and Aβ42 immunohistochemistry in the temporal cortex in case 2. (a) Aβ42-positive plaques. (b) Aβ40-positive plaques. Aβ40 rather than Aβ42 is predominantly deposited in the cerebellum. (c) There are no tau-positive lesions. (a) FCA3542 (Aβ42) immunostain, (b) FCA3340 (Aβ40) immunostain, (c) AT-8 immunostain. All scale bars = 200 μm.

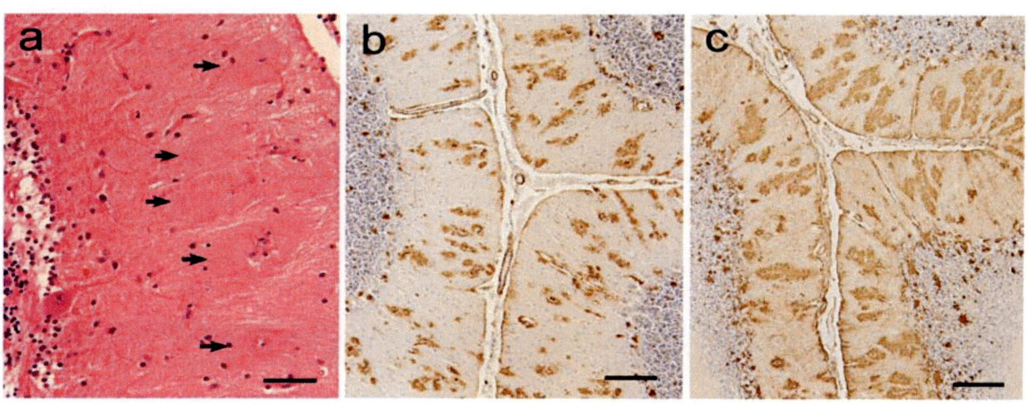

Figure 15. Plaques in the cerebellum in case 2. (a) Many homogeneous non-cored plaques visible with hematoxylin-eosin stain (arrows). (b) Aβ42-positive deposits in the cerebellum. (c) Aβ40-positive deposits in the cerebellum. Aβ40 rather than Aβ42 is predominantly deposited in the cerebellum, as well as in the cerebral cortex. (a) Hematoxylin-eosin stain, (b) FCA3542 (Aβ42) immunostain, (c) FCA3340 (Aβ40) immunostain. Scale bars = (a) 50 μm, (b, c) 200 μm.

Another intriguing feature was the almost complete absence of inflammatory response in the cerebral cortex. Few reactive astrocytes immunopositive for GFAP were found in the cortex in contrast to abundant Aβ deposits (Figure 13c). By contrast, astrocytic proliferation was evident only in the superficial cortical layer and subcortical white matter. Furthermore, no tau-positive lesion was encountered in any region (Figure 14c).

Genetic analysis using paraffin-embedded brain sections revealed no mutation in exons 3 to 12 of the PS1 gene, exons 3-12 of PS2 gene, or exons 16 and 17 of the APP gene, which included all coding regions. Apo E genotype was ε3/ε4.

Discussion

Since a report of CWP-AD due to the deletion of exon 9 of the PS1 gene in 1998 [4], about 20 novel mutations of the PS1 gene associated with CWP-AD have been reported [19-32]. In addition, several cases of CWP-AD lacking an obvious family history have been reported. Cases of CWP-AD with PS1 mutation usually present with initial symptoms in their thirties to fifties. Further, although rare, there are early-onset cases that develop their first symptoms at under 30 years of age [20,27,33]. On the other hand, some of the sporadic CWP-AD cases are late onset [18,34]. Dementia and spastic paraparesis are the most representative symptoms of CWP-AD [4,21], but the presentation of clinical phenotype of CWP-AD is not uniform. Indeed, the order of the development of dementia and spastic paraparesis is not necessarily consistent between cases with a same PS1 mutation in the same pedigree [4]. Further, there are cases that exhibit only dementia or only spastic paraparesis in one pedigree [23,31]. Sporadic CWP-AD cases often showed dementia but not spastic paraparesis [18,34]. In addition, several uncommon symptoms in CWP-AD have been described: morbid jealousy [31], severely stooped posture and kyphoscoliosis [28], low back pain (especially as an onset symptom) [35], hyperorality [28], diplopia and ocular movement disturbance [24], facial palsy [35], and ataxia [14,24,33,35]. Likewise, histopathological phenotypes showed some variation between cases even when they were from the same pedigree. For example, some cases carrying a mutation associated with CWPs had cored plaques but not CWPs [23]. The quantity of CWPs often differs between cases with the same mutation [23]. Also in the pedigree of case 1 presented in this paper, a demented relative with the PS1 gene mutation (case IV.1, see Figure 1) had many neuritic plaques in addition to a few CWPs that were found only in the hippocampus and insular cortex (personal communication from Dr. Kawakatsu, Department of Neuropsychiatry, Yamagata University). Coexistence of Lewy bodies with CWPs was described in at least two previous cases [18,32]. One of the cases reported by our group is a woman who was 45 years old at the time of death. This case initially developed personality change with disinhibition at age 34. Dementia and L-dopa-responsive parkinsonism were observed 5 years after the onset [18]. This case was clinically diagnosed as having Parkinson's disease with dementia. Postmortem examination disclosed numerous CWPs widespread in the cerebral cortex and Lewy bodies in the neocortex and substantia nigra. Another case was a 52-year-old man with a deletion in exon 12 of the PS1 gene [32]. The onset symptom was L-dopa-responsive parkinsonism, and dementia occurred subsequently. This case had CWPs, corticospinal tract involvement, and Lewy body pathology widespread in the cerebral cortex. The occurrence of NFTs was not severe, corresponding to Braak stage IV. At present, the frequency and significance of coexistence of Lewy bodies with CWPs are unclear.

To the best of our knowledge, the first description of CWPs is the 'plaque-like bodies' reported by Matsuoka et al. in Japanese in 1967 [35]. Recently, this case was reexamined with conventional histopathological and immunohistochemical methods by several researchers including our group, and the features of the plaques were verified to be consistent with those of what are now called CWPs [18,37]. In summary, this was a 36-year-old woman at the time of death with a clinical course of 8 years. Her initial symptom was dysarthria, hypersalivation, and pain in the left leg at age 28. Pain and motor disturbance occurred in the right leg also, and she could not walk at age 31. Thereafter, irritability, impulsivity, double vision, impairment of ocular movement, left facial palsy, muscle atrophy in the tongue, dysarthria, hearing loss on the right side, pyramidal signs, and cerebellar signs also occurred. Fasciculation, aphasia, apraxia, and agnosia were not noted. She showed dementia, and her IQ was 30 on the Wechsler-Bellevue Intelligence Scale. Brain weight was 1185g. Macroscopically, the bilateral frontal lobes, base of the pons, corpus callosum, and cerebral peduncle were atrophic. Microscopically, numerous CWPs were widespread in the cerebral cortex, basal ganglia, brainstem, cerebellum, and spinal cord. Many NFTs, corticospinal tract degeneration, and amyloid angiopathy were also encountered. We did not find any mutations of the PS1, presenilin-2, and amyloid precursor protein genes using paraffin-embedded brain sections [18,37], although the possibility that the present cases had a deletion or other mutation could not be excluded because neither frozen tissue nor lymphoblast lines was available. The apo E genotype was ε3/ε4. Interestingly, a concordant monozygotic sibling of this case also showed nystagmus, dysarthria, gait disturbance, increased deep tendon reflexes, and cerebellar ataxia at age 32. Pathological examination was not done. Her brother had motor disturbance in the bilateral lower extremities, but the details are not clear. Other early cases we know include a case reported by Mizushima et al. in 1974 (unfortunately, only a Japanese abstract was published in Shineki Kenkyu no Shinpo, volume 18, pages 206-7) and a case reported by Fukatsu et al. in 1980 [36]. The case reported by Mizushima et al. was a 37-year-old man at the time of death, with a clinical course of 11 years. The onset symptom was bradykinesia. Thereafter, memory impairment, masked face, disorientation, rigidity, and gait disturbance were observed. The family history was not described. CWPs, amyloid angiopathy, and pyramidal tract degeneration were revealed by recent postmortem reexamination [38]. Another case reported by Fukatsu et al. [36] was a 42-year-old man at the time of death, with a disease duration of 2.5 years. The initial symptom was low back pain and pain in the left leg. Reduced spontaneity, irritability, bradykinesia, memory impairment, and gait disturbance also developed during the course. Pathologically, numerous lesions, the now-called CWPs, widespread amyloid angiopathy, and NFT formation were disclosed.

Although many conventional histopathological and immunohistochemical characteristics of CWPs have been accumulated [22,39,40], we consider that the trend that cortical neurons and laminar structure are relatively better preserved in CWP-AD than in common AD may be a significant characteristic to understand the pathomechanism leading to CWP formation and cognitive impairment. Cortical neurons in CWP-AD are often considerably well preserved, being disproportional to the occurrence of abundant CWPs. The preservation of the cortical laminar structure may be associated with the minimal glial response in CWP-AD [4,34,40,41]. These features had been already noticed in 1967 by Matsuoka et al. [35] and Hayashi et al. [17], and Fujisawa also emphasized them in 1980 in association with a paper by Fukatsu et al. [36]. Although CWPs tend to displace surrounding normal structures, which was often noted in recent papers [34,40], the tendency may be associated with a well preserved laminar structure in the cerebral cortex. Only limited data concerning neuronal loss in CWP-AD are available. Ishikawa et al. [32] systematically examined neuronal loss in a case of CWP-AD associated with a PS1 mutation. This case had mild to moderate neuronal loss and severe amyloid angiopathy in the neocortex. Tau pathology was not severe, corresponding to Braak stage IV. On the other hand, severe neuronal loss has also been described in several previous cases of CWP-AD. Takao et al. [28] reported two CWP-AD cases with a G217D PS1 mutation that had severe neuronal loss in extensive regions, including the frontal, temporal, and cingulate cortices, amygdala, hippocampus, subiculum, entorhinal cortex, caudate nucleus, substantia nigra, and locus coeruleus. This case had numerous CWPs in the cerebral cortex and basal ganglia, as well as severe NFT formation, severe amyloid angiopathy, and a relatively small number of neuritic plaques throughout the cerebral cortex. Likewise, among six cases of CWP-AD described by Brooks et al. [31], one had severe neuronal loss in the cerebral cortex and hippocampus.

Although the factors determining the loss of neurons in the cerebral cortex in CWP-AD remain unclear, it is possible that the quantity of neuritic plaques and/or NFTs is associated with its severity. For example, Smith et al. [23] reported a PS1-linked pedigree that included cases having variable degrees of neuronal loss and CWPs. Among three cases for which detailed microscopic findings were described, widespread and marked neuronal loss was observed only in one case with severe NFT formation and frequent cored plaques. This case lacked CWP formation. Another case bearing CWPs, cored plaques (fewer than CWPs), and sparse NFTs showed less marked neuronal loss compared with the prior case. Interestingly, the last case with many CWPs but lacking cored plaques and significant NFTs showed no significant neuronal loss. This case presented with spastic paraparesis but not dementia. These findings are consistent with those in our cases presented in this paper. Namely, our case 1 had more neuritic changes including NFTs compared with case 2, and the neuronal loss in case 1 was more severe than that in case 2 (Table). It should be also emphasized that both our cases presented with severe dementia despite only slight neuronal loss in the cerebrum. Furthermore, it is noteworthy that one of our cases lacked tau pathology. These findings suggest the possibility that neuritic plaques, NFTs, and severe neuronal loss are not always necessary for the occurrence of cognitive decline in AD patients. Some researchers have demonstrated that intracellular Aβ accumulation is associated with the pathogenesis of AD including apoptosis [42-45]. Further accumulation of findings regarding other factors is awaited to explore potential therapeutic targets in the pathogenesis of AD.

ACKNOWLEDGEMENT

We would like to thank Mr. Y. Shoda and Ms. K. Suzuki (Tokyo Institute of Psychiatry) and Ms. M. Onbe (Department of Neuropsychiatry, Okayama University Graduate School of

Medicine, Dentistry and Pharmaceutical Sciences) for their excellent technical assistance and Mr. A. Sasaki for help with the production of the manuscript. This work was supported by a grant-in-aid for scientific research from the Ministry of Education, Culture, Sports, Science and Technology (14570957) and a research grant from the Zikei Institute of Psychiatry.

References

[1] Mirra, SS; Heyman, A; McKeel, D; Sumi, SM; Crain, BJ; Brownlee, LM; Vogel, FS; Hughes, JP; van Belle, G; Berg, L. The Consortium to Establish a Registry for Alzheimer's Disease (CERAD). Part II. Standardization of the neuropathologic assessment of Alzheimer's disease. *Neurology,* 1991, 41, 479-486.

[2] Hyman BT; Trojanowski JQ. Consensus recommendations for the postmortem diagnosis of Alzheimer disease from the National Institute on Aging and the Reagan Institute Working Group on diagnostic criteria for the neuropathological assessment of Alzheimer disease. *J Neuropathol Exp Neuro,* 1997, 56, 1095-1097.

[3] Arriagada, PV; Growdon, JH; Hedley-Whyte, ET; Hyman, BT. Neurofibrillary tangles but not senile plaques parallel duration and severity of Alzheimer's disease. *Neurology,* 1992, 42, 631-639.

[4] Crook, R; Verkkoniemi, A; Perez-Tur, J; Mehta, N; Baker, M; Houlden, H; Farrer, M; Hutton, M; Lincoln, S; Hardy, J; Gwinn, K; Somer, M; Paetau, A; Kalimo, H; Ylikoski, R; Poyhonen, M; Kucera, S; Haltia, M. A variant of Alzheimer's disease with spastic paraparesis and unusual plaques due to deletion of exon 9 of presenilin 1. *Nat Med,* 1998, 4, 452-455.

[5] Barelli, H; Lebeau, A; Vizzavona, J; Delaere, P; Chevallier, N; Drouot, C; Marambaud, P; Ancolio, K; Buxbaum, JD; Khorkova, O; Heroux, J; Sahasrabudhe, S; Martinez, J; Warter, JM; Mohr, M; Checler, F. Characterization of new polyclonal antibodies specific for 40 and 42 amino acid-long amyloid beta peptides: their use to examine the cell biology of presenilins and the immunohistochemistry of sporadic Alzheimer's disease and cerebral amyloid angiopathy cases. *Mol Med,* 1997, 10, 695-707.

[6] Tsuchiya, K; Ikeda, K; Uchihara, T; Oda, T; Shimada, H. Distribution of cerebral cortical lesions in corticobasal degeneration: a clinicopathological study of five autopsy cases in Japan. *Acta Neuropathol (Berl),* 1997, 94, 416-424.

[7] Tsuchiya, K; Ikeda, M; Hasegawa, K; Fukui, T; Kuroiwa, T; Haga, C; Oyanagi, S; Nakano, I; Matsushita, M; Yagishita, S; Ikeda, K. Distribution of cerebral cortical lesions in Pick's disease with Pick bodies: a clinicopathological study of six autopsy cases showing unusual clinical presentations. *Acta Neuropathol (Berl),* 2001, 102, 553-571.

[8] Tsuchiya, K; Nakayama, H; Haga, C; Oshima, K; Niizato, K; Arai, T; Matsushita, M; Akiyama, H. Distribution of cerebral cortical lesions in diffuse neurofibrillary tangles with calcification: a clinicopathological study of four autopsy cases showing prominent parietal lobe involvement. *Acta Neuropathol (Berl),* 2005, 110, 57-68.

[9] Tsuchiya, K; Piao, YS; Oda, T; Mochizuki, A; Arima, K; Hasegawa, K; Haga, C; Kakita, A; Hori, K; Tominaga, I; Yagishita, S; Akiyama, H; Takahashi, H. Pathological heterogeneity of the precentral gyrus in Pick's disease: a study of 16 autopsy cases. *Acta Neuropathol (Berl),* 2006, 112, 29-42.

[10] Yokota, O; Tsuchiya, K; Oda, T; Ishihara, T; Ishizu, H; de Silva, R; Lees, AJ; Kuroda, S; Akiyama, H. Amyotrophic lateral sclerosis with dementia: an autopsy case showing many Bunina bodies, tau-positive neuronal and astrocytic plaque-like pathologies, and pallido-nigral degeneration. *Acta Neuropathol (Berl),* 2006, 112, 633-645.

[11] Yokota, O; Tsuchiya, K; Uchihara, T; Ujike, H; Terada, S; Mafuyu, T; Kimura, Y; Ishizu, H; Akiyama, H; Kuroda, S. Lewy body variant of Alzheimer's disease or cerebral type Lewy body disease?: two autopsy cases of presenile onset with minimal involvement of the brainstem. *Neuropathology,* 2007, 27, 21-35.

[12] Hutton, M; Busfield, F; Wragg, M; Crook, R; Perez-Tur, J; Clark, RF; Prihar, G; Talbot, C; Phillips, H; Wright, K; Baker, M; Lendon, C; Duff, K; Martinez, A; Houlden, H; Nichols, A; Karran, E; Roberts, G; Roques, P; Rossor, M; Venter, JC; Adams, MD; Cline, RT; Phillips, CA; Fuldner, RA; Hardy, J; Goate, A. Complete analysis of the presenilin 1 gene in early onset Alzheimer's disease. *Neuroreport,* 1996, 7, 801-805.

[13] Wenham, PR; Price, WH; Blandell, G. Apolipoprotein E genotyping by one-stage PCR. *Lancet,* 1991, 337, 1158-1159.

[14] Kawakatsu, S; Suzuki, H; Totsuka, S. A case of familial Alzheimer's disease with G384A presenilin-1 mutation exhibiting pyramidal tract degeneration. *Neuropathology,* 2003, 23, A43.

[15] Iritani, S; Tsuchiya, K; Ikeda, K; Kosaka, K. Two autopsy cases with Alzheimer's disease indicating peculiar clinical and neuropathological findings (in Japanese). *Seishin Igaku (Clinical Psychiatry),* 1999, 41, 1061-1069.

[16] Oshima, K; Tsuchiya, K; Iritani, S; Niizato, K; Uchihara, T; Sizuki, K; Haga, C; Akiyama, H; Ikeda, K; Arai, H. Early-onset familial Alzheimer's disease with a presenilin-1 mutation (G384A) associated with spastic paraparesis and cotton wool plaques: an autopsy case report (in Japanese with English abstract). *Dementia Japan,* 2004, 18, 64-72.

[17] Hayashi, Y; Mii, T; Sudo, K. An autopsy case of presenile dementia with senile plaque-like changes (in Japanese with English abstract). *Shineki Kenkyu no Shinpo,* 1967, 11, 793-800.

[18] Yokota, O; Terada, S; Ishizu, H; Ujike, H; Ishihara, T; Namba, M; Hayashi, Y; Nishinaka, T; Namba, R; Nakashima, H; Ueda, K; Checler, F; Kuroda, S. Variability and heterogeneity in Alzheimer's disease with cotton wool plaques: a clinicopathological study of four autopsy cases. *Acta Neuropathol (Berl),* 2003, 106, 348-356.

[19] Kwok, JB; Taddei, K; Hallupp, M; Fisher, C; Brooks, WS; Broe, GA; Hardy, J; Fulham, MJ; Nicholson, GA; Stell, R; St George Hyslop, PH; Fraser, PE; Kakulas, B; Clarnette, R; Relkin, N; Gandy, SE; Schofield, PR; Martins, RN. Two novel (M233T and R278T) presenilin-1 mutations in early-onset Alzheimer's disease pedigrees and

preliminary evidence for association of presenilin-1 mutations with a novel phenotype. *Neuroreport,* 1997, 8, 1537-1542.

[20] Houlden H; Baker, M; McGowan, E; Lewis, P; Hutton, M; Crook, R; Wood, NW; Kumar-Singh, S; Geddes, J; Swash, M; Scaravilli, F; Holton, JL; Lashley, T; Tomita, T; Hashimoto, T; Verkkoniemi, A; Kalimo, H; Somer, M; Paetau, A; Martin, JJ; Van Broeckhoven, C; Golde, T; Hardy, J; Haltia, M; Revesz, T. Variant Alzheimer's disease with spastic paraparesis and cotton wool plaques is caused by PS-1 mutations that lead to exceptionally high amyloid-beta concentrations. *Ann Neurol,* 2000, 48, 806-808.

[21] Verkkoniemi, A; Somer, M; Rinne, JO; Myllykangas, L; Crook, R; Hardy, J; Viitanen, M; Kalimo, H; Haltia, M. Variant Alzheimer's disease with spastic paraparesis: clinical characterization. *Neurology,* 2000, 54, 1103-1109.

[22] Mann, DM; Takeuchi, A; Sato, S; Cairns, NJ; Lantos, PL; Rossor, MN; Haltia, M; Kalimo, H; Iwatsubo, T. Cases of Alzheimer's disease due to deletion of exon 9 of the presenilin-1 gene show an unusual but characteristic beta-amyloid pathology known as 'cotton wool' plaques. *Neuropathol Appl Neurobiol,* 2001, 27, 189-196.

[23] Smith, MJ; Kwok, JB; McLean, CA; Kril, JJ; Broe, GA; Nicholson, GA; Cappai, R; Hallupp, M; Cotton, RG; Masters, CL; Schofield, PR; Brooks, WS. Variable phenotype of Alzheimer's disease with spastic paraparesis. *Ann Neurol,* 2001, 49, 125-129.

[24] O'Riordan, S; McMonagle, P; Janssen, JC; Fox, NC; Farrell, M; Collinge, J; Rossor, MN; Hutchinson, M. Presenilin-1 mutation (E280G), spastic paraparesis, and cranial MRI white-matter abnormalities. *Neurology,* 2002, 59, 1108-1110.

[25] Shibuya, M; Tachikawa, H; Yagishita, S; Tabira, T; Tanahashi, H; Ogawa, Y; Shinohara, Y. An autopsy case of atypical Alzheimer's disease with spastic paraparesis and cotton wool plaques in association with presenilin 1 gene novel mutation. *Neuropathology,* 2002, 22, A38.

[26] Kwok, JB; Hallupp, M; Badenhop, RF; Schofield, PR; Halliday, GM; Brooks, WS; Dolios, G; Murayama, O; Takashima, A; Vickers, J; Gandy, SE. Presenilin-1 mutation (L271V) results in altered exon 8 splicing and Alzheimer's disease with non-cored plaques and neuritic dystrophy. *Neurobiol Aging,* 2002, 23, s277.

[27] Moehlmann, T; Winkler, E; Xia, X; Edbauer, D; Murrell, J; Capell, A; Kaether, C; Zheng, H; Ghetti, B; Haass, C; Steiner, H. Presenilin-1 mutations of leucine 166 equally affect the generation of the Notch and APP intracellular domains independent of their effect on Abeta 42 production. *Proc Natl Acad Sci U S A,* 2002, 99, 8025-8030.

[28] Takao, M; Ghetti, B; Hayakawa, I; Ikeda, E; Fukuuchi, Y; Miravalle, L; Piccardo, P; Murrell, JR; Glazier, BS; Koto, A. A novel mutation (G217D) in the presenilin 1 gene (PSEN1) in a Japanese family: presenile dementia and parkinsonism are associated with cotton wool plaques in the cortex and striatum. *Acta Neuropathol (Berl),* 2002, 104, 155-170.

[29] Takao, M; Ghetti, B; Piccardo, P; Koto, A. Clinical and neuropathologic phenotype of Alzheimer's disease associated with CWPs and PSEN1 mutations. *Neuropathology,* 2003, 23, A52.

[30] Kwok, JB; Halliday, GM; Brooks, WS; Dolios, G; Laudon, H; Murayama, O; Hallupp, M; Badenhop, RF; Vickers, J; Wang, R; Naslund, J; Takashima, A; Gandy, SE; Schofield, PR. Presenilin-1 mutation L271V results in altered exon 8 splicing and Alzheimer's disease with non-cored plaques and no neuritic dystrophy. *J Biol Chem,* 2003, 278, 6748-6754.

[31] Brooks, WS; Kwok, JB; Kril, JJ; Broe, GA; Blumbergs, PC; Tannenberg, AE; Lamont, PJ; Hedges, P; Schofield, PR. Alzheimer's disease with spastic paraparesis and 'cotton wool' plaques: two pedigrees with PS-1 exon 9 deletions. *Brain,* 2003, 126, 783-791.

[32] Ishikawa, A; Piao, YS; Miyashita, A; Kuwano, R; Onodera, O; Ohtake, H; Suzuki, M; Nishizawa, M; Takahashi, H. A mutant PSEN1 causes dementia with Lewy bodies and variant Alzheimer's disease. *Ann Neurol,* 2005, 57, 429-434.

[33] Murrell, J; Evans, RM; Boyer, PJ; Piccardo, P; Towfighi, J; Ghetti, B. Alzheimer disease with onset in adolescence due to a novel mutation in *presenilin 1* (L166P). *J Neuropathol Experimental Neurol,* 2000, 59, 466.

[34] Le, TV; Crook, R; Hardy, J; Dickson, DW. Cotton wool plaques in non-familial late-onset Alzheimer disease. *J Neuropathol Exp Neurol,* 2001, 60, 1051-1061.

[35] Matsuoka, T; Miyoshi, K; Saka, K; Kawagoe, T; Nishikiori, T; Suzuki, S; Hirabayashi, M; Shisozuka, T; Suda, K; Aoki, A; Shimokawa, K; Shiraki, H. A case of encephalopathy with plaque-like bodies; neurofibrillary changes; angiopathy and amyotrophic lateral sclerosis-like lesions (in Japanese with English abstract). *Shinkei Kenkyu no Shinpo,* 1967, 11, 801-811.

[36] Fukatsu, R; Ikeda, T; Ueno, T; Tanabe, M; Honma, H; Kimura, N; Takahata, N. An unusual case of presenile dementia with numerous argentophilic plaques and severe amyloid vascular changes. *Shineki Kenkyu no Shinpo,* 1980, 24, 271-282.

[37] Tabira, T; Chui, DH; Nakayama, H; Kuroda, S; Shibuya, M. Alzheimer's disease with spastic paresis and cotton wool type plaques. *J Neurosci Res,* 2002, 70, 367-372.

[38] Nakayama, H; Arima, K; Mizushima, S; Chui, DH; Tabira, T. An autopsy case of juvenile Alzheimer's disease with cotton wool plaques. *Neuropathology,* 2001, 21, A32

[39] Uchihara, T; Nakamura, A; Nakayama, H; Arima, K; Ishizuka, N; Mori, H; Mizushima, S. Triple immunofluorolabeling with two rabbit polyclonal antibodies and a mouse monoclonal antibody allowing three-dimensional analysis of cotton wool plaques in Alzheimer disease. *J Histochem Cytochem,* 2003, 51, 1201-1206.

[40] Verkkoniemi, A; Kalimo, H; Paetau, A; Somer, M; Iwatsubo, T; Hardy, J; Haltia, M. Variant Alzheimer disease with spastic paraparesis: neuropathological phenotype. *J Neuropathol Exp Neurol,* 2001, 60, 483-492.

[41] Yokota, O; Terada, S; Ishizu, H; Ishihara, T; Ujike, H; Nakashima, H; Nakashima, Y; Kugo, A, Checler, F; Kuroda, S. Cyclooxygenase-2 in the hippocampus is up-regulated in Alzheimer's disease but not in variant Alzheimer's disease with cotton wool plaques in humans. *Neurosci Lett,* 2003, 343, 175-179.

[42] Mochizuki, A; Tamaoka, A; Shimohata, A; Komatsuzaki, Y; Shoji, S. Abeta42-positive non-pyramidal neurons around amyloid plaques in Alzheimer's disease. *Lancet,* 2000, 355, 42-43.

[43] Chui, DH; Dobo, E; Makifuchi, T; Akiyama, H; Kawakatsu, S; Petit, A; Checler, F; Araki, W; Takahashi, K; Tabira, T. Apoptotic neurons in Alzheimer's disease frequently show intracellular Abeta42 labeling. *J Alzheimers Dis,* 2001, 3, 231-239.

[44] Ohyagi, Y; Asahara, H; Chui, DH; Tsuruta, Y; Sakae, N; Miyoshi, K; Yamada, T; Kikuchi, H; Taniwaki, T; Murai, H; Ikezoe, K; Furuya, H; Kawarabayashi, T; Shoji, M; Checler, F; Iwaki, T; Makifuchi, T; Takeda, K; Kira, J; Tabira, T. Intracellular Abeta42 activates p53 promoter: a pathway to neurodegeneration in Alzheimer's disease. *FASEB J,* 2005, 19, 255-257.

[45] Oakley, H; Cole, SL; Logan, S; Maus, E; Shao, P; Craft, J; Guillozet-Bongaarts, A; Ohno, M; Disterhoft, J; Van Eldik, L; Berry, R; Vassar, R. Intraneuronal beta-amyloid aggregates, neurodegeneration, and neuron loss in transgenic mice with five familial Alzheimer's disease mutations: potential factors in amyloid plaque formation. *J Neurosci,* 2006, 26, 10129-10140.

In: Alzheimer's Disease Research Trends
Editor: A.P. Chan, pp. 117-146
ISBN 978-1-60021-712-8

Chapter VI

ALZHEIMER'S DISEASE

Maria Luiza Mamede-Rosa

INTRODUCTION

Alzheimer's disease (AD) is a devastating and always fatal degenerative disorder of the brain, the most prominent form of dementia among the main types currently defined. Dementia itself is an acquired impairment in intellectual abilities that affects memory, language, visuospatial skills, cognition, emotion and personality. Although mild cognitive losses occur as part of the normal ageing process, the cognitive impairment observed in demented patients is both qualitative and quantitatively more severe. The AD process involves the progressive degeneration of synapses and neurons in brain regions that play fundamental roles in learning and memory, including the hippocampus, entorhinal cortex, basal forebrain, amygdala, frontal cortex, and inferior parietal cortex.

It has been estimated that approximately 50 million people around the world are currently affected by AD with a probable prevalence of 3% in subjects aged 65-74, 19% in those aged 75-84, and 47% in those over 85. Ageing itself is the most important risk factor for AD. Thus, with the continuing exponential increase of the aged population, the incidence of AD is expected to increase significantly in the next decades.

AD is classified into familial and sporadic forms, and exhibits both early-onset (less than 65 years of age) and late-onset (over 65 years of age). It has been shown that there is a correlation between the age of onset of clinical symptoms and the severity of the disease; hence, older patients tend to have a slower disease progression and less severe pathology at death.

Diagnosis of AD cannot be made certain in life and the confirmation is only possible by morphological and histological examination of the brain at autopsy.

NEUROPATHOLOGY

The neuropathological hallmarks of AD were described by the German neuropathologist Alois Alzheimer about 100 years ago, and are characterized by the presence of extracellular β-amyloid deposits (senile plaques) and intracellular tau protein aggregation (neurofibrillary tangles) in the brain. Only about 10 years ago, the neurotoxicity of the β-amyloid peptide was first described. The β-amyloid peptides are overproduced in AD and aggregate spontaneously to a neurotoxic form that attacks neurons in the central nervous system (CNS), leading them to become dysfunctional and, eventually, to death.

The tau protein is involved on the stabilization of microtubule structure and function in the cell. The function of the microtubule is to make the transport of proteins along the axons (axonal transport), which is very important for the survival of the cell. Thus, any impairment of this transport may affect the survival of the nerve cell. The tau protein, when abnormally phosphorilated, accumulates and forms paired helical filaments known as neurofibrillary tangles.

Both senile plaques and neurofibrillary tangles have been used as markers for the diagnosis of AD in *post-mortem* brain. Figure 1 illustrates these histological features.

Morphological changes also occur in the AD brain, which are characterized by cortical atrophy, widened cortical sulci and ventricular dilation. Figure 2 shows a brain with these characteristics from a patient who had AD.

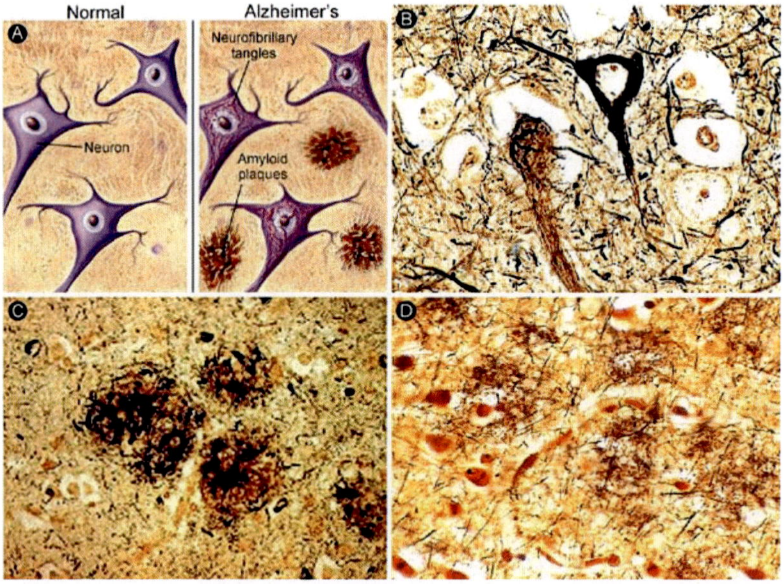

Figure 1. Histological features of Alzheimer's disease. A- a schematic picture of the differences between normal neurons (left, absence of senile plaques and neurofibrillary tangles) and neurons in AD (right, presence of extracellular senile plaques and intracellular neurofibrillary tangles). B- neurofibrillary tangles stained with Bielschowsky silver stain. C- neuritic plaques stained with Bielschowsky silver stain. D- diffuse plaques stained with Bielschowsky stain.

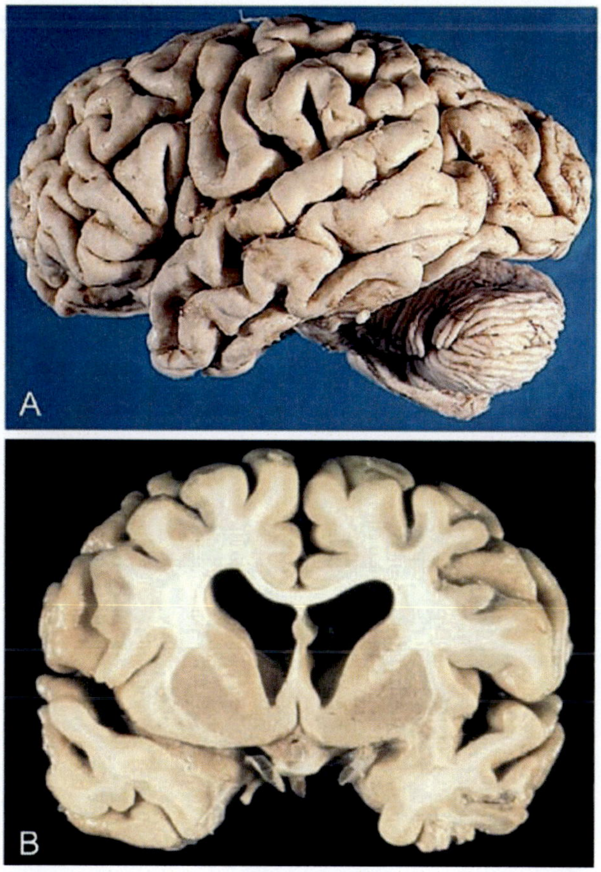

Figure 2. Morphological features of the Alzheimer's disease brain. A- the external appearance shows diffuse atrophy and widened cortical sulci. B- the brain was cut to show the dilated ventricles.

Regional Progression

Pathological changes follow a regional pattern in relation to the progression of the disease. At early stages, accentuated degeneration begins in the hippocampal formation and temporal cortex (Brodmann areas 20-22), then the degenerative process spreads diffusely across the entorhinal cortex to the inferior and superior frontal cortex (areas 8-12), the superior and inferior parietal cortex (areas 39 and 40), and the posterior cingulated gyrus (area 23). Only at advanced stages, motor and sensorimotor cortices (pre- and post-central gyri), anterior cingulated gyrus (area 24) and occipital cortex (areas 17 and 18) are affected. Figure 3 shows a schematic diagram of the regional progression of the disease and a picture of the human brain with the proposed areas involved in AD according to Brodmann's map.

There is a hypothesis that the distribution of neurodegeneration in AD results from the spread of the pathology via known neuroanatomical pathways. This spreading is predicted to occur preferentially in a retrograde direction, which is assumed to be more rapid. However, it does not mean that anterograde spread does not occur.

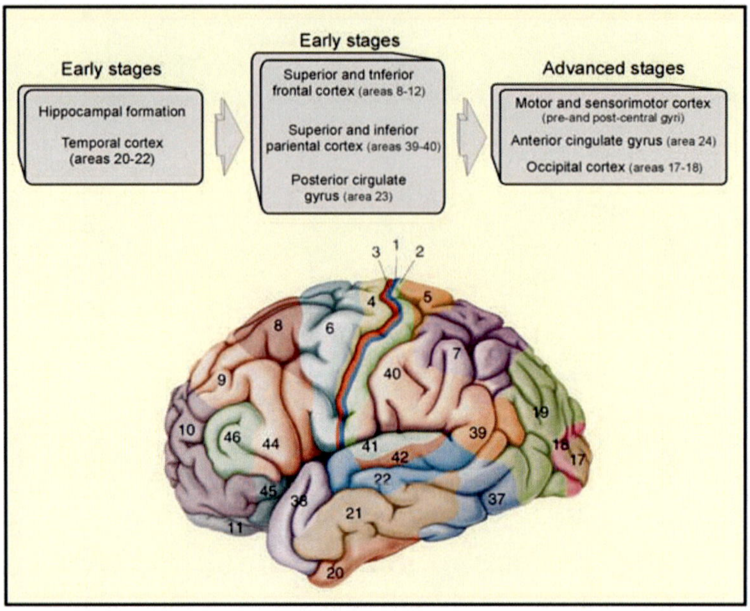

Figure 3. Schematic representation of brain areas predicted to be involved in AD. A- diagram of the regional progression of the pathology. B- picture of the human brain showing the Brodmann's areas.

NEUROTRANSMISSION

Many pathways selectively vulnerable to AD pathology utilize specific neurotransmitters. Senile plaques and neurofibrillary tangles have been associated mainly with degeneration of the basal forebrain and cholinergic deficit. For this reason, in clinical practice the treatment of AD is directed to acetylcholine (ACh) neurotransmission, using basically cholinesterase inhibitors (ChEIs).

In addition to ACh, some other neurotransmitter systems and mechanisms have extensively been reported to be involved in the pathophysiology of AD such as glutamate, norepinephrine, serotonin, peptides, oxidative stress, tau protein, β-amyloid peptide, apoE, and presenilin, among others. The cholinergic pathways are affected first, consistently, and with destruction of function. However, neuronal cell loss is also observed in cell bodies and dendrites of glutamatergic neurons in the cortex and hippocampus. A better knowledge of the mechanisms underlying this disorder is essential for the development of prevention and therapy, necessary to improve the quality of life of our ageing society.

The aims of the present chapter are: i) to make some theoretical considerations about those mechanisms, ii) to present the current therapy to the treatment of AD, and iii) to discuss the correlation of multiple mechanisms underlying the pathology of AD. Specifically related to the last one, the clear understanding of those correlations may be useful for improving the treatment of AD in the future, probably by using mix pharmacotherapeutic approaches directed to multiple targets.

ACETHYLCOLINE

For many years, the cholinergic hypothesis of AD has been the basis of AD research. The simultaneous discovery by Bowen and colleagues, Davies and Maloney and Perry and colleagues of the cholinergic deficit, approximately 30 years ago, became a landmark in the research of AD and since then has provided accumulated evidence for the development of a variety of compounds that lead to an improvement of cholinergic neurotransmission, which would be expected to stabilize the disease symptomatically.

The neurotransmitter ACh is synthesized from choline and acetyl-CoA by an enzyme called choline acetyltransferase (CAT). In the synaptic cleft, ACh may trigger its effects by interacting with two subtypes of receptors, muscarinic (mAChRs) or nicotinic (nAChRs). The ACh neurotransmitter is degraded in the synaptic cleft by the enzyme acetylcholinesterase (AChE). The mAChRs belong to a family of G-protein coupled receptors and the nAChRs belong to a family of ligand gated ion channels. Both receptors participate in many important functional processes in the brain, including learning, memory and cognitive functions. Figure 4 shows a cholinergic synapse with various steps involved in neurotransmission.

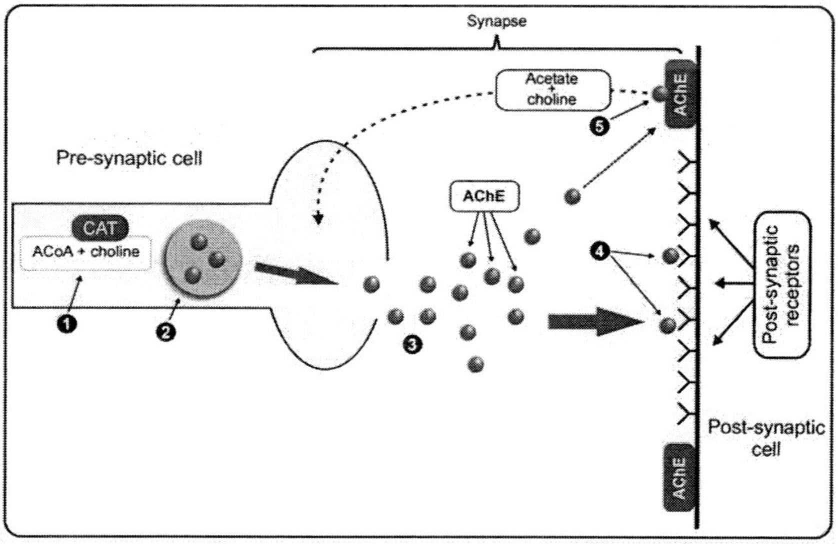

Figure 4. Schematic representation of an acetylcholine (ACh) synapse with the main steps involved on the neurotransmission. On the pre-synaptic neuron: 1) synthesis of ACh; 2) storage of ACh in vesicles. On the synaptic cleft: 3) releasing of the neurotransmitter by exocitosis; 4) interaction of the neurotransmitter with the receptors located on the post-synaptic neuron membrane; 5) enzymatic degradation of ACh by cholinesterases (AChE) located on the post-synaptic neuron membrane.

In AD, the levels of choline acetyltransferase and both ACh receptors are markedly reduced with a loss of cholinergic neurons and functions. Before been associated to AD, the enzyme choline acetyltransferase and the number of choline acetyltransferase-positive nerve cells were found to decrease approximately 4 times during normal ageing. Subsequently, the synthesis of ACh was reported to be reduced by 50% in AD brains, as compared to normal aged brains, and atrophy of cholinergic nerve cells was described in the nucleus basalis

(Meinert). The total number of AchRs, as well as specific subtypes are differently decreased in different areas of the brain. The deficit in learning and memory induced by cholinergic deficit shows the importance of this neurotransmitter system to cognitive processes.

Both choline acetyltransferase and AChE decrease very late in the progression of AD. However, if the synthesis of ACh is highly reduced even in normal concentrations of the synthesizing enzyme, the amount of ACh released in the synaptic cleft is also reduced. In addition, the degrading enzyme is still there, what contributes to an additional reduction of the neurotransmission in the remaining cholinergic neurons. The intervention on the decline in cholinergic neurotransmission, or the supplementation of ACh could be simple therapies for treating AD patients.

Apart from degrading the ACh neurotransmitter, the enzyme AChE is able to promote the formation of Aβ plaques, and Aβ in turn, reduces degradation of AChE, a mechanism that facilitates the aggregation of this peptide. Thus, AChE inhibition provides neuronal protection by both facilitating ACh neurotransmission and modulating the APP processing. This is supported by the demonstration that galantamine, an AChE inhibitor, reduces the cellular death induced by Aβ in the human neuroblastoma cell line.

B-Amyloid

The brain of patients with AD is characterized by two neuropathological features: i) the extracellular deposition of β-amyloid as senile plaques, and also often in the walls of cerebral and meningeal blood vessels and, ii) the intracellular accumulation of hyperphosphorylated tau protein as neurofibrillary tangles. β-amyloid and tau are altered, or shift their location within the cell in AD. These events are often accompanied with loss of neurons and synapses.

Although senile plaques and neurofibrillary tangles are undoubtedly the histopathological hallmarks of AD, it is important to take in mind some particular characteristics of both, when analyzing post-morten brain tissues. Senile plaques involve neuronal processes, including axons and are, therefore, more anatomically divergent than neurofibrillary tangles, i.e. single neurons in brain areas or nuclei may have branching axons projecting to widely different destinations. Neurofibrillary tangles, considered as a marker of cell soma involvement in AD, cannot be only associated to neurodegeneration. Neuronal loss can occur without neurofibrillary tangles formation. In the hippocampus for example, significant shrinkage is a universal phenomenon reported in dentate gyrus and adjacent CA fields in advanced AD, but only CA fields show neurofibrillary tangles. In addition, neurofibrillary tangles are not specific to AD, but occur in a variety of neurodegenerative processes such as non-demented elderly subjects, frontotemporal dementia, Pick's disease, and amyotrophic lateral sclerosis, among others, suggesting that neurofibrillary tangles are secondary events before being AD causative.

B-Amyloid Precursor Protein (APP)

The central core of senile plaques consists of an insoluble deposit of a 39-43 amino acid peptides (~ 4-kDa) known as β-amyloid protein or Aβ. Aβ is derived from a set of larger (~120-kDa) integral transmembrane glycoproteins, collectivelly known as β-amyloid precursor protein (APP) through cleavage by proteases referred to as secretases.

APP is encoded by a single gene on the long arm of chromosome 21, which has 18 exons. APP consists of a single transmembrane-spanning domain, a large extracellular N-terminus and a short intracellular C-terminus. Figure 5 shows a schematic structure of the APP in the cell membrane. The region Aβ of APP corresponds to amino acids 11-15 of the transmembrane domain and 28 amino acids of the extracellular domain. At least 10 isoforms of APP are derived from various mRNAs by the alternative splicing of the APP gene. Three major isoforms of APP are known to contain Aβ, APP770 (full-length APP), APP751 (minus exon 8), and APP695 (minus exons 7 and 8). Both APP751 and APP770 contain a sequence of 56 amino acids, encoded by exon 7, showing a close similarity to the family of Kunitz's protease inhibitors (KPI) and are often referred as KPI-containing APP (APP-KPI). Exon 8 encodes the MRC-OX2 domain (OX2). Figure 6 shows a scheme with the main isoforms of APP.

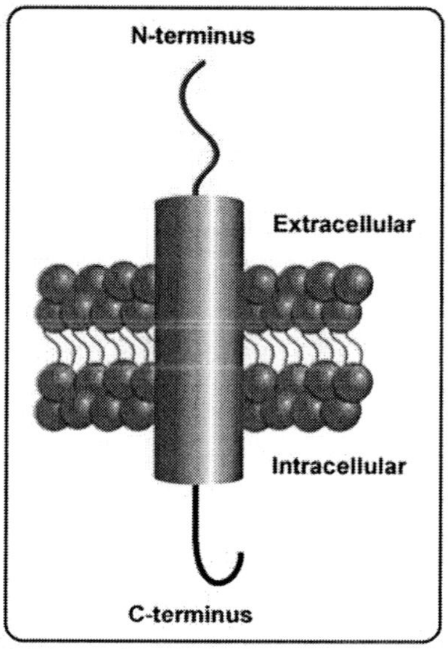

Figure 5. Amyloid precursor protein (APP) in the cell membrane. The scheme shows a transmembrane spanning protein with a single transmembrane-spanning domain, a large extracellular N-terminus and a short intracellular C-terminus.

APP Distribution

The APP is synthesized by most cell types and is abundantly expressed in many different tissues within the body (central and peripheral tissues) at all stages of life. The multiple transcripts of APP (mRNAs) are expressed differentially in terms of localization and relative abundance. Within the brain, APP isoforms are expressed in a cell type-specific manner, with APP695 being synthesized primarily, but not exclusively in neurons, and APP-KPI, predominantly in astroglial cells, suggesting that the β-amyloid can arise from non-neuronal cells. The APP695 protein and mRNA are expressed from the early stages of development, increase during synaptogenesis in the processes of neurite outgrowth and cell targeting, and in the maintenance of the functional integrity of synapses in the mature brain. During the period of maximal synaptogenetic activity, the distribution of APP is more homogeneous throughout the cell compartments to facilitate the formation of contacts between the neurons. However, during the period of synapse maturation and consolidation, APP appears to be gradually enriched in synaptosomal compartments, indicating important functional roles of APP in synaptic regions of the adult brain. In culture, APP695 has been shown to enhance the proliferation of neural stem cells. However, in all stages of development, the concentration of APP-KPI mRNAs is lower in the brain, as compared to peripheral tissues. In cortical neurons specifically, APP751 is the predominant isoform of APP-KPI.

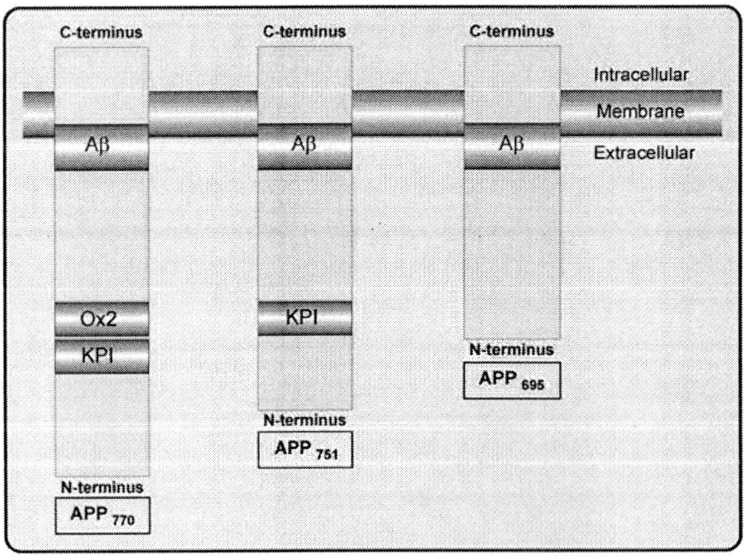

Figure 6. Schematic diagram of the three main APP isoforms, generated by alternative splicing. The β-amyloid (Aβ) domain is shown to share an extracellular fragment and a fragment within the membrane. See details on the text. *KPI* - Kunitz-type protease inhibitor; *OX2* - MRC-OX2 domain.

APP, Aβ and AD

The APP gene has been the subject of numerous studies on neurodegenerative processes specially AD, and the findings are conflicting, with increases, decreases, and no change. The expression of APP is not per se a pathological event. The hypothesis that β-amyloid deposition in AD was caused by simple overexpression of APP, as it is thought to be the case in Down's syndrome has proved to be wrong. A number of changes has been shown for one or more APP mRNAs, in one or more regions of the AD brain but the findings are inconsistent. The variation does not correlate with age, *post mortem* interval or β-amyloid deposition, but APP mRNAs are affected by premorten course (agonal state), which explain some of the variability observed among individuals.

Several studies have shown a decrease in both APP695 and APP-KPI mRNAs in the frontal cortex in AD. However, these APP isoforms do not change in the hippocampus in AD, and no relationship has been seen between the abundance of APP mRNAs in this area and the severity of the disease, suggesting that major changes in APP mRNA expression do not occur in the hippocampus in AD. It is important to identify whether the abundance of a specific APP mRNA predicts that of the encoded protein and, if so, whether any particular APP transcript is of special relevance as an amyloidogenic precursor.

β-amyloid deposits are found in several brain areas, such as the amygdala, hippocampus and neocortex in AD, and have been associated with synaptic contacts on dendrites in diffuse plaques and with dystrophic neurites, astrocytic processes and microglia in more mature plaques. Degeneration of synapses is believed to occur early in the disease process and to correlate strongly with cognitive deficits. Altered APP processing can impair synaptic functions, such as the long-term potentiation of the hippocampal synaptic transmission, a cellular mechanism that is considered as a basic mechanism for learning and memory. Aβ impairs synaptic function in vivo, as indicated by the memory impairment in rats following injection of Aβ into the hippocampus.

Plaques of Aβ have been associated with APP-KPI isoforms, APP-KPI protein and mRNA being preferentially up-regulated in AD with the APP751 isoform demonstrating greater amyloidogenesis. The APP751/695 ratio is specifically increased in AD, suggesting that alterations in the balance between KPI- and non-KPI-containing APP splice variants may lead to accumulation of Aβ. An autoregulatory process may explain this differential splicing in response to cellular stress. For example, higher expression of APP751 has been reported to suppress expression of both APP770 and APP695, and the production of Aβ1-42 is higher in cells expressing APP751, as compared to cells expressing APP695. Based on these evidence, it is possible to conclude that the increased ratio of APP751/695 in AD is not merely due to a decrease in neurons expressing APP695, but rather to a specific increase in the potentially amyloidogenic splice variant. This is particularly very interesting when considering the processing of APP (Box 1), as it has been reported that cells expressing APP751 make proportionally less sAPPα and P3, and more sAPPβ and Aβ1-42, indicating that the expression of the KPI domain reduces cleavage by α secretase. Thus, the level of expression of the APP-KPI in the brain is probably an important factor influencing the development of AD in a way that changes the specific species of Aβ which are secreted.

Evidence supporting this is the demonstration that in the AD brain, APP-KPI (specifically APP751) accumulates in areas vulnerable to degeneration, such as the cortex and hippocampus. Considering that APP751 is particularly amyloidogenic, its accumulation may be an important pathogenic event in AD.

The alterations in APP processing seen in AD contribute with an additive mechanism to the development of the disease. The protein sAPP is known to have neuroprotective effects by several mechanisms including its ability to stabilize cellular Ca2+ homeostasis (neurotoxicity to ions Ca2+ will be further discussed). Besides, it is able to protect neurons against excitotoxic injury and Aβ toxicity, and also to regulate learning and memory processes in the hippocampus. Thus, the decreased levels of sAPP that occur in AD, contribute to the altered Ca2+ homeostasis and neuronal degeneration, as a consequence of the reduction on neuroprotection.

Aβ And Glial Cells in AD

Neurons are not the only cell type in the brain that is affected in AD. Although the research has been widely focused on the role of neurons with regard to Aβ deposition, vulnerable brain regions also exhibit activated microglial cells and astrocytes often associated with amyloid deposits. The presence of reactive astrocytes surrounding senile plaques, and the association of a number of astrocyte-derived proteins such as S100-β, α 1 anti-chymotrypsin and apolipoprotein E in and surrounding the plaque core, indicate that glial cells respond to Aβ and may play a role in the pathogenesis of AD. Indeed, a wealth of evidence indicates that glial cells may trigger similar mechanisms to neurons in response to stress conditions. For example, in a culture of human astrocytes, an increase in the APP-KPI mRNA expression was induced by a heat shock (a model of cellular stress) and was specific for the APP751 splice variant, with a decrease in APP770 and no change in APP695 mRNA. In addition, the heat shock induced changes in the APP processing with an increase in the β-secretase processing. These findings demonstrate that the response of astrocytes to cellular stress may occur by a shift in the expression and processing of APP towards a potentially amyloidogenic route. Thus, the astrocytes may be involved in pathological processes like AD, leading to an increase in APP-KPI expression and, consequently, to deposition of Aβ. However, additional mechanisms and different types of glial cells appear to contribute to the development of AD.

Each type of glial cell express APP and presenilins, mainly PS1 and are therefore subject to adverse effects of altered APP processing and PS1 mutations in AD. (I would recommend a look at the subtopic about presenilin and apolipoprotein below, before continuing this reading). The resultant form of APP and the mutant forms of PS1 induce alterations in Ca^{2+} homeostasis that have specific effects in each type of glial cell. For example, Aβ increases intracellular Ca^{2+} levels in astrocytes that activate these cells, leading to the propagation of Ca^{2+} signals. Because the astrocytes transfer signals to neurons that modulate their activity and survival, the alteration in astrocytes Ca2+ homeostasis may contribute to neuronal death in AD.

In oligodendrocytes, mutant forms of PS1 are expressed in AD. These forms induce alterations in Ca^{2+} homeostasis that may contribute to white matter damage seen in this pathology. Experimental findings show that PS1 mutants induce learning and memory deficits, suggesting that white matter damage contributes to cognitive dysfunction in AD.

In microglia, Aβ increases Ca^{2+} influx activating these cells, and mutations of PS1 alter Ca^{2+} homeostasis that induces an increase in inflammatory cytokines.

Apolipoprotein E and Presenilin

Apolipoprotein E (ApoE), presenilin 1 (PS1) and presenilin 2 (PS2) have also been reported to contribute to AD.

Apolipoproteins are known for their well established role in taking cholesterol from the blood into the cells. ApoEs exist in different isoforms, which are related to increased or reduced risk for atherosclerotic cardiovascular disease and AD. ApoE mRNA is expressed in both neurons and astrocytes and is particularly elevated in astrocytes in AD, which shows a positive correlation with the gliosis that occurs in the disease. However, ApoE mRNA increases more than glial fibrillary acidic protein (GFAP) mRNA in AD, suggesting that the enhanced ApoE expression in this disease is not entirely due to gliosis. Several studies report that ApoEs have a neurotoxic fragment and that the mechanism involves an increase in Ca2+ influx. In contrast to this effect, ApoEs were shown to modulate Ca^{2+} homeostasis through the interaction with sAPP. This interaction enhances the ability of sAPP to reduce intracellular $Ca^{2}+$ levels. Other findings suggest that ApoEs can stabilize the concentration of $Ca^{2}+$ through their antioxidant effects, as ApoEs were shown to protect cultured cells from cell death induced by either hydrogen peroxide or Aβ. According to the mechanism of action, the different isoforms of ApoEs are more or less effective. A better understanding of how ApoEs modulate cellular Ca^{2+} homeostasis is important to understand how the neurodegenerative cascade in AD may be affected.

PS1 and PS2 are integral membrane proteins widely expressed in many different cells types. In the brain, neurons contain high levels of PS1 and PS2 but they are also seen in glial cells. PS1 contributes to the complex of proteins required for the activity of γ secretase during the processing of APP, and is of exceptional importance for this enzyme activity. PS1 and PS2 have shown to play a role in the pathogenesis of AD, where the mutations within these genes are the most common genetic cause identified in familial AD (FAD). PS1 mutations account for many more cases of FAD than the PS2 mutations do, and the pathogenic mechanism has showed that the mutations in the forms of PS1 induce alterations on the cellular Ca^{2+} homeostasis. Overexpression of those forms of PS1 has been identified in cultured neural cells from FAD brain tissue. In these cells they have increased the amount of Ca^{2+} released from endoplasmatic reticulum (ER) that resulted in increased levels of cytoplasmic Ca^{2+}. These neurons have showed more vulnerability to excitotoxicity and apoptosis. The mechanism about how the PS1 mutants alter the regulation of ER Ca^{2+} stores is not clear yet. It may involve an intracellular secondary mechanism.

Ab and Neurotransmitter Systems in AD

It is well known that a consistent feature of AD is the degeneration of cholinergic neurons which leads to a deficit in acetylcholine transmission and then causes subsequent impairment of learning, memory and cognitive functions. However, in addition to ACh, multiple neurotransmitter systems appear to be disturbed in the AD brain. It has been demonstrated for example, that Aβ induces degeneration of cholinergic neurons via glutamate NMDA receptors, subsequent $Ca2^{+}$ entry and activation of the neuronal nitric oxide synthase (nNOS), which shows that various neurotransmitter systems contribute to this mechanism of injury.

In addition, choline acetyltransferase, somatostatin and substance P have been reported to disappear in the areas of senile plaque, and accumulate in the dystrophic neurites, in and around amyloid cores in several brain areas such as the cortex, hippocampus, amygdala, olfactory bulb, forebrain, and basal ganglia, among others. Thus, Aβ amyloidosis may disrupt multiple neurotransmitter systems, through the focal disappearance of neurotransmitters and abnormal formation of distrophic neurites. These pathological changes are directly correlated with the progressive cognitive impairment in AD.

The appearance of dystrophic neurites containing neurotransmitters in the AD brain precedes that of those containing paired helical filaments (neurofibrillary tangles), suggesting that Aβ amyloidosis induces the formation of dystrophic neurites containing neurotransmitters, and then causes subsequent alterations, such as tautopathy. This is supported by the demonstration that the cholinergic deficit in the cortex coincides with Aβ deposition in the earliest stage of AD, where β-amyloid can impair the coupling of muscarinic acetylcholine receptors to the GTP-binding proteins. Accumulation of Aβ for longer periods may develop and spread these focal changes throughout the cortices and induce tautopathy, including neurofibrillary tangles. This cascade of events may underlie the pathological role of Aβ amyloidosis in AD, resulting in neuronal loss.

Additional Roles of APP

Until recently, it was believed that deposition of Aβ was involved in the physiological and pathological responses of the brain under various neurodegenerative conditions, but it has now been shown that Aβ is produced under normal circumstances in healthy cells in vitro, and is detected in the cerebrospinal fluid of healthy individuals. Additionally, APP-KPI mRNAs are increased in aged animals without developing Aβ deposits or senile plaques. The basic biochemical pathways to the APP processing show the general importance of the APP processing and of the amyloid proteins in the physiology of the cell. Thus, a variety of functions may be attributed to the original APP and Aβ in the neurons. It has been hypothesized for example, that APP can be a neurotrophic factor, a cell adhesion molecule, a modulator for neuronal responsiveness to glutamate, or can be involved in several neurotransmitter systems in the brain.

The large variety of physiological roles attributed to APP has led to the suggestion that different forms of APP participate in different functions. It is also important to mention that there is evidence supporting the involvement of APP in other functions in the brain, in addition to its involvement with AD.

If we consider for example, the mechanisms underlying the responses to different stressful stimuli in brain areas including the amygdala, hippocampus and the cortex, among others, a body of evidence supports the involvement of several neurotransmitters such as dopamine, serotonin, glutamate and nitric oxide (NO). Specifically related to NO, it is a non-conventional neurotransmitter formed by nNOS and proposed to participate in physiological and pathological processes in the brain. Restraint stress has been shown to activate putative neurons producing NO in the amygdala. We found an increase in nNOS mRNA expression in the medial amygdala after restraint stress in rats. Reported evidence shows the involvement of β-amyloid plaques with the NO system in the brain, i.e. nNOS is activated by Aβ, NO is released by astrocytes surrounding Aβ plaques, and NO contributes to neuronal alterations induced by Aβ. In addition, we have recently demonstrated that restraint stress has induced an increase in the APP695 splice variant mRNA expression, but not in the APP-KPI mRNA expression in the basolateral amygdala. Taking together, the findings lead to speculate that APP may be involved in the stressful responsiveness mechanisms in the amygdala, by regulating the NO neurotransmission. However, it is important to mention that the basolateral and lateral amygdala are affected by both AD and Down Syndrome with high reduction in volume, more than 50% of neuronal loss and severe amyloidosis, suggesting that different APP isoforms may have different roles, on the same brain area.

At the same time, an APP isoform may exert different functions as it has been demonstrated that APP695 is involved in either the neurotoxic or neuroprotective effect of glutamate by regulating NMDA or non-NMDA receptors. It has been shown that APP695 increases the intracellular Ca2+ concentration and the neuronal death induced by glutamate in cultured hippocampal cells, effects blocked by NMDA and non-NMDA antagonists. However, APP695 reduces the NMDA doses for promoting the survival of cerebellar neurons in culture.

The body of evidence contributes strongly to the idea that APP isoforms play different roles in an adult brain, contributing to the plasticity of the CNS.

GLUTAMATE

Classification and Properties of Glutamate Receptors

Glutamate (Glu) is the principal excitatory neurotransmitter in the central nervous system (CNS), and is involved in both physiological functions and pathological processes of the brain, by interacting with pharmacologically distinct receptors. Physiological functions include neuronal differentiation and synapse consolidation during the development, activity-dependent forms of synaptic plasticity, and long-term potentiation. In pathological processes, glutamate is involved in stress, ischemia, schizophrenia, epilepsy, and Parkinson's, Alzheimer's and Huntington's diseases, among others.

Two major groups of glutamate receptors have been described, the metabotropic (mGluR) and ionotropic (iGluR). The mGluR represents a subgroup of receptors linked to intracellular secondary signaling, coupled to G-protein, and is classified in eight subtypes (mGluR1-8), subdivided into three groups: group I (mGluR1 and 5), coupled to phospholipase C-polyphosphoinositide hydrolysis; group II (mGluR 2 and 3) and group III (mGluR 4, 6, 7 and 8), both negatively coupled to adenyl cyclase, or linked to ion channels. The iGluR represents channels of membrane with selective ionic permeability, particularly to ions calcium (Ca^{2+}) and is classified by its selective affinity for specific agonists in NMDA (N-methyl-D-aspartate), AMPA (α-amino-3-hydroxy-5-methylisoxazole-4-propionic acid) and KA (kainate). AMPA and KA are also classified as non-NMDA receptors and are often called together as AMPA/KA receptors. At least thirteen genes of iGluR have been cloned with each subtype presenting a specific profile of distribution and pharmacological properties.

There are seven subunits of NMDA receptors, NR1, NR2A-D and NR3A-B. NR1 is encoded by a single gene, which, via alternative splicing of the RNA, generates eight different receptor proteins. In contrast, each of the NR2 and NR3 subunits is encoded by a different gene. The NMDA receptors are blocked by Mg^{2+} ions at resting conditions, but it is removed by the membrane depolarization. The AMPA receptors exist in four different subunits, GluR1-4 or GluR A-D derived from a single gene. Each of those generates two different isoforms of proteins (flip and flop) with distinct properties, by alternative splicing. The KA receptors are found in five subunits, GluR5-7 (receptors of low affinity) and KA1-2 (receptors of high affinity), encoded by different genes.

The iGluRs are ligand-gated ion channels formed by complexes of subunits proteins. Different assemblies of subunits and isoforms confer distinct permeability and pharmacological and functional properties to these receptors. Figure 7 shows a schematic representation of the iGluR subtype.

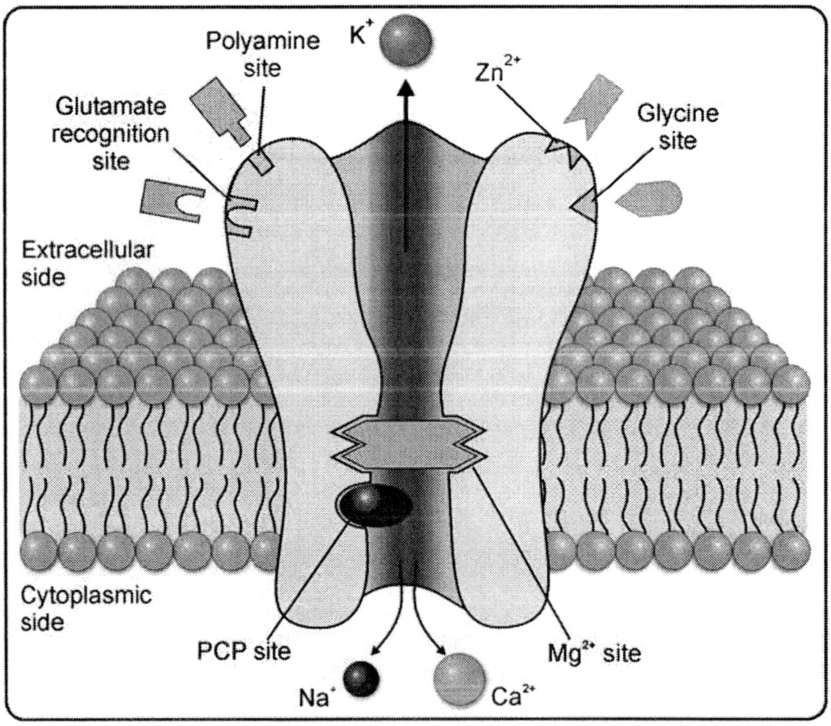

Figure 7. The scheme shows an ionotropic glutamate receptor (iGluR) in the cell membrane, represented specifically by the NMDA receptor. Note: 1) different subunits composition form the channel; 2) the presence of the agonists binding sites in different subunits; 3) the presence of a number of binding sites for modulators. See details in the text.

TOXICITY

The pionnering work of Olney, about 30 years ago, suggested a role for glutamate on the pathophysiology of brain diseases. Overactivation of glutamatergic neurotransmission may lead to excitatory neurotoxicity (excitotoxicity), a cellular event that has been largely linked to neurodegenerative conditions. The concentration of Glu in the synaptic cleft at resting conditions is around 0.6 μM, but exceeds 10 μM during the synaptic transmission. The termination of the excitatory action of Glu is mediated by a high-affinity uptake system on both pre- and post-synaptic neurons and adjacent glial cells. Because the uptake mechanisms remove Glu from the synaptic cleft, they mask its neurotoxic potential.

The toxicity of Glu is principally mediated by Ca^{2+} influx. An overactivation of Glu receptors induces an immediate intracellular Ca^{2+} overload that initiates a secondary cascade of events leading, at the end, to neuronal death. Alterations in the cellular Ca^{2+} homeostasis occur in various neurodegenerative disorders including Alzheimer's, Parkinson's and Huntington's diseases, ischemic stroke, and amyotrophic lateral sclerosis. The factor(s) that initiate the neurodegenerative cascade may differ among these disorders. However, some cellular and molecular mechanisms are relevant to all of them. For example, oxidative stress and metabolic impairment contribute to the alteration in neuronal Ca^{2+} homeostasis, which likely leads to synaptic dysfunction and excitotoxic and/or apoptotic death of vulnerable neuronal populations.

TOXICITY AND NMDA RECEPTORS

Among all groups of GluR, the NMDA is the most studied regarding its involvement on the excitotoxicity induced by glutamate. NMDA receptors are localized on the post-synaptic membrane of excitatory synapses and exhibit a higher permeability to Ca^{2+} than AMPA or KA receptors do. They also possess a higher capacity to induce excessive Ca^{2+} influx and trigger the degenerative cascade. In cultured neurons, cell death can be prevented by blocking NMDA receptors or by removing Ca^{2+} from the growth medium. Thus, NMDA receptors could be a target for the inhibition of the neuronal excitotoxicity that occurs in several neurodegenerative disorders and, consequently, an alternative pharmacotherapeutic approach to the treatment of AD.

In agreement with this, several characteristics of NMDA receptors make them a good target for using drugs with the aim of modulating neurodegenerative processes. NMDA receptors are assembled as tetrameric or pentameric complexes containing NR1, NR2, and NR3 subunits. The NR1 subunit contains the glycine-binding site, and the NR2 subunits contain the glutamate-binding site. Functional receptors contain at least two NR1 subunits and two NR2 (A-D) subunits, implying a minimum of 4 subunits. The type of NR2 subunit determines the agonist affinity, channel conductance, and sensitivity to the Mg^{2+} block, among others. The NR3 subunits can assemble with NR1-NR2 complexes to depress the responses to NMDA receptors. The activation of NMDA receptors requires the co-incident binding of both neurotransmitters Glu and glycine, and there is evidence for at least six other distinct functional subcomponents of the NMDA receptors, each with discrete ligand binding domains. This multiplicity of ligand binding sites indicates that NMDA receptors can be a suitable target for distinct and complex pharmacological modulations. However, the physiologic activation of the NMDA receptors is necessary for a number of normal functions, including cognition and memory. Thus, the activity of these receptors should be finely modulated.

TOXICITY AND AMPA/KA RECEPTORS

A characteristic of many neurological diseases is a selective pattern of neurodegeneration. For example, while hippocampal pyramidal neurons degenerate preferentially in ischemia and epilepsy, these neurons and basal forebrain cholinergic neurons are preferentially injured in AD, and spinal motoneurons are the target for degeneration in amyotrophic lateral sclerosis (ALS). Although there is some knowledge about the pathogenic mechanisms of these diseases, there is little understanding of the basis for the selective neuronal loss. Thus, in addition to crucial factors for cell loss in particular conditions, such as loss of blood flow in ischemia or genetic mutations associated with AD and ALS, the selectivity of neuronal loss that occurs, probably reflects factors that are particular to the cell or its immediate environment.

As mentioned before, most studies of the potential neurotoxicity mediated by glutamate have focused on the highly Ca^{2+}-permeable and widely distributed NMDA receptors. However, the widespread distribution of these receptors is incoherent with the induction of very selective patterns of cell loss. The opposite characteristics presented by AMPA/KA receptors, such as restricted distribution and selective Ca^{2+} permeability make them possible candidates for that, contributing to selective injury in neurodegenerative disorders.

Similarly to NMDA, AMPA/KA receptors are heteromeric complexes of GluR1-4 subunits for AMPA or GluR5-7, KA1 and KA2 subunits for KA. The subunits are differently permeable to Ca^{2+}, with GluR2 subunit being completely impermeable to the ion. Thus, different assemblies of subunits confer distinct Ca^{2+} permeability to these receptors, particularly by the presence of GluR2 subunit, which determines reduction in such permeability.

As AMPA/KA channels may be impermeable to Ca^{2+}, the mechanisms underlying their neurotoxicity are unclear. However, it has been demonstrated that subpopulations of neurons in the CNS possess AMPA or KA receptors that are directly permeable to Ca^{2+} ions. For example, it has been found that spinal motoneurons and basal forebrain cholinergic neurons have Ca^{2+}-permeable AMPA/KA receptors that result from low levels of GluR2, and that these neurons display preferential vulnerability to injury.

Toxicity caused by activation of Ca^{2+}-permeable AMPA/KA receptors appear to occur through various mechanisms, such as triggering the degenerative cascade that results from oxidative stress, similarly to the mechanism triggered by overactivation of NMDA receptors. However, other features of Ca^{2+}-permeable AMPA/KA receptors make them particularly suited for triggering injury in diseases. A selective reduction in the synthesis of GluR2 might occur after transient global ischemia or epilepsy that results in increased number of Ca^{2+}-permeable AMPA/KA receptors. The consequent increase in Ca^{2+} influx through these channels results in a loss of Ca^{2+} homeostasis, and contributes to the delayed neurodegeneration seen in these conditions. Specifically related to AD and consistent with this hypothesis, a decrease in the GluR2 levels has been reported in pyramidal neurons in this pathology, and in aging.

It is important to mention that not all neurons that possess Ca^{2+}-permeable AMPA/KA receptors are equally prone to degenerate into disease. It means that the vulnerability of neurons that possess these receptors is probably modulated by additional factors. In fact, it has been seen that many neurons have a remarkable ability to adapt to an increased number of Ca^{2+}-permeable channels that they possess, as it has been seen that they are resistant to injury resultant from a high Ca^{2+} influx through these channels.

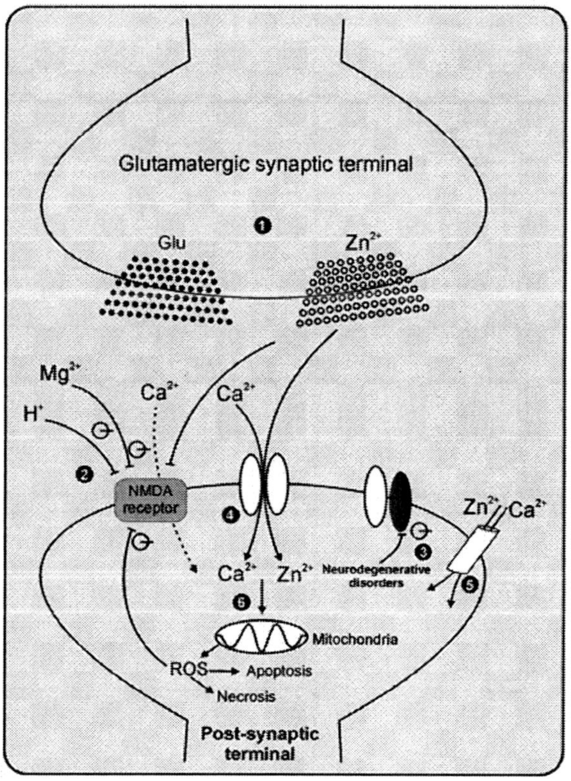

Figure 8. Schematic representation of injury mechanisms induced by glutamate (Glu) and zinc (Zn^{2+}) through Ca^{2+}-permeable AMPA or kainate receptors (Ca^{2+}-permeable AMPA/KA). These mechanisms are predicted to mediate selective neurodegeneration. 1) co-releasing of Glu and Zn^{2+} at glutamatergic synapse; 2) NMDA channels are inhibited by Mg^{2+}, ROS, Zn^{2+} (inhibition of Ca^{2+} influx, broken line); 3) specific neurodegenerative disorder (i.e. Alzheimer's disease or ischemia or epilepsy) induces selective downregulation of GluR2 subunit (in black) resulting in increased numbers of Ca^{2+}-permeable AMPA/KA; 4) the Ca^{2+}-permeable AMPA/KA receptor channels are highly permeable to Zn^{2+} as well as to Ca^{2+}; 5) voltage-sensitive Ca^{2+} channels (VSCC) are permeable to Zn^{2+} but contribute with less influx because they are mostly extrasynaptic; 6) Ca^{2+} and Zn^{2+} influx result in mitochondrial dysfunction and ROS generation which leads to either necrosis or apoptosis. Modified from Weiss and Sensi, 2000.

Contributing to the hypothesis of the involvement of AMPA/KA receptors on the mechanisms underlying selective neurodegeneration, several studies have demonstrated that the divalent cation Zn^{2+} permeates Ca^{2+}-permeable AMPA/KA receptors channels with particular ease, and induces neuronal injury. In ischemia or epilepsy, ions Zn^{2+} stored in synaptic vesicles of excitatory neurons are rapidly released at high concentrations, translocate across the synapse, and accumulate in postsynaptic neurons. Neurons that accumulate Zn^{2+} are strongly correlated to those that degenerate. The mechanisms through which Zn^{2+} entry into neurons through Ca^{2+}-permeable AMPA/KA receptors triggers injury appear also to involve oxidative stress, as this effect has shown to be attenuated by antioxidants. This is compatible with the oxidative tissue damage and mitochondrial dysfunction seen in ischemia, AD and SLA. Indeed, mitochondrial disruption that results from the divalent cation influx through Ca^{2+}-permeable AMPA/KA receptors channels, could feed into either acute necrotic cell death pathways or apoptotic cell death pathways that are more applicable to neurodegenerative conditions. Figure 8 shows a schematic synapse with the Ca2+-permeable AMPA/KA receptors triggering a mechanism of injury.

Metabotropic Receptors and AD

In the previous paragraphs regarding the glutamatergic neurotransmission mediated by ionotropic receptors, the neurotoxic effects of glutamate induced by overactivation of those receptors was mainly discussed. However, an opposite effect has been reported for glutamatergic neurotransmission mediated by metabotropic receptors. Through these, glutamate acts as a neuroprotetor instead of a neurotoxic agent, associated with an altered APP processing.

In the processing of APP, the interaction of glutamate with metabotropic receptors leads to activation of a signalling cascade involving activation of protein kinase C (PKC) which promotes the release of sAPPα. This mechanism shows that the activation of metabotropic receptors triggers the anti-amyloidogenic pathway of the APP processing. This signalling system involving activation of PKC coupled to sAPPα release has been seen in hippocampal and cortical brain slices.

As mentioned before, it is well known that astrocytes express APP, secrete Aβ and are associated with neuritic plaques formation. These cells express a number of receptors coupled to ion channels and second messengers. It has been specifically demonstrated that metabotropic receptors agonists increase the secretion of sAPPα following the activation of the PKC-signalling cascade in these cells.

The findings suggest the involvement of metabotropic receptors on the complex mechanisms triggered by glutamate in AD, possibly mediating a modulation.

Oxidative Stress and Neurotransmitter Systems in AD

Before looking at the following topics regarding the involvement of oxidative stress on the mechanism triggered by ACh and Glu in AD, it is recommended to look at Box 2 where the oxidative stress mechanism is briefly described.

Acetylcholine

Since the AChRs are protein receptors that locate in cellular membrane, the modification of the membrane lipid structure surrounding the receptors, or the oxidation of the protein receptors themselves by the attack of free radicals, could be involved on mechanisms leading to ACh deficit in AD. Indeed, considerable evidence shows that oxidative stress underlies a reduction of the ACh neurotransmission mediated by both nAChR and mAChR in AD, through a distinct mechanism. It has been demonstrated for example, a significant increase in the lipid peroxidation correlated with a decrease of a specific nAChR protein subunit in the temporal cortex of AD patients. Because no difference has been seen in the protein peroxidation, the mechanism concerning the deficit of nAChR in AD may involve a disturbance of the cellular membrane integrity, resulting from the lipid peroxidation. It has also been demonstrated that mAChR is inactivated by a low molecular weight (LMW) endogenous inhibitor which blocks the binding of either the agonist or antagonist to the receptor, and is significantly increased in the frontal cortex of patients with AD. The LMW endogenous inhibitor requires free radicals for its action. Natural antioxidants such as myricetin and quercetin, antioxidants such as vitamin E and flavonoid constituents of Ginkgo biloba, and pyrophosphate analogs have been found to protect the mAChR from the inactivation by the endogenous inhibitor. These compounds will likely prove to be protective in other systems that are susceptible to oxidative stress. Thus, antioxidants and pyrophosphate analogs may have therapeutic potential for the treatment and prevention of any disorders involving oxidative stress such as AD.

Increasing evidence support the involvement of a combination of events including the cholinergic system, oxidative stress, and APP processing in the pathology of AD. For example, Aβ generates free radicals contributing to the lipid peroxidation that, in turn, induces a decrease of nAChRs. Free radicals also contribute to the inactivation of mAChRs by the LMW endogenous inhibitor. Because the normal processing of APP, as well as the reduction of the tau protein phosphorilation is promoted by the mAChR stimulation, its inactivation induces an increase in both the Aβ deposition and the neurofibrillary tangles formation. Thus, the combination of therapies including antioxidants, AChRs agonists and AChEIs may be more effective in slowing the progression of AD.

Glutamate

The degeneration induced by Glu may primarily involve the activation of catabolic enzymes that degrade neuronal structural proteins and cause cytoskeletal breakdown. High intracellular Ca^{2+} concentrations may activate the Ca^{2+}-dependent protein kinases that lead to hyper-phosphorylation of cytoskeletal proteins, including tau and ubiquitin, constituents of neurofibrillary tangles. These mechanisms have been confirmed in AD, considering that increased levels of Ca^{2+} have been associated with increased levels of the Ca^{2+}/calmodulin-dependent protein kinase in neurons containing neurofibrillary tangles.

Glutamatergic function has also been related to oxidative stress associated with Aβ peptide in AD. The increased levels of intracellular Ca^{2+} induced by overstimulation of Glu receptors cause alterations in the APP processing with increased production of Aβ. The aggregation of Aβ results in neuronal degeneration and death by promoting apoptosis and excitotoxicity. During the process of self-aggregation, Aβ generates hydrogen peroxide and hydroxyl radical, a reactive oxygen species (ROS) that induces membrane lipid peroxidation which can disrupt the Ca^{2+} homeostasis. The peptide Aβ may also affect the Ca^{2+} homeostasis by potentiating the activation of voltage-dependent Ca^{2+}channels. Thus, Aβ causes an increase in intracellular Ca^{2+} levels and enhance the Ca^{2+} influx, as a consequence of the Glu receptors activation.

In the AD brain, lipid peroxidation is prominent in neurons associated with Aβ deposits. The involvement of these multiple mechanisms working together on the neuronal degeneration is supported by the ability of the antioxidants vitamin E and glutathione to treat oxidative stress induced by hyperactivity of glutamate receptors and to protect neurons from the Aβ toxicity, respectively.

Alzheimer's Disease Therapy

A decade ago, there was no effective therapeutic agent for amelioration of the symptoms of AD. As modest as the benefits of the current treatment are, they nevertheless represent a major step in the pharmacotherapy of AD.

The target mechanism is to block the destruction of the neurotransmitter ACh by AChE. Drugs acting as cholinesterase inhibitors (ChEIs) lead to an increase in the levels of ACh in the synaptic cleft, stabilizing the neurotransmission. ChEIs are the standard therapy for the treatment of patients with AD and are a class of drugs approved by the Food and Drug Administration (FDA) for the treatment of this condition. The presence of amyloid deposits and neurofibrillary tangles is associated with loss of cholinergic neurons in the AD brain, and there is emerging evidence that much of the neurotoxicity of AD may be reversed by ChEIs. The major therapeutic effect of these drugs in AD patients is the maintenance of a higher level of the cognitive function that implies not only a slowing of the disability, but also a delay in the disease progression.

Cholinesterases

There are two different cholinesterases in the body, AChE and butyrylcholinesterase (BuChE). They differ genetically, structurally, and kinetically. In the normal brain, the AChE activity is 99% of all cholinesterase activity of the brain, while the BuChE activity is only 1%. However, in the brains of patients with AD, the AChE activity decreases progressively with dementia while the BuChE activity increases. The corresponding ratio in advanced AD is 65% and 35% suggesting that BuChE may replace AChE in hydrolysing ACh at this stage of the disease. This hypothesis is supported by the presence of BuChE in neuritic plaques and neurofibrillary tangles in AD. Clinical evidence suggests that both cholinesterases may contribute to the progression of AD, as patients show cognitive benefit when AChE and BuChE are inhibited.

Cholinesterase Inhibitors

Four ChEIs have been approved by the FDA, tacrine, donepezil, rivastigmine, and galantamine. The FDA approvation requires significant drug-placebo difference for measures of cognition and global changes. The drug-placebo difference observed in clinical trials is the difference between the deterioration of the placebo group and the improvement, stabilization or reduced deterioration of the group receiving the active agent. Tacrine was the first agent approved specifically for the AD therapy, but after being associated with hepatotoxicity, it has rarely been used. Donepezil (Aricept), rivastigmine (Exelon), and galantamine (Reminyl) have comparable efficacy without inducing hepatic injury and are in widespread clinical use. Each of those is considered a first-line drug. They represent different classes of ChEIs with different pharmacological properties and half-lives. Donepezil has a longer half-life and is metabolized via hepatic cytochrome P450 enzymes. Rivastigmine and galantamine have shorter half-lives, galantamine being metabolized as donepezil while rivastigmine is metabolized by esterases and its product excreted in the urine.

The ChEIs present inhibition selectivity for AChE or BuChE. Donepezil and galantamine are selective AChE inhibitors, whereas rivastigmine inhibits both enzymes. It has been described that galantamine is a relatively weak AChE inhibitor. However, it is also an allosteric-potentiating ligand for the nAChRs that leads to an increased presynaptic release of ACh and therefore enhances cholinergic neurotransmission. Positive allosteric modulators bind to a site on the nAChR, different from the binding site of its natural agonist, ACh, and amplify the actions of ACh at postsynaptic and presynaptic nAChRs. The positive allosteric effect of galantamine on nAChR compensates for its weak AChE inhibition. Galantamine can be described as belonging to two classes of drugs, ChEI and nicotinic-receptor agonist. Although galantamine itself cannot elicit ionic currents across nAChR sites, it potentiates the receptor's responsiveness to ACh.

In this context, it has been mentioned before that the number of AChRs is reduced in the AD brain and that these receptors are important for learning and memory functions. Considering that galantamine is a selective nAChRs agonist, the enhancement of nicotinic neurotransmission may be a promising approach to the treatment of AD. Its action on nAChRs may be the source of therapeutic efficacy rather than the cholinergic enhancement resulting from cholinesterase inhibition.

The benefits provided by ChEIs therapy are modest and are associated with quality-of-life improvement for patients and their caregivers. ChEIs enhance the ability to perform activities of daily living (ADL), reduce behavioral disturbances, and stabilize cognitive impairment, decrease caregiver's stress, and delay the first entry into a nursing home. ChEIs allow patients with AD to live longer in the community, with associated personal, social, and economic benefits. More than symptomatic relief and delay of disease progression, these improvements offer hope to AD patients, their physicians, and their caregivers. Although the 3 ChEIs in common use differ in their pharmacodynamic properties, mechanisms of action, and adverse-effect profiles, none of them is more efficacious or effective than the others.

Treatment with ChEIs is indicated for symptoms of mild to moderate AD. However, galantamine and donepezil show sustained efficacy in patients with moderate to severe AD.

Despite the fact that many clinical studies have been performed in a short-term range, a real long-term study analyzing the long-term efficiency of these drugs anti-dementia is still missing. The efficiency of conservative treatment strategies of AD by using AChEIs has been recently questioned. It is not clear whether these compounds indeed increase the life span of patients with AD. Although new clinical studies and other research strategies are in the developmental stage, an effective long-term treatment of AD is still distant.

NMDA Receptor Antagonist

Because the degeneration of pathways mediated by glutamate occurs early in the disease, before the deficit of ACh neurotransmission, a novel strategy for pharmacotherapeutic intervention in AD could be the inhibition of this early event. Thus, a non-competitive NMDA antagonist with low-affinity for the receptor has been developed, memantine, a drug that is constantly present in the synaptic cleft and penetrates slowly into the NMDA receptors, leaving only a small proportion of the receptors available to participate in synaptic transmission. It is a very interesting drug because it blocks the excitotoxicity mediated by the overstimulation of NMDA without blocking the physiological activation of the receptor. Specifically, it appears that it does not interfere with the acquisition or processing of cognitive information. Thus, memantine is an ideal drug to block NMDA because it only affects pathophysiological conditions.

The clinical use of memantine for the treatment of AD was approved in 2002/2003. However, it is effective in moderate and severe cases of AD but not in the early process of the disease, when it is still really possible to slow the progression of the disease. The treatment with memantine has shown that the drug is able to improve symptoms and reduce deterioration in patients with moderate to severe AD. It is good for example, to delay cognitive and functional decline without significant adverse effects. In addition, memantine is a well tolerated drug.

Low-affinity antagonists like memantine are promising in the treatment of AD as it has been predicted that by delaying the mean onset of AD for 5 years, it would be possible to reduce approximately 50% of the number of individuals with AD.

Combination of AChEI and NMDA Receptor Antagonist

Consistent evidence suggests the concomitant involvement of distinct mechanisms in AD, such as cholinergic and glutamatergic ones. For example, damage of cholinergic neurons can lead to nuclear fragmentation and apoptotic cellular death; overstimulation of glutamate receptors induces an excessive Ca^{2+} influx that leads to neuronal death; memantine can protect cholinergic neurons against the excitotoxic destruction induced by glutamate; and the ChEIs donepezil and galantamine have shown to be efficacious concerning the excitotoxicity induced by glutamate. Thus, it has recently been tested the combination of memantine with donepezil in AD patients, and this therapy has shown greater efficacy than the efficacy of donepezil alone. Although memantine is not approved for the treatment of mild AD, patients with moderate impairment may benefit from the addition of memantine to ChEIs. Considering the involvement of multiple complex mechanisms in the pathophysiology of AD, the combination of therapies can be an effective approach to the treatment of this disease.

Future Perspectives for the Treatment of AD

Apart from the current pharmacological interventions in the treatment of AD, basically AChEIs and NMDA receptor antagonist, a number of investigations continue to be done with the aim to improve those therapies. Among them, researchers have been trying to improve their understanding about the basic mechanisms involved on the pathophysiology of the disease. As many details become clear, as many targets for interventions are possible. On the following topics, some findings from these investigations will be discussed.

Modulation of NMDA Receptors by Polyamines in AD

Polyamines (spermine) are organic molecules present in the brain, involved on the modulation of various cellular functions such as cellular growth and differentiation, programmed cell death, inhibition of membrane permeability, and regulation of gene expression, among others. They also affect ion channels, particularly the NMDA receptor. Distinct binding sites of polyamines have been identified in the NMDA receptor and their effects are dependent on the subunit composition of the NMDA receptor (see Figure 7). The polyamine binding causes an increase in the NMDA receptor activity, in part by enhancing the potentiation mediated by glycine of the NMDA receptor activation to glutamate.

The synthesis of polyamines is activated in the brain of patients with AD. The levels of spermidine, the precursor of spermine, are increased in the temporal cortex of these patients, suggesting that stimulation of NMDA receptors would be also increased in this region. Thus, variations in the NMDA receptor composition may underlie the local vulnerability of neurons to excitotoxicity, by contributing to the interaction of high concentrations of polyamines that result in augmented Ca^{2+} influx. It is not clear whether the observed differences occur in response to the disease or are pre-existent, and thus underlie the pathogenic cascade.

Again, increasing evidence shows how complex is the mechanism underlying the neurodegeneration in AD. For example, the interaction of the NMDA receptor and Aβ may be neurotoxic, as Aβ1-42 can increase extracellular spermine levels, which would thereby activate NMDA receptors. The degeneration caused by Aβ has been partially related to the excessive activation of NMDA receptors. These findings support previous observations of co-localization of glutamatergic neurons with pathological alterations (plaques of Aβ and neurofibrillary tangles) in the post-morten AD brain tissue.

Thus, it is possible that a drug acting as inhibitor of the polyamine binding site may be an alternative approach for improving the treatment of AD. This kind of drug would interfere with the NMDA receptor activation directly by itself, and indirectly by blocking the Aβ action.

Ca^{2+} Homeostasis

As discussed previously, excitotoxicity induced by intracellular Ca^{2+} overload is involved in many neurodegenerative processes like AD, what suggests a potential benefit of drugs that suppress Ca^{2+} influx. However, these drugs may also compromise the normal functions of neurons that rely on Ca^{2+} influx. It is particularly important in chronic neurodegenerative disorder such as AD which typically has a course of many years and, therefore, requires continuous treatment with the drug.

Another approach to treat AD by stabilizing Ca^{2+} homeostasis is to introduce a diet with reduced caloric intake, as it has recently suggested that dietary restriction can stabilize neuronal Ca^{2+} homeostasis and protect neurons against excitotoxicity and apoptosis. In addition, dietary restriction has been shown to enhance learning and memory during aging, and can protect synapses against insults relevant to AD.

Finally, dietary restriction can enhance the hippocampal neurogenesis that has been impaired by alterations in the Ca^{2+} homeostasis in AD, suggesting that the stimulation of neurogenesis may be another strategy for preventing and treating AD.

Ca^{2+}- Zn^{2+} Permeable AMPA/KA Receptors

As previously discussed, these specific iGluRs appear to be involved on the mechanisms underlying the selective neurodegeneration that occurs in neurodegenerative processes (see Figure 8). Based on that, a Ca2+- Zn2+ permeable AMPA/KA receptor central model could have implications for AD disease therapy, as well as for other neurodegenerative diseases, by suggesting new targets for intervention. These might include for example the channels themselves, determinants of their synthesis, Zn^{2+}, and ROS.

Aβ, Oxidative Stress and Inflammation

Among all potential roles postulated for Aβ in the pathogenesis of AD, it is believed that it induces oxidative stress and inflammation in the brain. For example, Aβ induces the production of hydrogen peroxide and lipid peroxide in neurons, and superoxide and proinflammatory cytokines in astrocytes and microglial cells.

It has been demonsrated that intracerebroventricular injections of Aβ1-42 in rats and mice induce an increase in interleukin-1 (IL-1) in the hippocampus, what is known to inhibit long-term potentiation in this area, leading to learning and memory impairment. These abnormalities are accompanied by both a decrease in cortical acetylcholine levels and an increase in the glial fibrillary acidic protein (GFAP) in the hippocampus.

Antioxidant agents have been used to protect against cytotoxicity in vivo, as well as learning and memory deficits induced by Aβ. In addition, antioxidants such as α-tocopherol and anti-inflammatory drugs such as indometacin are able to slow the progression of AD. Thus, drugs having both antioxidant and anti-inflammatory activities should be ideal for protection against the oxidative stress and inflammation induced by Aβ.

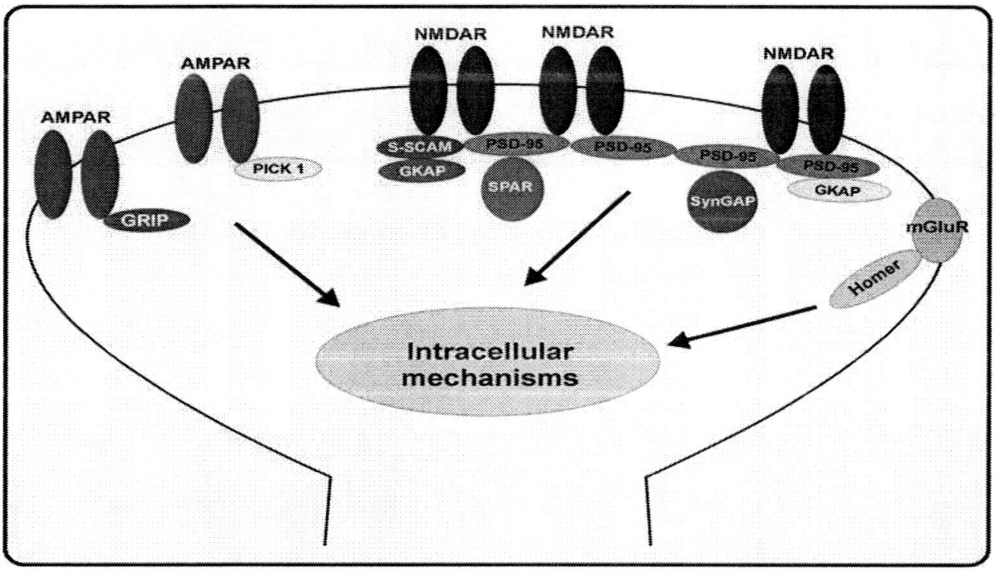

Figure 9. NMDA receptor-PSD95 complex and AMPA receptor binding proteins. PSD- postsynaptic density, represents proteins located beneath postsynaptic membranes; Homer- products of three genes (Homer 1-3); GKAP- consisted of four members (GKAP1-4), C-terminal of GKAP binds to the PDZ domain that binds to the GK domain of PSD-95; S-SCAM- contains 5 or 6 PDZ domains and 1 GK domain- binds to GKAP and PSD-95; Syn GAP- a Ras GTPase-activating protein (GAP)- binds to the PDZ domain of PSD-95; SPAR- a Rap GTPase-activating protein (GAP)- binds to the GK domain of PSD-95; GRIP/PICK1- PDZ-containing proteins- binds mainly in GluR2 and GluR3. Modified from Tashiro and Yuste, 2003.

NMDA Receptors and Membrane-Associated Proteins

Another functional characteristic of the NMDA receptors is that they interact with numerous membrane-associated proteins which contain multiple protein-protein interacting domains and are highly expressed in neurons. These interactions appear to affect the functional properties of the receptors, by triggering distinct secondary intracellular mechanisms. Figure 9 shows a simple scheme with the predicted diversity of interactions between GluRs and membrane-associated proteins. It has been demonstrated for example that a membrane-associated protein links a specific intracellular protein to the NMDA receptor and that this interaction may underlie the excitotoxicity seen in Huntington's disease. Thus, studies of the diversity of possible interactions may be useful, as they provide the information required for the design and synthesis of novel drugs modulating specific NMDA functions, by interfering with specific interactions.

Concluding Remarks

Based on what was presented in this chapter, only few drugs have been currently used to treat Alzheimer's disease and they are usually directed to two main targets: AChE and NMDA receptors. However, a number of other possibilities aimed at different mechanisms as new therapeutic targets have also been searched for with the objective of finding ways to improve the quality of life of AD patients.

Box 1

Processing of Amyloid Precursor Protein (APP)

APP is normally processed through consecutive cleavage events that constitute two different pathways, the amyloidogenic pathway (with plaque formation) and the anti-amyloidogenic pathway (with no plaque formation). On the amyloidogenic pathway, APP is firstly cleaved by β secretase to produce a large N-terminal secreted fragment (sAPPβ) and a C-terminal 99 amino acid (C99) fragment of APP beginning at Aβ1. Subsequent cleavage of C99 within its transmembrane domain by γ secretase generates and releases Aβ protein (Aβ40 or Aβ42) that forms senile plaques, as well as generates APP intracellular domain. The longer Aβ42 has a greater propensity to self-aggregate and is more toxic to neurons than the shorter Aβ40. On the anti-amyloidogenic pathway, APP is firstly cleaved by α secretase within the Aβ protein domain to produce a slightly longer N-terminal secreted fragment (sAPPα) and a C-terminal 83 amino acid (C83) fragment of APP beginning at Aβ17. C83 is also subsequently cleaved by γ secretase, releasing an approximately 3-kDa fragment of Aβ (P3) and APP intracellular domain. Because this pathway inhibits Aβ generation, there is no plaque formation. Figure 8A shows a scheme of the APP processing with the cleavage sites for the secretases within APP sequence.

The pathways, amyloidogenic or anti-amyloidogenic, involved on the processing of APP may be useful as potential targets for the treatment of AD. The development of drugs that increase the activity of α secretase, or that inhibit the activity of both β and γ secretases may improve the pharmacotherapeutic approaches to the treatment of this dementia.

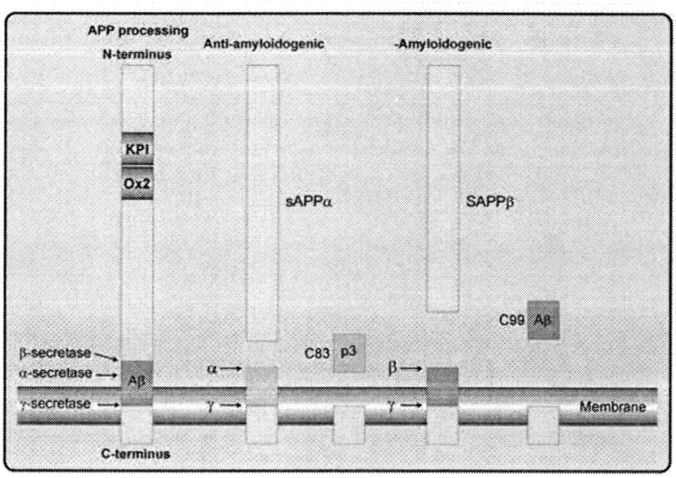

Figure 8A. Schematic representation of the amyloid precursor protein (APP) processing. The processing is divided into an amyloidogenic pathway and an anti-amyloidogenic pathway. In each pathway the APP is cleaved by specific proteases (secretases) generating distinct products. See details on the text.

Box 2

Oxidative Stress

Oxidative stress describes the biochemical consequences of an imbalance in the production of free oxygen and nitrogen radicals and the highly reactive detoxification of these molecules. In normal situations, reactive radicals have important physiological functions. However, in situations of oxidative stress there is an intracellular accumulation of these destructive molecules that lead to structural modification of DNA, proteins (formation of protein carbonyl), and lipids (lipid peroxidation). Under physiological conditions, nerve cells can prevent or counteract the pathological accumulation of these free radicals, but when this ability is impaired, destructive oxidation occurs in the cell. The high number of polyunsaturated fatty acids in the membranes and the low potential of regeneration make the neurons particularly sensitive to oxidation. Figure 8B shows a simple scheme of the cascade of events involved in oxidative stress.

Several investigations have shown the involvement of oxidative stress in neurodegenerative processes, but AD is the most intensively studied with respect to the impact of oxidative stress on the nerve cell death. Marker molecules of oxidations have been identified in the AD brain, such as increased levels of both lipid peroxidation products and formation of protein carbonyl. More recently, oxidation of carbohydrates has also been identified in AD. The importance of oxidative stress in the pathogenesis of AD has also been demonstrated by the neuroprotector effect of antioxidant compounds in this disease.

Antioxidant compounds may act through different mechanisms and are classified as: i) direct antioxidants – tocopherols (vitamin E), flavonoids, carotene, and others; ii) indirect antioxidants – ion chelators, oxidase inhibitors, $Ca2^{+}$ antagonists, glutamate receptor antagonists, cyclooxygenase inhibitors, and others; iii) metabolic antioxidants – glutathione, ubiquinone, carnitine, and others. Vitamins E and C are the focus of the most studies. While vitamin E, known as α-tocopherol, is a lipophilic antioxidant that protects lipophilic structures such as cell membranes against oxidative stress, vitamin C is the counterpart that acts in hydrophilic environment.

Clinical studies in AD patients have shown that the combined treatment with vitamin E and vitamin C reduces the prevalence and incidence of AD. However, the use of either vitamin E or vitamin C supplements alone does not show protective effect. The use of combined vitamin supplements for the prevention of AD needs intensive studies.

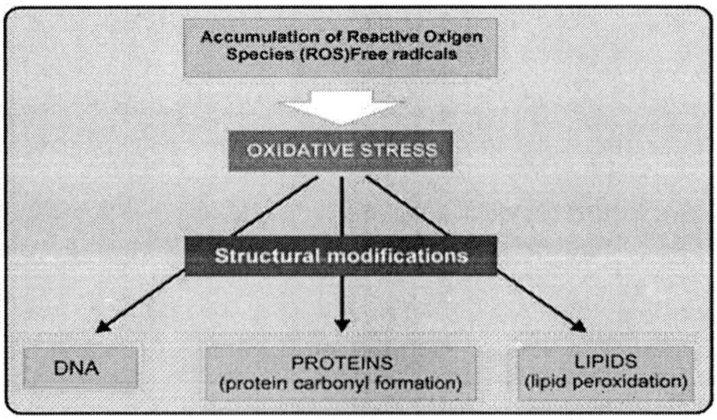

Figure 8B. A schematic hierarchical diagram of oxidative stress mechanisms that might result in cellular injury by necrosis or apoptosis.

REFERENCES

Baltimore: Lippincott Williamns andandandand Wilkins, 2001.

Bear MF, Connors BW, Paradiso MA. *Neuroscience : Exploring the brain*, 2nd edition.

Bettler B, Mulle C. Review: neurotransmitter receptors II AMPA and kainate receptors. *Neuropharmacology 34*:123-139, 1995.

Blanchard BJ, Chen A, Rozeboom LM, Stafford KA, Weigele P, Ingram VM. Efficient reversal of Alzheimer's disease fibril formation and elimination of neurotoxity by a small molecule. *Proc Natl Acad Sci 101*:14326-14332, 2004.

Bowen DM, Smith CB, White P, Davison AN. Neurotransmitter-related enzymes and indices of hypoxia in senile dementia and other abiotrophies. *Brain 99*:459-496, 1976.

Cummings JL. Use of cholinesterase inhibitors in clinical practice. *Am J Geriatr Psychiatry 11*:131-145, 2003.

Davies AP, Moloney AJF. Selective loss of cholinergic neurons in Alzheimer's disease. *Lancet ii*:1403-1404, 1976.

Fawcett JR, Bordayo EZ, Jackson K, Liu H, Peterson J, Svitak A, Frey II WH. Inactivation of the human brain muscarinic acetylcholine receptor by oxidative damage catalysed by a low molecular weight endogenous inhibitor from Alzheimer's brain is prevented by pyrophosphate analogs, bioflavonoids and other antioxidants. *Brain Res 950*:10-20, 2002.

Harrison PJ, Wighton-Benn WH, Heffernan JM, Sanders MW, Pearson RCA. Amyloid precursor protein mRNAs in Alzheimer's disease. *Neurodegeneration 5*:409-415, 1996.

Hynd MR, Scott HL, Dodd PR. Glutamate-mediated excitotoxicity and neurodegeneration in Alzheimer's disease. *Neurochem Intern 45*:583-595, 2004.

Ho L, Fukuchi K, Younkin SG. The alternatively spliced Kunitz protease inhibitor domain alters amyloid β protein precursor processing and amyloid β protein production in cultured cells. *J Biol Chem 271*:30929-30934, 1996.

Mattson MP, Chan SL. Neuronal and glial calcium signaling in Alzheimer's disease. *Cell Calcium 34*:385-397, 2003.

Mayer ML, Armstrong N. Structure and function of glutamate receptor ion channels. *Annu Rev Physiol 66*:161-181, 2004.

Olney JW. Brain lesion, obesity and other disturbances in mice treated with monosodium glutamate. *Science 164*:719-721, 1969.

Ozawal S, Kamiya H, Tsuzuki K. Glutamate receptors in the mammalian central nervous system. *Prog Neurobiol 54*:581-618, 1998.

Pearson RCA. Cortical connections and the pathology of Alzheimer's disease. *Neurodegeneration 5*:429-434, 1996.

Pearson RCA, Powell TPS. The neuroanatomy of Alzheimer's disease. *Rev Neurosci 2*:101-122, 1989.

Perry EK, Perry RH, Blessed B, Tomlinson BE. Neurotransmitter enzyme abnormalities in senile dementia: CAT and GAD activities in necropsy tissue. *J Neurol Sci 32*:247-265, 1977.

Pietrzik C, Behl C. Concepts for the treatment of Alzheimer's disease: molecular mechanisms and clinical application. *Int J Exp Path 86*:173-185, 2005.

Prybylowski K, Wenthold RJ. *N*-Methyl-D-aspartate receptors: subunit assembly and trafficking to the synapse. *J Biol Chem 279*:9673-9676, 2004.

Racchi M, Govoni, S. Rationalizing a pharmacological intervention on the amyloid precursor protein metabolism. *Trends Pharmacol Sci 20*:418-423, 1999.

Rosa MLNM, Guimarães FS, Oliveira RMW, Padovan CM, Pearson RCA, Del Bel EA. Restrain stress induces β-amyloid precursor protein mRNA expression in the rat basolateral amygdala. *Brain Research Bulletin 65*:69-75, 2005.

Rosa MLNM, Guimarães FS, Pearson RCA, Del Bel EA. Effects of single or repeated restraint stress on GluR1 and GluR2 flip and flop mRNA expression in the hippocampal formation. *Brain Res Bull 59*:117-125, 2002.

Rosa MLNM, Jefferys JGR, Sanders MW, Pearson RCA. Expression of mRNAs encoding flip isoforms of GluR1 and GluR2 glutamate receptors is increased in rat hippocampus in epilepsy induced by tetanus toxin. *Epilepsy Res 36*:243-251, 1999.

Shepherd CE, Bowes S, Parkinson D, Cambray-Deakin M, Pearson RCA. Expression of amyloid precursor protein in human astrocytes *in vitro*: isoform-specific increases following heat shock. *Neuroscience 99*:317-325, 2000.

Stanbridge MDJB. Pharmacotherapeutic approaches to the treatment of Alzheimer's disease. *Clin Ther 26*:615-630, 2004.

Tan S, Wood M, Maher P. Oxidative stress induces a form of programmed cell death with characteristics of both apoptosis and necrosis in neuronal cells. *J Neurochem 71*:95-105, 1998.

Weiss JH, Sensi SL. Ca^{2+}-Zn^{2+} permeable AMPA or kainate receptors: possible key factors in selective neurodegeneration. *Trends Neurosci 23*:365-371, 2000.

Yu W-F, Nordberg A, Ravid R, Guan Z-Z. Correlation of oxidative stress and the loss of the nicotinic receptor alpha4 subunit in the temporal cortex of patients with Alzheimer's disease. *Neurosci Lett 338*:13-16, 2003.

In: Alzheimer's Disease Research Trends
Editor: A.P. Chan, pp. 147-173

ISBN 978-1-60021-712-8

Chapter VII

Volumetric Hippocampal Differences Affect fMRI Differences in the Brain Functional Activation for Alzheimer´s Disease Patients During Memory Encoding

Alfonso Barrós-Loscertales[1,*], Vicente Belloch-Ugarte[2], Rosella Mallol[3], María-Dolores Martínez-Lozano[3], Cristina Forn[1], Maria-Antònia Parcet[1], Salvador Campos[2] and César Ávila[1]

[1]Dept. Psychology, Universitat Jaume I, 12080 Castellón, Spain;
[2]ERESA, Hospital Arnau de Vilanova, Calle San Clemente, 14. 46015 Valencia, Spain;
[3]Neurology Unit, Hospital La Magdalena, Calle Partida Bovalar s/n, 12004 Castellón, Spain.

Abstract

Patients with Mild Cognitive Impairment (MCI) have the hallmark clinical feature of memory impairment beyond that expected for age and education, yet are not demented. Using fMRI, we studied differences in activation of bilateral mesial temporal structures between 9 MCI patients, 10 probable Alzheimer's disease patients and 11 healthy elders during a picture encoding memory task and a naming task at the level of random effects. A predefined masked region of interest including bilateral hippocampus, parahippocampus, posterior cingulate, and fusiform and lingual gyrus was applied for both paradigms. Within-group analyses showed main activations in the posterior cingulate, parahippocampus, and the lingual and fusiform gyrus for the three groups

* Correspondence concerning this article should be addressed to Alfonso Barrós-Loscertales, Dpto. Psicología FCHS. Campus Riu de Sec Universitat Jaume I, 12080 Castellón, Spain. Tel: 0034 (964) 72 9696; Fax: 0034 (964) 72 9267; e-mail: barros@psb.uji.es.

differently distributed during the memory encoding task; while the naming task showed its main activations in the fusiform gyrus among other activations throughout the occipito-temporal gyri in the lingual gyri and the mesial temporal lobe (MTL). Furthermore, the three groups differed in the magnitude of these activations with controls showing more activation than patients, and the MCI group presenting a higher activation than the AD group during both paradigms. These differences increased for the memory encoding paradigm when contrasts among groups were controlled by the hippocampal volume, but this did not occur during the naming paradigm. We may conclude that the differential brain activation in the MTL related to memory encoding among these groups of patients may be biased by hippocampal volumes. Therefore, individual volume differences may blur contrasts of functional activations depending on the functional task.

Keywords: Alzheimer´s disease, functional neuroimaging, hippocampus, volumetry, memory and dementia.

Introduction

Mild cognitive impairment (MCI) has been proposed and commonly accepted as a diagnostic entity within the continuum of cognitive decline toward Alzheimer's Disease (AD) in old age (Grundman et al., 2004; Petersen, 2004) and defined as a prodromal phase to AD (Almkvist et al., 1998). However, the reliable detection of AD at early stages of the disease remains a challenge. It has been shown that MCI patients progress to AD at a rate of approximately 12% per year (Petersen et al., 1999), although it has also been shown that some MCI patients never decline to dementia. However, MCI diagnostic criteria seem to represent a transitional state between normal aging and AD.

AD and the most common forms of MCI are mainly characterized by an episodic memory impairment (Petersen, 2004) defined as a deficit in acquisition, temporary storage and retrieval of explicit facts and events (Squire & Zola-Morgan, 1991). Moreover, patients with AD and MCI characteristically show early pathological alterations in the mesial temporal lobe (MTL) system. Episodic memory problems in MCI have been linked to the hippocampus compared to nonmemory problems (Grundman et al., 2004), while memory and nonmemory cognitive impairments in probable AD are better described by the hierarchical progression of tau lesions which spread along the temporal lobe to other posterior areas (Chetelat & Baron, 2003). In this sense, naming difficulties have already been reported in MCI or at the early stages of AD (Petersen et al., 1999; Bennet et al., 2002; Grundman et al., 2004; Dudas et al., 2005), showing a strong and positive correlation with dementia severity, drawing a continuum in its evolution (Backman et al., 2004), or indicating an increased risk of developing AD in healthy elders (Howieson et al., 2003). Previous studies showed that confrontation naming involves the fusiform gyrus within the occipito-temporal cortex (Martin, 2000; Bookheimer et al., 1995; Martin et al., 1996; Murtha et al., 1999), an early involved neuroanatomical landmark affected by the disease.

New neuroimaging techniques have focused research on early AD markers. Functional and structural neuroimaging techniques show brain functional differences between these preclinical and clinical stages of the disease (Dickerson et al., 2004; 2005; Johnson et al.,

2004; 2006; Ries et al., 2006). The convergence and consistency of imaging results from multiple studies is required for these results to be accepted. Some authors have highlighted the fact that a malfunction of the MTL should precede the structural changes in the MTL system, so functional neuroimaging would be an earlier marker of AD than structural deficits (Dickerson et al., 2004; Machulda et al., 2003; Rombouts et al., 2000). On the other hand, early structural changes have been shown through volumetry in MCI and AD on MTL (Pennanen et al., 2004; Jack et al., 1999; DeToledo-Morrell et al., 2004; Bottino et al., 2002; Erten-Lyons et al., 2006; Chetelat & Baron 2003), measures that have been shown to correlate with a poorer performance in neuropsychological memory tests (Petersen et al., 2004). Otherwise, other studies showed early structural changes in healthy elders (Meyer et al., 1994) with no relation to neuropsychological test performance (Tisserand et al., 2000). Therefore, it seems that previous studies on brain differences did not show a straightforward congruency on function-structure related changes in the continuum to AD.

Functional measures of changes may be complicated by the presence of cortical and subcortical atrophy (Sandstrom et al., 2006). Then, we may consider whether functional and structural differences should be studied separately or simultaneously. In this sense, the clinical importance of linking anatomical and functional measures has been suggested to study cognitive impairment and the early diagnosis of AD (Maestú et al., 2006, Chetelat & Baron 2003).

The study of memory function in AD throughout fMRI highly depends on the applied paradigm (see Ries et al., 2006). Previous studies of memory function by means of fMRI applied face-name association encoding tasks (Sperling et al., 2003; Dickerson et al., 2005; Sandstrom et al., 2006), or picture encoding tasks (Rombouts et al., 2000; Iadaka et al., 2001). In the present research, we used a memory-encoding task to investigate the differences in brain functioning between early AD, MCI and healthy controls. This task consisted in displaying pictures at a fixed rate of presentation for later recall once the scanner session was finished. Previous studies that used complex picture-encoding tasks in healthy subjects proved to lead to a bilateral activation in the parahippocampus (PH), fusiform gyrus (FG) and hippocampal formation (Detre et al., 1998; Rabin et al., 2004; Small et al., 1999). Studies involving patients with AD and MCI have revealed a reduced activation of the left MTL structures when comparing AD and MCI with controls (Johnson et al., 2004; Machulda et al., 2003; Rombouts et al., 2000). However, no differences between groups were seen in one study (Machulda et al., 2003) when comparing AD and MCI patients, while a higher bilateral activation in MCI was revealed in another study (Dickerson et al., 2005). On the other hand, other functional tasks may involve temporal lobe structures early affected by the disease. In this sense, we also used a confrontation naming task. The brain functional domain involved in confrontation naming may be explained by a wide network (Grossman et al., 2004). However, naming difficulties in AD have been explained by a semantic deficit (Laatu et al., 2003) and the fusiform gyri have been specifically involved in semantic processing (Murtha et al., 1999). In this function, previous results have shown a reduced bilateral activation in the fusiform giri in high genetic risk subjects for AD (Smith et al., 1999). Atrophy in the left temporal lobe has also been related to naming deficits in AD (Grossman et al., 2004; Brambati et al., 2006). However, literature show that fMRI studies in temporal lobe activation during confrontation naming in AD are not as common as memory studies

MTL is a target structure in MCI and AD functional and structural studies, although the heterogeneity of activation paradigms and methodological analyses make it difficult to find communality among them. Likewise, structural atrophy has not been commonly considered by analyzing functional differences. This fact is of most importance in brain-template analyses since it has been shown that individual variations in neuroanatomical structures may persist after anatomical normalization (Juch et al., 2005; Toga & Thomson, 2001; Krishnan et al., 2006). Specifically, recent results showed that template-based ROIs fMRI measures of functional activation are confounded by hippocampal atrophy in the MCI population (Sandstrom et al., 2006). This effect may be explained by decreased normalization accuracy in memory-impaired subjects and its related atrophy in the hippocampus and MTL (Krishnan et al., 2006). Therefore, although it is assumed that spatial normalization sufficiently accounts for individual differences in the size/shape of homologous regions across subjects, the degree to which this assumption is valid for a given group will determine the power to detect group activations due to signal averaging (Krishnan et al., 2006), which directly affect group differences.

The purposes of this study were: a) to assess functional differences in MTL among MCI and AD patients during a memory-encoding task to study the structural effect of hippocampal volume across individuals as a confounder; and b) to specifically show that this effect is related to memory encoding and not to another functional task, such as naming which is early related to the clinical manifestation of the disease. Therefore, we hypothesized that the introduction of the individual hippocampal volumes would increase functional differences among a control group, and two separate MCI and AD patient groups. Moreover, this effect would not be found in group differences for a naming task.

Methodology

Subjects

Thirty subjects participated in this study: 11 healthy elders, 9 patients with MCI and 10 patients with early AD (Table 1). All subjects were recruited from the Neurology Service at La Magdalena Hospital and the Neuropsychology Service at the Universitat Jaume I, Castellón. All experimental procedures complied with the guidelines of the ethical research committee at the Universitat Jaume I. Written informed consent was obtained from every subject or their appropriate proxy prior to participation.

Selection for the participant group was made after careful neurological and neuropsychological assessment. The neuropsychological test battery involved Digit Span, Similarities, Vocabulary, Boston Naming Test (BNT) and Block Design of the WAIS-III; Luria's Watches test, and Poppelreuter´s Overlapping Figure test. In order to homogenize the sample, memory impairment was only evaluated using the Spanish version of the CVLT: all MCI and AD patients obtained scores of 1.5 SD below the mean in the CVLT. Results of neuropsychological tests for controls, MCI and AD patients are presented in Table 1.

Criteria for the diagnosis of cognitively normal control subjects were: 1) no active neurological or psychiatric disorders; 2) if medical problems were present, the illnesses or their treatments did not interfere with cognitive functioning; 3) a normal neuropsychological exam; 4) no psychoactive medication; and 5) intact ability to perform normal daily activities.

The clinical criteria for the diagnosis of MCI were: 1) a memory complaint, corroborated by an informant; 2) objective memory impairment for age and education (a score of 1.5 SD below the mean on the California Verbal Learning Test; CVLT); 3) largely normal general cognitive functioning as indexed by normal scores on Vocabulary (scores of 9 or above), Block Design (7 or above) and Luria's Watches (3 or above), BNT (compared to the age matched population; Lezack, 2001); 4) essentially intact ability to perform normal daily activities; 5) Clinical Dementia Rating (score equal to 0.5).

Finally, the diagnosis of probable AD was made according to the criteria for probable AD developed by the research group from NINCDS-ADRDA (McKhann et al., 1984).

Table 1. Demographic data, results of neuropsychological tests, hippocampal volumetry (mean±SD), and comparisons between the three groups: controls, Mild Cognitive Impairment (MCI) and Alzheimer´s Disease (AD) patients

TEST	Control (N=11)	MCI (N=9)	AD (N=10)	Control vs MCI	Control vs AD	MCI vs AD
Age	70.27±3.58	73.33±4.55	71.5±4.35	NS	NS	NS
M/F	8/3	2/7	1/9	P=0.025	P=0.004	NS
Years of education	11.1±3.09	9.77±2.11	10±2.11	NS	NS	NS
Handedness R/L	10/1	9/0	10/0	NS	NS	NS
CDR	0±0	0.5±0	0.95±0.15	P < 0.001	P < 0.001	P < 0.001
Vocabulary (WAIS)	15±3.12	10.50±1.87	10.38±2.5	P=0.01	P=0.004	NS
Digit Span, standard (WAIS)	12.73±2.24	10.33±2.10	10.30±1.16	NS	NS	NS
CVLT, 1ST trial	6.15±1.90	2.33±1.41	1.70±1.25	P < 0.001	P < 0.001	NS
CVLT, 5th trial	13.82±2.10	6.11±3.29	5.00±1.63	P < 0.001	P < 0.001	NS
CVLT, free recall	12.45±3.04	1.89±1.62	0.20±0.63	P < 0.001	P < 0.001	NS
WAIS, Similarities	15.55±2.30	10.00±2.40	8.10±1.52	P < 0.001	P < 0.001	NS
Poppelreuter´s test	10±0	9.89±0.33	9.40±0.84	NS	P=0.041	NS
Luria's Watches	4±0	3.67±0.71	2.00±1.33	NS	P < 0.001	P < 0.001
Boston Naming Test	53.09±5.37	42.56±5.46	33.56±10.21	P=0.01	P < 0.001	P<0.05
Block Design (WAIS)	13.73±2.10	11.33±2.69	8.20±2.66	NS	P < 0.001	P=0.044
Right Hippocampus Volume	2.70±0.38	1.81±0.47	1.47±0.42	P < 0.001	P < 0.001	NS
Left Hippocampus Volume	2.43±0.29	1.78±0.51	1.37±0.31	P < 0.001	P < 0.001	P<0.05

M = male; F = female; R = right-handed; L = left-handed; CDR = Clinical Dementia Rating; WAIS = Wechsler Adult Intelligence Scale; CVLT = California Verbal Learning Test; NS = non-significant difference, SD = standard deviation.

Magnetic Resonance Imaging Procedures

Blood oxygenation level-dependent (BOLD) fMRI data were acquired on a 1.5T General Electric system. Subjects were placed in a supine position in the MRI scanner. Their heads were immobilized with cushions to reduce motion artifacts. The stimuli were directly presented using goggles Visuastim XGA (Resonance Technologies, Inc). Vision correction was used when necessary.

One functional imaging run sensitive to blood oxygenation level-dependent (BOLD) contrast was collected for each subject during task performance using a 1.5-T GE (Milwaky, WI) scanner (T2*- weighted echo-planar imaging, matrix size128×128, FOV 24 cm. TE= 40ms, TR=3000; thickness=5mm; gap=2mm) were positioned perpendicular to the hippocampus and covering the hippocampal formation and the parahippocampus. A whole brain high resolution 3D-Gradient Echo (FSPGR) T1-weighted anatomical reference scan was acquired during the same scanning session (TE=4.2 ms, TR=11.3 ms, FOV 24 cm; matrix=256×256×124, 1.4 mm-thick coronal images).

fMRI: Memory Activation Paradigm

The memory paradigm was designed to emphasize MTL activation related to the encoding of new complex picture scenes. The task was programmed using Presentation software (v0.70). A blocked task-activation paradigm lasting 6 minutes was employed, alternating between 30 sec. baseline conditions and 30 s experimental conditions. During each block of the experimental condition, 10 new photographs were presented at a rate of one every 3 seconds (display lasting for 2500 ms and 500 ms ITI) for a total of 60 photographs viewed during the entire scanning run. A black screen was shown during ITI. The photographs consisted of outdoor scenes compiled for this purpose from personal collections and the Internet, although care was taken to avoid pictures of famous buildings or monuments that would be differentially recognized by participants. We used a non-recognizable stimulus for the control task following the original procedure (Detre et al., 1998), thus simplifying the task and avoiding confusion in the impaired subjects (Machulda et al., 2003). This stimulus was a single distorted, pixelated picture in which the pixels of a photograph were randomly reshuffled to make the original image unrecognizable. This image was repeated at the same rate (2500 ms with an ITI of 500 ms) as the photographs in the activation task. The pixelated image controlled for basic aspects of visual processing such as luminance and color level proportion but did not control for specific aspects of feature detection and object recognition. Participants were instructed to attend to the presented pictures during the scanning session for subsequent recognition testing. No response was required during the paradigm from the subject to avoid task complexity in impaired patients compared to control. Prior to the scanning session, all subjects completed training that included an overview of a 2-minute version of the encoding task with new pictures that were not included afterwards in the scan session or in the recognition memory test conducted after the scan session.

Following a previous study (Detre et al., 1998), subjects were tested for recognition memory in a forced choice format outside the scanner approximately 30 minutes after the memory task was completed. This consisted of a run of 32 pictures including eight photographs that had been previously presented during the scanning session and 24 new photographs. Recognition scores (RS) were calculated by applying this formula: RS = (Hits-(FA/3)), where FA stood for false alarms.

fMRI: Naming Paradigm

All subjects performed a naming fMRI activation paradigm after the memory-encoding paradigm. They were carefully instructed to name silently when they showed a line drawing picture during the activation blocks and to just look at straight lines during control blocks. A blocked task-activation paradigm lasting 6 minutes was employed, alternating between 30 sec baseline conditions and 30 sec experimental conditions. During each activation task, 15 line drawing pictures were presented at a rate of 1 every 2 seconds, lasting for 500 ms and a 1500 ms ITI, for a total of 90 pictures viewed during the entire scanning run. The line-drawing pictures selected were objects and animals compiled from Snodgrass and Vanderwart (1980) collection based on frequency parameters. The paradigm was composed by high frequency line-drawings and low frequency line-drawings conditions alternated with control conditions (according to previous Spanish norms; Sanfeliu & Fernandez, 1996), starting with a high frequency run after first control condition. However, results related to frecuency effect will not be presented since exceed our purposes.

Prior to the scanning session all subjects completed training on a reduced version of the fMRI task. The training session was done speaking overtly to control execution and difficulties in patient groups, though it had been previously tested in the neuropsychological evaluation by the administration of the BNT.

Calculating Volume of Hippocampi

Tracing of the hippocampi was done by a single tracer, blinded to the clinical data of the studied subjects. The volumes were traced from 1.4 mm thick contiguous coronal images oriented perpendicularly to the long axis of the hippocampus. The tracing was done manually with the VOXAR program (v4.2 Manufacturer, Location). The volumes of the hippocampus were measured starting from their initial appearance below the amygdala, and ending posteriorly in the section where the crura of the fornices depart from the lateral wall of the lateral ventricles. Once the ROI has been traced, the software calculates the volume for each structure by computing the number of voxels for each image that has been traced. The intraclass correlation coefficients for intrarater reliability were 0.97, measured from 15 subjects. For data presentation purposes, the volumes reported herein are normalized to the intracranial volume according to the formula: (volume/intracranial volume)×1000. To compute intracranial volume, the inner table of the cranium was traced in consecutive coronal sections spanning the entire brain.

Statistical Analysis

Behavioral Analysis

Statistical analysis of neurological and neuropsychological results was conducted using the SPSS package (v11.0). An analysis of variance (ANOVA) was specifically conducted for each neurological and neuropsychological test, and differences between the means of the three groups were assessed by a post-hoc Bonferroni test (Table 1).

Common fMRI Analysis

MRI images were processed using the SPM2 software (Wellcome Department of Cognitive Neurology, London). After realignment of functional scans and co-registration with the anatomical scan using 12 parameter affine transformations, images were normalized (Montreal Neurology Institute, MNI coordinates), and smoothed with a 12 mm Gaussian kernel. The data for each participant were modeled using a box-car design convolved with the canonical hemodynamic response function. Motion correction parameters from realignment were included as regressors of non-interest at this first level and a high-pass filter was applied (128 s.).

A two-level random-effect analysis was performed. Contrasts of parameter estimates were calculated to produce a contrast image for each subject in each paradigm (memory and naming). Activation at the within-group level was checked and reported for whole volume analysis without mask restriction ($p < 0.001$, uncorrected). Differences between groups were studied using a mask based on the WFU-PickAtlas 1.03 tool (Maldjian et al., 2003; 2004) using the Talairach and Tournoux (1998) coordinate system. This predefined region was selected from previous research on mesial temporal lobe and its functionally related functions (Avila et al., 2006; Bookheimer et al., 2000; Machulda et al., 2003; Rabin et al., 2004; Sperling et al., 2003 b), and included the left and right hippocampus, parahippocampus, fusiform gyrus, posterior cingulate (PC) and lingual gyri (LG). The mask was drawn in MNI space without any dilation, thus allowing voxel-by-voxel comparisons among groups. Hypothesis about group differences were assessed within the mask using one-factor ANOVA ($p < 0.005$, uncorrected) with at least 10 continuous active voxels to avoid spike activations. Because of significant differences in gender distribution between groups, the same analyses were run including this variable as a covariate for both paradigms. These analyses were not included in the final report since the inclusion of gender as a covariate did not show any significant effect.

A further ANCOVA analysis ($p < 0.005$, uncorrected) was also carried out to investigate between-group differences including total hippocampal volume as a covariate to test structural effects on functional activation during both tasks separately. As this particular manipulation was not made in previous studies, we will report results both including and not including the covariate in order to contrast them. Coordinates for peak significant activation in each predefined region in all analyses were converted from the standard MNI coordinate system in SPM2 to Talairach coordinates (http://www.mrccbu.cam.ac.uk/Imaging/Common/mnispace.html) and localized using the neuroanatomical atlas by Talairach and Tournoux (1998).

Memory fMRI Specific Analysis

Correlations within-group and across subjects were done to study the relation between volumetry and functional activation. Since volumetry was focused on both hippocampi, functional measure of mean activation in separated left and right hippocampi were extracted from each subject. The area of activation used to determine subject specific mean ROI activation was defined from Marsbar [v 0.38] predefined MNI_ROIs for both hippocampi separately. We chose to define the area of activation for each subject from standard space by three fold: firstly, analysis were planned for voxel wise statistics to contrast among groups, that is, after normalization; therefore, mean activation was extracted from normalized ROIs. It may present a potential confound since brain standardization system may be vulnerable to atrophy-related variability (Krishnan et al., 2006), but ROI placement encapsulated the hippocampus in every subject as we visually inspected. Secondly, individual hippocampal areas defined from volumetry were not applicable to SPM analysis, and its application supposed an analysis in a different space of reference from that conducted at functional level. Then thirdly, to define the region from activation at a reference group (controls) may introduce other bias toward the group of reference. Another alternative, as location of the maximum voxel was tested and it consistently increased statistical significance compared to mean ROI activation for every contrasts (correlations within-groups and across subjects). Finally, it was discarded due to arise new issues on this particular measure application, and its relative contribution on general results.

Results

Neuropsychological Data

Table 1 shows demographic and neuropsychological data for each group. Gender distribution was different between the control and AD groups ($p < 0.05$), but no group differences were found with regard to age and education. Gender was introduced as a covariate in all contrasts with no significant effect on differences ($p > 0.1$). As expected, the results of the neuropsychological evaluation showed differences in verbal learning and long-term recall between patients and controls. Importantly, the mean scores of MCI patients were within the normal limits in different non-memory tests, such as Digit Span, Luria's Watches, Poppelreuter's test, Similarities, Vocabulary, BNT and Block Design. When the groups were compared, controls outscored AD and MCI patients in most of the tests, and MCI had significantly higher scores than AD in Luria's Watches, BNT and Block Design (see Table 1).

Hippocampal Volumes

A 2×3 mixed model ANCOVA was run to investigate differences in hippocampal volumes between groups using laterality as a within-subjects factor (left vs. right) and group (control, MCI or AD) as a between-group factor. Total intracranial volume and gender were introduced as covariates. The analyses only yielded a main effect for groups [$F(2.27) = 19.25$, $p < 0.001$]. Comparisons between groups revealed that AD and MCI had smaller hippocampi than controls, and that MCI had a greater left hippocampus than AD patients (Table 1).

fMRI: Memory Paradigm

Post-scan recognition testing showed that healthy elders, MCI and AD had a mean RS score of 3.36, 1.28 and 1.03, respectively. The difference between control elders and the AD patient group was significant ($p < 0.05$). However, there were no significant differences between the MCI group and the other two groups ($p > 0.05$). As no responses were recorded during scanning, we made individual analyses of t-map images in order to ensure that all participants showed significantly activated voxels within the predefined masks of the hippocampal formation and parahippocampus (threshold; $p < 0.001$).These individual analyses demonstrated that most of the participants showed activation in these regions. However, two MCI patients and one AD patient showed no activation in predefined regions at the specified threshold. They were excluded from the study and not included in the sample description.

Our first interest was to test which areas were activated by each group during the memory-encoding paradigm. Within-group analyses using a one-sample t test revealed that the local maximum of signal increase ($p < 0.001$; uncorrected) yielded bilateral activations in the fusiform gyri of the MTL for the three groups (Table 2, Figure 1). Healthy elders and MCI patients (but not AD patients) also showed activation bilaterally in the PH (Table 2). Finally, only the control group presented bilateral activation in the hippocampus. An analysis of another activation showed local maxima distributed differently in the posterior cingulate and lingual gyrus in the three groups (see Table 2; Figure 1).

Table 2. fMRI analysis of active brain areas during memory encoding paradigm in each group

GROUP	Area of activation	Hemisphere	x	y	z	Z score	Cluster size
Control	PH /FG/PC/LG/Hippocampus	L	-28	-46	-14	5.02	2457
	PH/FG/PC/LGl/Hippocampus	R	36	-40	-24	4.05	1324
MCI	PH /FG/LG/PC	L	-26	-52	-10	5.55	881
	FG/ LG/ PC/ PH	R	30	-58	-12	5.13	1281
AD	FG/ PG/ LG	R	32	-42	-22	4.06	625
	FG	L	-40	-60	-16	3.20	11
	LG	L	-20	-68	-10	3.36	32
	PC	R	16	-60	14	3.46	28

Local maximums are reported at cluster level (MNI coordinate system) for each active region and others within the cluster. Results reported in each group for one-sample t-test ($p<0.001$; uncorrected). AD, Alzheimer´s disease; MCI, Mild Cognitive Impairment; ROI, region of interest; LG, lingual gyrus; FG, fusiform gyrus; PC, posterior cingulate; PH, parahippocampus; L, left hemisphere; R, right hemisphere.

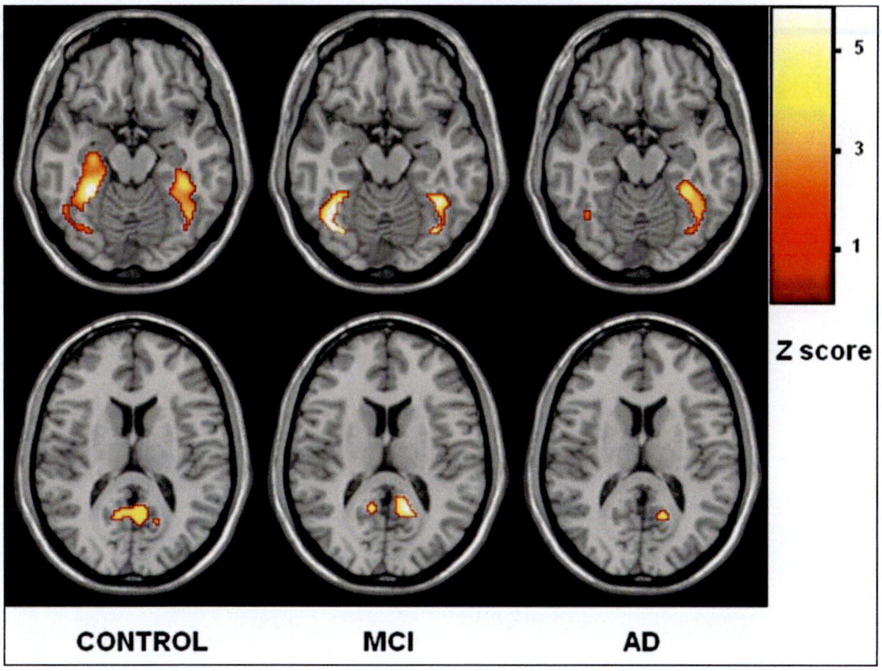

Figure 1. Average brain activation during encoding of complex picture scenes. Axial brain slices in standard MNI space (first raw at z = -17; second row at z = 12). Images are displayed using the neurological convention (left is left). Results from a one-sample t-test (p<0.001, uncorrected), shown according to Z-score color scale (right side), as an example of activation in each group: control, Mild Cognitive Impairment (MCI) and Alzheimer´s Disease (AD) groups.

Our second objective was to study brain functional differences between groups to identify areas of reduced activation during encoding in the memory-impaired groups of MCI and AD. Firstly, between-group differences were studied using one-factor ANOVAs ($p < 0.005$, uncorrected) in the predefined mask (Table 3; Figure 2, top). As expected, healthy elders showed a greater activation throughout the PH, LG and PC bilaterally, and in the left FG and hippocampus than AD patients. Differences between the control and the MCI patient groups were restricted to the left PH, FG, and bilateral LG and PC. Finally, differences between the MCI and AD patient groups were found in the bilateral PH and left hippocampus (Table 3).

Finally, we studied a possible effect of hippocampal volume on functional differences between groups. Hippocampal volume differences had been identified among our groups at the native space. We expected an effect of volume differences in brain activation, although brain normalization was supposed to eliminate structural differences in memory-impaired subjects. When functional activation was corrected for total hippocampal volume, demeaned for each group (ANCOVA; $p < 0.005$, uncorrected), differences in between-group contrasts were extended to other regions (see Table 3 and Figure 2, bottom row). Thus, the control group showed higher activations in the hippocampus and FG bilaterally than AD patients besides those previously reported. Controls presented higher activations extended to the right FG than MCI patients. Finally, MCI showed higher activations extended to PC bilaterally and left FG, in addition to the right LG and hippocampus, than AD patients. No differences were found between groups when opposite contrasts (AD>Control; AD>MCI; and MCI>Control) were defined. Therefore, group differences were increased by eliminating a possible effect of structure over functional activation. Furthermore, possible interactions between volume and functional activation were explored at a voxel level within the predefined masked ROIs. No significant cluster of activation (k=10, p<0.005 uncorrected) was found to show an interaction between structure and function. Hence, hippocampal volume showed to increase functional differences between groups, which may be statistically explained by a reduction of the error variance.

Table 3. Contrast results of fMRI between groups during the memory encoding task without controlling (A) and controlling (B) by total hippocampal volume.

CONTRAST	Area of activation	H	x	y	z	Z score	Cluster size
A							
Control>AD	FG/LG/PC/ PH/Hippocampus	L	-26	-50	-14	4.66	1954
	LG/PC	R	12	-64	2	3.37	471
	PH	R	12	-36	-6	2.95	27
Control>MCI	LG/FG/ PC/ PH	L	-20	-60	-2	3.59	566
	LG/PC	R	8	-62	8	3.00	206
	PH	L	-18	-28	-12	2.78	20
MCI > AD	PH	R	14	-36	4	3.08	20
	Hippocampus/PH	L	-28	-38	0	2.85	28
B							
Control/AD	PC	L	-2	-32	22	3.76	20
		R	4	-32	22	3.27	39
	PH /LGl/FG/ Hippocampus	L	-26	-46	-12	4.59	2871
	PH/LG/ FG/Hippocampus	R	14	-34	0	3.96	722
Control>MCI	LG/ PC/ FG/ PH	L	-22	-62	-2	3.79	1627
	FG/LG/PC	R	40	-42	-24	3.17	91
MCI > AD	LG	R	18	-64	-10	2.93	70
	PC	L	-2	-32	22	3.50	28
		R	4	-32	22	3.67	63
	PH	R	14	-35	5	4.14	81
	PH/Hippocampus	R	30	-18	-22	3.02	103
	PH/FG	L	-24	-24	-28	2.93	11
	Hippocampus/PH	L	-22	-38	-6	3.50	408

Areas included in each significant cluster and its local maxima are reported (MNI coordinate system) for more accurate activation description. Results are reported in each contrast for one-factor ANOVA (p<0.005; uncorrected) and ANCOVA (p<0.005; uncorrected). AD, Alzheimer´s disease; MCI, Mild Cognitive Impairment; ROI, region of interest; LG, lingual gyrus; FG, fusiform gyrus; PC, posterior cingulate; PH, parahippocampus; L, left hemisphere; R, right hemisphere.

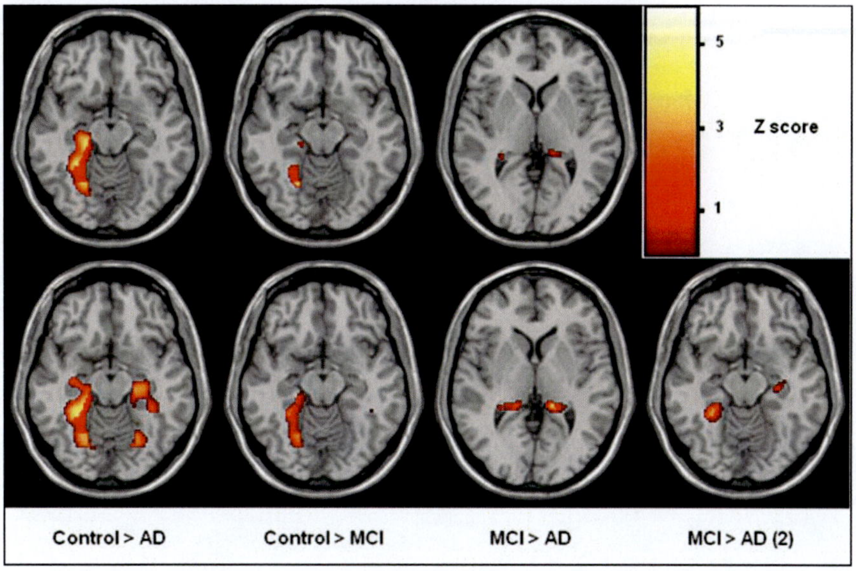

Figure 2. Contrast images for memory encoding of complex scenes among groups without hippocampal volume (A) (left+right) and with it as covariate (B). Axial brain slices in standard MNI space. Images are displayed using the neurological convention (left is left). Results from one-way ANOVA (A) and ANCOVA (B) (p<0.005, uncorrected), shown according to Z-score color scale (right side), for each contrast: control vs Alzheimer´s Disease (AD) groups (z =-11); control vs. Mild Cognitive Impairment (MCI) groups (z = -11); and MCI vs. AD groups [z = 2 and -11(2)].

Table 4. Results of fMRI analysis for average brain activations in each group during the naming task

GROUP	Area of activation	Hemisphere	x	y	z	Z score	Cluster size
Control	Fusiform gyrus	L-BA19	-38	-70	-20	4.60	716
		L-BA37	-46	-62	-24	4.10	
		L-BA37	-44	-56	-14	3.98	
		R-BA37	42	-58	-24	4.32	345
		R-BA20	32	-42	-24	3.50	
MCI	Fusiform gyrus	L-BA37	-42	-62	-16	4.42	184
	Occipital lobe	R	34	-68	-20	4.37	319
		R-BA37	40	-62	-20	4.25	
	Fusiform gyrus	R-BA20	32	-42	-22	4.22	
	Middle temporal gyrus	R	48	-62	4	3.29	27
AD	Fusiform gyrus	L	-30	-62	-16	3.36	12
	Fusiform gyrus	R-BA37	40	-46	-24	3.91	29

Local maximums are reported at voxel level (MNI coordinate system) for more accurate activation description. Results reported in each group for one-sample t-test (p<0.001; uncorrected). AD, Alzheimer´s disease; MCI, Mild Cognitive Impairment; L, left hemisphere; R, right hemisphere.

fMRI: Naming Paradigm

The confrontation naming task was also analyzed to study the functional activation in each group. Image analysis was based on a voxel-by-voxel statistical test of whole volume analysis. Figure 3 shows group effects for the naming task when compared to the control task with main local maximum in the fusiform gyri for all groups after a one-sample t-test ($p<0.001$, uncorrected). Other local maximas were located along the occipito-temporal gyri in the lingual gyri and the medial temporal lobe for some groups (see Table 4).

When differences between groups were contrasted to study areas of reduced activation in MCI and AD patients, main differences between groups in the left fusiform gyrus (ANOVA; $p<0.005$, uncorrected) along the occipito-temporal sulcus (Table 5; Figure 4) were located. It was only when the control group was compared to MCI that the former showed a higher activation in the lingual gyri. Another local maxima was located in the left inferior parietal temporal lobe (BA 40) when the control group was compared to both patient groups.

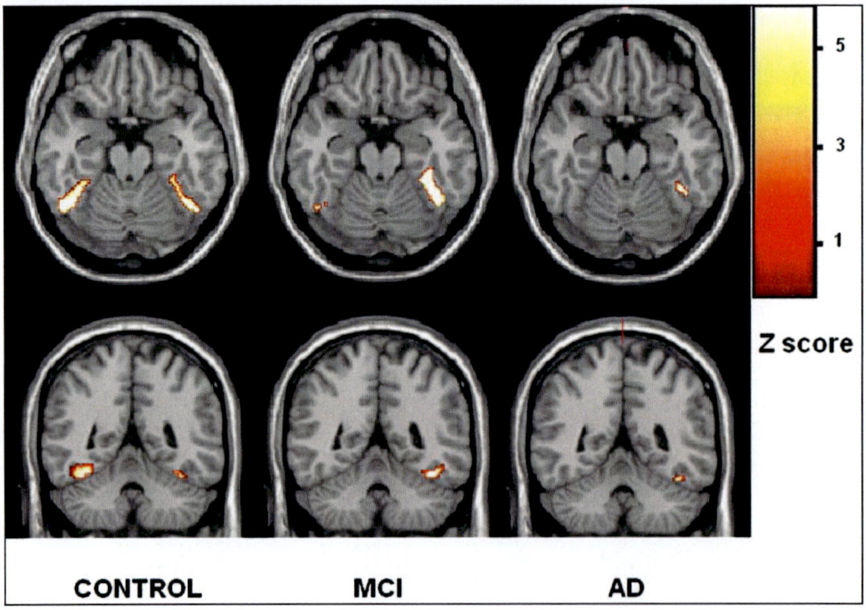

Figure 3. Average brain activation during confrontation naming. Axial and coronal brain slices in standard MNI space (first raw at z = -20; second row at y = -48). Images are displayed using the neurological convention (left is left). Results from a one-sample t-test ($p<0.001$, uncorrected), shown according to Z-score color scale (right side), as an example of activation in each group: control, Mild Cognitive Impairment (MCI) and Alzheimer´s Disease (AD) groups.

Memory fMRI Activation and Volumetric Results

We analyzed the relationships of the functional, structural MRI variables. Functional activation was measured as the mean activation within both the left and right hippocampi. Activation was measured from a predefined MNI_ROI. All correlation analyses were considered with a bilateral level of significance. Within individual subjects, the group analysis of correlation among these variables was not found to be significant, except for the AD group, specifically between the volume and mean activation in the right hippocampus ($r=-0.75$, $p<0.01$) during encoding (Figure 5). There were correlations between the mean activation in the left hippocampus and the bilateral hippocampal volume (left: r=0.44, p=0.016; right: r=0.39, P=0.035) across the entire group of 30 subjects, while there was no correlation between the right mean activation and the hippocampal volume (P>0.1). In an ANCOVA model, there was a main significant effect of group (P=0.023), but there were neither a main effect of the covariate (p>0.1) nor the interaction term was significant (P>0.1) on the right hippocampal activation using the template-based analysis. Likewise, there was a main significant effect of group (P=0.044) on the left hippocampal mean activation, but there were neither a main effect of the covariate (p>0.1) nor the interaction term was significant (p>0.1).

Table 5. Contrast results of fMRI between groups during the confrontation naming task

CONTRAST	ROI area	H	x	y	z	Z score	Cluster Size
Control > MCI	Fusiform Gyrus	L-BA37	-22	-52	-14	3.07	23
	Lingual gyrus	L	-18	-70	-16	2.90	18
		L-BA19	-16	-48	-6	3.01	13
		L-BA19	-12	-70	-10	2.72	
	Inferior parietal gyrus	L-BA40	-58	-36	32	4.09	82
		R-BA40	60	-30	38	2.99	10
Control > AD	Fusiform gyrus	L-BA20	-38	-36	-20	3.25	51
		L	-42	-44	-16	2.66	
	Inferior parietal lobule	L-BA40	-60	-36	30	3.03	14
MCI > AD	Fusiform gyrus	L	-44	-46	-14	2.98	12

Local maximums are reported at voxel level (MNI coordinate system) for more accurate activation description. Results reported in each group for one-sample t-test (p<0.005; uncorrected). Analysis restricted to the predefined bilateral ROIs. AD, Alzheimer´s disease; MCI, Mild Cognitive Impairment; L, left hemisphere; R, right hemisphere.

CONCLUSION

The present study has shown relevant differences between controls and patients with AD and MCI in the activation of the MTL structures while encoding complex scenes. Moreover, functional differences are also shown between these same groups during a confrontation naming task. However, the three groups differed as regards to the magnitude of these activations, with controls presenting more activation than patients and the MCI group showing a greater activation than the AD group. Furthermore, the extension and significance of these differences increased for the memory-encoding task when controlling for hippocampal atrophy. However, this did not apply for confrontation naming contrasts among groups. These results may have important implications on AD research through neuroimaging techniques.

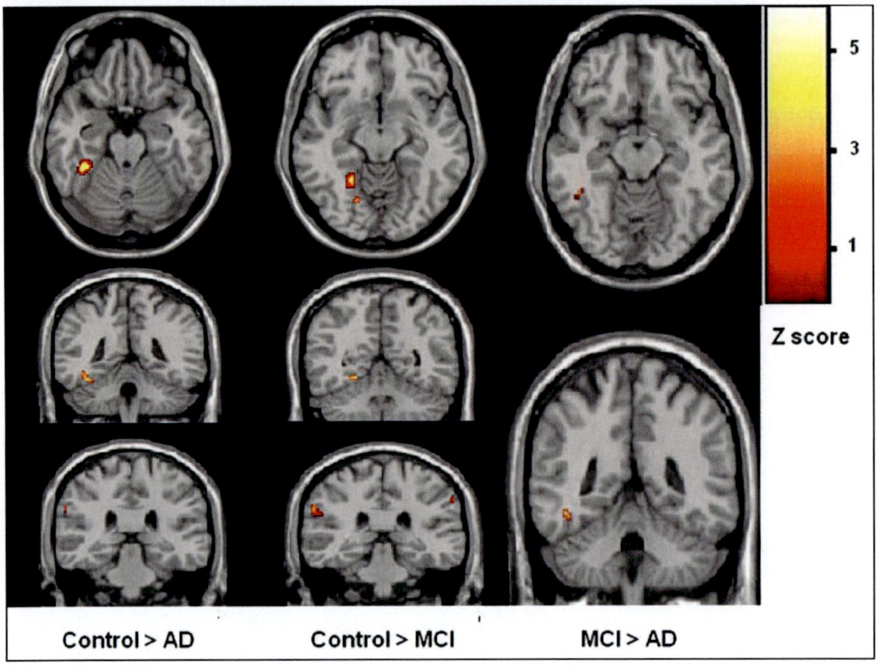

Figure 4. Axial and coronal brain slices in standard MNI space. Images are displayed using the neurological convention (left is left). Results from one-way ANOVA ($p<0.005$, uncorrected), shown according to Z-score color scale (right side), for each contrast: control vs Alzheimer´s Disease (AD) groups (z=-20, y=-45, y=-31, from firt to third raw); control vs. Mild Cognitive Impairment (MCI) groups (z=-11; y=-55 ;y=-30, from the first to the third raw); and MCI vs. AD groups (z = -15; y= -45; for the two raws respectively).

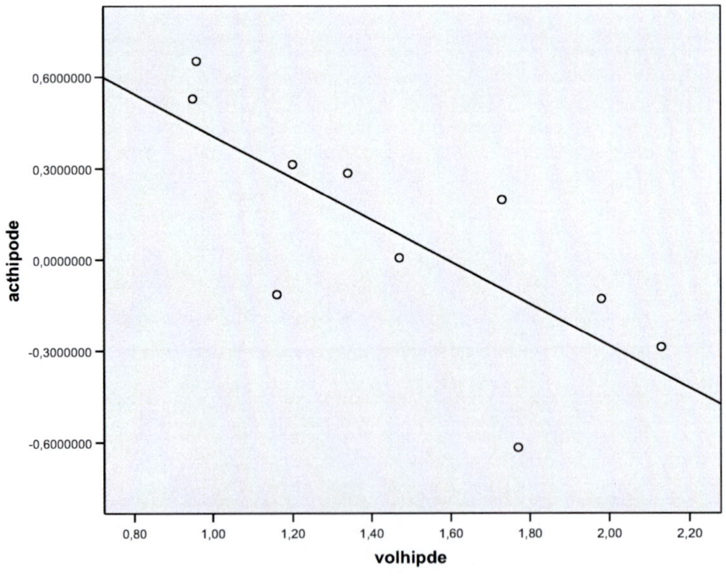

Figure 5. Correlation of right hippocampal activation in a template-space based ROI with right hippocampal volume in subjets with MCI during memory encoding.

Functional Activation During Memory Encoding in MCI and AD

Separate analyses of the three groups during the memory-encoding task yielded a bilateral activation of the MTL structures (Table 2, Figure 1). These results confirmed previous studies showing posterior MTL activation bilaterally in healthy and neurologically-impaired subjects (Chein & Schneider, 2003; Detre et al., 1998; Machulda et al., 2004; Rabin et al., 2004; Rombouts et al., 2004), which extended from the visual association areas (i.e. lingual gyrus) into the MTL. FG and PH are final routes of the inferior occipito-temporal ventral stream system that extract highly specific information about what visually encountered objects are (Ungerleider & Mishkin, 1982). Studies have shown the involvement of FG (Kirchhof et al., 2000; Kuskowski et al., 1999; Sperling et al., 2003 b; Wagner et al., 1998), PH (Burgess, 2002) and the posterior cingulate (Johnson et al., 2006; Ranganath et al., 2005; Ries et al., 2006) in the encoding and retrieval success of information, as well as in the hippocampus. Our results not only showed the activation of this area in each group, but also its differential functioning among the groups during memory encoding. Our groups of patients with MCI and AD, characterized by a memory impairment, showed decreased activation in these areas while encoding pictures. Thus, memory problems may be spread to other memory-related structures along the MTL beyond the hippocampus.

The hippocampus receives most of its inputs from the PH, with which it is reciprocally connected (Rabin et al., 2004). The right PH was proposed as being involved in the integration of all visuo-spatial features of visual stimuli. Meanwhile, the left PH is thought to be involved in the verbal integration of these same stimuli within a larger prefrontal-medial temporal circuit (Fernandez & Tendolkar, 2002; Simons & Spiers, 2003; Ungerleider & Mishkin, 1982; Kirchhoff et al., 2000). This circuit also included the posterior cingulate (Duvernoy, 1998; Johnson et al., 2006; Ranganath et al., 2005; Ries et al., 2006). Our analysis showed a pattern of differential activations between the control group, and the MCI and AD patients groups in these same areas in the MTL, as in previous studies (Johnson et al., 2004; 2006; Machulda et al., 2003). Furthermore, other studies have revealed an increased activation in MCI patients when compared with the controls in the MTL structures (i.e. hippocampus) (Dickerson et al., 2005) and in people at risk of AD (Bookheimer et al., 2000). These differences will be commented below under the inclusion of structural atrophy as an important variable to measure functional activation in memory-impaired populations.

Visual encoding of complex scenes has been related to bilateral MTL functional activation (Golby et al., 2001). This task seems to be well suited to study bilateral MTL activation and possible functional asymmetries (Avila et al., 2006). Although asymmetries were not directly studied in this research, our results seemed to be in agreement with the lateralized progression of tau lesions (Chetelat & Baron, 2003) from the left to the right hemisphere. These asymmetries may be related to a deficit in the verbal coding of stimuli (Hodges et al., 1992) at the cognitive level. This is congruent with the verbal memory dysfunction (CVLT) revealed in our MCI and AD patients, and with a lower execution in other verbal tasks (Vocabulary, Similarities and BNT) in AD, when compared to MCI, during the neuropsychological evaluation. A hypothesized hierarchical progression during the continuum to AD in brain atrophy and the cognitive dysfunction may also be related to the functional differences found in our research on the functional activation during confrontation naming.

Functional Activation During Confrontation Naming in MCI and AD

FMRI results during confrontation naming demonstrated the activation of the brain areas in the occipito-temporal cortex in elders, and in MCI and AD patients. These activations showed that confrontation naming produced main activations in the bilateral fusiform gyrus, while differences among groups focused on the left fusiform gyrus. Previous results on naming had shown the bilateral implication of fusiform gyrus (Bookheimer et al., 1995; Martin et al., 2000; Murtha et al., 1999), and others revealed a left lateralization (Zelkowick et al., 1998). A general lateralization of functional activation during confrontation naming is of particular interest in AD. Its manifestation has shown its relation to dementia severity (Backman et al., 2004), and even a relation to an increased risk to develop AD (Howieson et al., 2003).

The effect of a semantic memory deficit (Laatu et al., 2003) has been mainly considered through the presence of naming difficulties in MCI and early manifestations of AD (Petersen et al., 1999; Bennet et al., 2002; Grundman et al., 2004; Dudas et al., 2005). Likewise, confrontation naming difficulties have been identified as a symptom of semantic memory deficit (Martin, 2000).

From our study we may conclude that functional differences in confrontation naming in the continuum from MCI to AD might be related to a left fusiform dysfunction. Furthermore, this may be associated with an early manifestation of a semantic deficit related to the reduced activation in the fusiform gyrus in the light of other studies. These evidences may be extracted, for instance, from repetition priming effect studies. This effect showed a decreased activation in the right fusiform gyrus through the repetition of the same stimuli with the same visual properties, whereas the left fusiform gyrus is particularly sensitive to the repetition of a similar stimulus by manipulating general/semantic features (Dehaene et al., 2002; Garoff et al., 2005). In this sense, the role of the left fusiform gyrus would be more related to semantic processing, whereas the right fusiform gyrus would be more highly associated with visual recognition. In parallel, a higher activation on the left fusiform gyrus was observed (Murtha et al., 1999; Price et al., 2005) when studies contrasted a more pure semantic task to test the fusiform role in semantic processing. Therefore, our results may reveal a semantic deficit related to naming difficulties in MCI and AD when compared to healthy elders. Moreover, this deficit may be related to a reduced functionality of the left fusiform gyrus. Once again, the biological reason for this reduced functionality in the left fusiform gyrus may be the hierarchical progression of tau lesions which spread along the temporal lobe (Chetelat & Baron, 2003). However, settling this functional consideration specifically to the fusiform gyrus in AD may generate as much discussion as unveiling an explanation for the functional differences in the inferior parietal lobe among our groups. Hence, further research will be necessary to clarify these conclusions.

fMRI and Volumetric Data Joined Effects in MCI and AD

The hippocampus is a key structure for understanding encoding/retrieval processes. In recent years, a considerable amount of research has related AD with the atrophy of the hippocampus and surrounding areas (Zakzanis et al., 2003). In the present study, we have adopted a relatively new approach to investigate structure-function relationships. As expected, our three groups differed in their hippocampus volume, and we used this atrophy as a covariate in the analyses of functional differences with a whole brain voxel-wise analysis approach. With this approach, we have studied truly functional differences that cannot be attributed to structural differences when compared to others which sought a direct relation by correlating volume atrophy and CBF changes (Johnson et al., 2000), or only compared to differences in voxel based morphometry (VBM) for a particular ROI (Johnson et al., 2004). This specific analysis sought to remove the hippocampal volume as a potential source of bias in the functional activation. Therefore, this group analysis increased statistical power by decreasing the size of the mean square against which the effects are tested. This reduced variance error and the increased between-group differences, which were noted while encoding pictures (see Figure 2), extended these differences to the hippocampus. Importantly, our research group has found that the same strategy did not significantly modify brain activations in a naming paradigm, which suggests hippocampal atrophy may only modulate brain activations of hippocampus-related episodic memory functions". A similar result was observed by Maestú et al. (2006) in an magnetoencephalography (MEG) study, who reported that hippocampal atrophy (measured by spectroscopy) improves the value of MEG regional activation in predicting individual scores in cognitive and functional measures. Therefore, it is possible to conclude the significance of considering volumetric and functional measures when studying group differences.

Previous results (Bookheimer et al., 2000; Dickerson et al., 2004; Dickerson et al., 2005; Machulda et al., 2003) along with our own may draw a explanatory model of compensatory activations between the left and right hippocampus. The right hippocampus compensated the left dysfunction and atrophy in MCI, increasing its activation over healthy subjects (Dickerson et al., 2004) at the onset of MCI. Advanced stages of the disease may maintain this pattern of compensatory activation, but atrophy does not allow for functional compensation (Johnson et al., 2000; Machulda et al., 2003). Thus, although higher activation may be related to increased neuronal atrophy, it may not compensate cognitive deficits. This unfit compensatory activation at the MTL may be inferred from the AD intra-group negative correlation among these variables shown in our study. However, it should be pointed out that this hypothesis has been previously suggested (Bookheimer et al, 2000; Dickerson et al., 2004; Dickerson et al., 2005; Bondi et al., 1997), but discussed by others as a confound rather than a real effect if they are based on template-based studies (Sandstrom et al., 2006). Sandstrom et al. (2006) showed this same negative correlation between atrophy and functional activation in a larger MCI sample. We did not found this effect on MCI, although our reduced sample size might account for this.

Differences between memory-impaired groups increased their extension and significance in memory-encoding activation when a control for hippocampal atrophy was applied in our study. This effect may be methodologically considered in two ways simultaneously (Oaks et al., 2006): a) the extent to which a functional activation can be reliably explained by underlying anatomical differences; and b) the extent to which a functional activation cannot be attributed to anatomical difference, and is thus likely due to the functional difference alone. In this sense, it has been pointed out that atrophy may confound functional differences when analyzed in a template-based ROI analysis (Sandstrom et al., 2006). These effects may be explained by the wrong assumption on the account of anatomical differences by normalization (Krishnan et al., 2005), as previously pointed out. Other than a voxel-wise analysis, we also performed a ROI analysis after normalization. We measured the mean activation within the standardized hippocampus ROI (Marsbar v0.38) and correlated it to within-group volumes. We only found a negative correlation in the AD group to the right hippocampus, similar to that reported by Sandstron et al. (2006) in MCI. However, we did not find that same correlation in MCI patients ($p<0.1$). Furthermore, we found a cross-group correlation of the left hippocampal activation to bilateral hippocampal volume separately. The effect of these correlations across groups would lead us to expect to see a large reduction in the error variance after controlling for hippocampal volume, which actually happened. On the other hand, the within-group correlation between AD and the ROI mean activation should not be considered as a confounding effect in the absence of interaction between groups and the covariate. However, no interaction was noted at either the template ROI level or the voxel-wise analysis. Furthermore, even in the case that the correlated right hippocampal volume would have accounted for the variance of group differences, we may be eliminating true differences between groups in the absence of interaction.

In summary, our study of brain atrophy of the hippocampus on memory-impaired subjects was firstly focused on the introduction of the hippocampal volume as a covariate in an ANCOVA. Hippocampal volume measures in the native space have revealed differences among our groups. The purpose of this analysis was to test the possible effect of volume differences on brain activation contrasts among groups. Therefore the analysis showed us an increase in brain activation differences among groups, which extended deeper into the MTL in the hippocampus (Table 3; Figure 2). Our interpretation of these results was that, although brains had been normalized, individual differences in native brain atrophy reduce error variance and increase functional differences. This interpretation would reflect the importance of accounting for hippocampal atrophy in memory-impaired subjects in order to test for real functional differences. However, interactions between groups and atrophy should also be considered in order to evaluate this real functional difference, which is not commonly performed in a joint fashion. Although further research is needed to elucidate the origin of these effects, it might increase neuroimaging methodological accuracy on AD research, or new findings in this field and the related functional research associated with structural variations might arise.

LIMITATIONS

Some limitations of this study should be mentioned. Firstly, the sample size was small, which may directly affect the observation of some group effects. However, we used an extended neuropsychological battery to diagnose the classification and sample description that may be considered for future comparisons of our group results with other studies. A second problem was that we did not directly assess the response during the memory paradigm, and therefore cannot guarantee that all the subjects were fully attending the stimuli. This would also have an effect on recognition scores. Nonetheless, the use of goggles connected to a desktop computer during the presentation of pictures made on-task distraction more unlikely since the pictures presented were the only visual stimuli within the subject's visual field. It has also been proven that goggles produce more consistent BOLD signal activations than projectors (Engström et al., 2005). Moreover, from our experience (Avila et al., 2006) and from other studies (Detre et al., 1998; Dickerson et al., 2005; Duvernoy, 1998; Rabin et al., 2004), the scene memory encoding paradigm produces a strong individual activation bilaterally in the MTL. This allowed this paradigm to be applied to the study of memory lateralization in epilepsy (Avila et al., 2006; Haxby et al., 2001; Golby et al., 2003; Dickerson et al., 2004; Detre et al., 1998; Duvernoy, 1998; Rabin et al., 2004; Simons & Spiers, 2003) because it produces a bilateral activation of the MTL (Simons & Spiers, 2003; Golby et al., 2001). Hence, the only way we considered it possible to test for the participants' implication in the task was to evaluate for individual activations within the MTL, and every subject in our analysis showed such activations. Nevertheless, there may be some doubt as to the level of processing involved in such activation. In this regard, the use of a perceptual control condition, consisting of a single, repeated pixelated image compared to the complex picture encoding task, may be questioned. A control task in which novel or repeated scenes were compared to the encoding task, as has been previously applied in healthy adults (Golby et al., 2001; Sperling et al., 2003), may be more likely to isolate activation due to memory. However, previous studies that applied this paradigm with similar samples (Dickerson et al., 2005; Machulda et al., 2003; DeToledo-Morrell et al., 2004) or different populations (Garoff et al., 2005; Chein & Scheneider., 2003; Dickerson et al., 2005; Detre et al., 1998; Duvernoy et al., 1998; Rabin et al., 2004), used this control condition arguing that certain confusion may exist in impaired subjects, and MTL activation was maximized and covert encoding was avoided, respectively. This consideration regarding the confrontation naming task may be performed through the use of a low-level baseline; besides, its effects have been considered (Price et al., 2005). However, functional activation and differences between groups were found in brain areas related to semantic processing and naming. Thirdly, the use of block designs may be problematic since it does not allow for a post-hoc classification of trials. Event-related designs have been useful to investigate the brain area involved in successful and unsuccessful encoding (Iidaka et al., 2001; Ungerleider et al., 1982). Despite this advantage of event-related designs, it should be borne in mind that their capacity to detect brain areas involved in a cognitive process (Sperling et al., 2006; Huettel et al., 2004), and probably to detect between-group differences, is lower than that of block designs. Finally, there was a significant difference in gender distribution between groups. Although its effect was covariated out, its effects elimination as a categorical variable may be questioned. Moreover, gender effects on AD functional and structural differences should be carefully considered (Callen et al., 2004; Salat DH et al., 1999).

Acknowledgment

We thank the subjects who participated in this study. The paper also benefited from the comments on statistical issues of Wesley Moons. This study was supported by a grant from the Spanish Ministry of Work and Social Affairs (IMSERSO; E-17 UJI) and a grant from the Spanish Ministry of Health (PI021756). Alfonso Barros-Loscertales was supported by a grant from the Conselleria de Empresa, Universidad y Ciencia from the Comunidad Valenciana.

References

Almkvist, O., Basun, H., Backman, L., Herlitz, A., Lannfelt, L., Small, B., Viitanene, M., Wahlund, L.O., & Winblad, B. (1998) Mild cognitive impairment--an early stage of Alzheimer's disease? *J. Neural. Transm., 54*, 21-29.

Avila, C., Barrós-Loscertales, A., Forn, C., Mallol, R., Parcet, M.A., Belloch, V., Campos, S., Feliu-Tatay, R., Gonzalez-Darder, J.M. (2006) Memory lateralization with two fMRI tasks in patients with lesion in the temporal lobe. *A.J.N.R, 27*, 498-503.

Backman, L., Jones, S., Berger, A.K., Laukka, E.J., Small, B.J. (2004) Multiple cognitive deficits during the transition to Alzheimer´s disease. *J Intern Med, 256*, 195-204.

Bennett, D.A., Wilson, R.S., Schneider, J.A., Evans, D.A., Beckett, L.A. Aggarwarl, N.T., Barnes L.L., Fox J.H., & Bach, J. (2002). Natural history of mild cognitive impairment in older persons. *Neurology, 59*, 198-205.

Bondi, M.W., Houston, W.S., Eyler, L.T., & Brown, G.G. (2005). fMRI evidence of compensatory mechanisms in older adults at genetic risk for Alzheimer disease. *Neurology, 64*, 501-508.

Bookheimer, S.Y., Zeffiro, T.A., Blaxton, T., Gaillard, W. & Theodore, W. (1995). Regional cerebral blood flow during object naming and word reading. *Human Brain Mapping, 3*, 93-106.

Bookheimer, S.Y., Strojwas, M.H., Cohen, M.S., Saunders, A.M., Pericak-Vance, M.A., Mazziotta, J.C. & Small, G.W. (2000). Patterns of brain activation in people at risk for Alzheimer´s disease. *N Engl J Med, 343*, 450-456.

Bottino, C.M., Castro, C.C., Gomes, R.L., Buchpiguel, C.A., Marchetti, R.L., Neto, M.R. (2002). Volumetric MRI measurements can differentiate Alzheimer's disease, mild cognitive impairment, and normal aging. *Int Psychogeriatry, 14*, 59-72.

Brambati, S.M., Myers, D., Wilson, A., Rankin, K.P., Allison, S.C., Rosen, H.J., Miller, B.L., & Gorno-Tempini, M.L. (2006). The anatomy of category-specific object naming in neurodegenerative disease. *Journal of Cognitive Neuroscience 18*, 1644-1653.

Burgess, N. (2002). The hippocampus space and viewpoints in episodic memory. *Q. J. Exp. Psychol. A., 55*, 1057-1080.

Callen, D.J., Black, S.E., Caldwell, C.B., Grady, C.L. (2004) The influence of sex on limbic volume and perfusion in AD. *Neurobiol Aging, 25*, 761-770.

Chein, J.M., & Schneider, W.(2003) Designing effective fMRI experiments. In *Handbook of neuropsychology: Vol. 9: Plasticity and rehabilitation*, J. Grafman and I.H. Robertson, eds. Elsevier, Amsterdam. The Netherlands, pp 299-326.

Chetelat, G., & Baron, J.C. (2003). Early diagnosis of Alzheimer's disease: contribution of structural neuroimaging. *Neuroimage, 18*, 525-541.

Dehaene, S., Naccache, L., Cohen, L., Bihan, D.L., Mangin, J.F., Poline, J.B., Riviere, D. (2001). Cerebral mechanisms of word masking and unconscious repetition priming. *Nat Neurosci, 4*, 752-758.

DeToledo-Morrell, L., Stoub, T.R., Bulgakova, M., Wilson, R.S., Bennett, D.A., Leurgans, S., Wuu, J., Turner, D.A. (2004). MRI-derived entorhinal volume is a good predictor of conversion from MCI to AD. *Neurobiol Aging, 25*, 1197-1203.

Detre, J.A., Maccotta, L., King, D., King, D., Alsop, D.C., Glosser, G., D'Esposito, M., Zarahn, E., Aguirre, G.K., French, J.A. (1998). Functional MRI lateralization of memory in temporal lobe epilepsy. *Neurology, 50*, 926-932.

Dickerson, B.C., Salat, D.H., Bates, J.F., Atiya, M., Killiany, R.J., Greve, D.N., Dale, A.M., Stern, C.E., Blacker, D., Albert, M.S., Sperling, R.A. (2004) Medial temporal lobe function and structure in mild cognitive impairment. *Ann Neurol, 56*, 27-35.

Dickerson, B.C., Salat, D.H., Greve, D.N., Chua, E.F., Rend-Giovannetti, E., Rentz, D.M., Bertram, L., Mullin, K., Tanzi, R.E., Blacker, D., Albert, M.S., Sperling, R.A. (2005). Increased hippocampal activation in mild cognitive impairment compared to normal aging and AD. *Neurology, 65*, 404-411.

Dudas, R.B., Clague, F., Thomson, S.A., Graham, K.S., Hodges, J.R. (2005). Episodio and semantic memory in mild cognitive impairment. *Neuropsicología, 43*, 1266-1276.

Duvernoy, H. (1998), *The human Hippocampus, 2nd Ed.* Sringer-Verlag, Berlin.

Engström, M., Ragnehed, M., Lundberg, P. (2005) Projection screen or video goggle as stimulus modality in functional magnetic resonance imaging. *Magnetic Resonance Imaging, 23*, 695-699.

Erten-Lyons, D., Howieson, D., Moore, M.M., Quinn, J., Sexton, G., Silbert, L,, Kaye, J. (2006). Brain volume loss in MCI predicts dementia. *Neurology* 2006, 66, 233-235.

Fernandez, G., Tendolkar, I. (2002) Imaging cognitive function of the parahippocampal region. In M. Witter and F Wouterlood, eds. *The parahippocampal region.* Oxford University Press. Oxford pp. 255-270.

Garoff, R.J., Slotnick, S.D., Schacter, D.L. (2005). The neural origins of specific and general memory: the role of the fusiform cortex. *Neuropsychologia, 43*, 847-59.

Golby, A.J., Poldrack, R.A., Illes, J., Chen, D., Desmond, J.E., Gabrieli, J.D. (2003). Memory lateralization in medial temporal lobe epilepsy assessed by functional MRI. *Epilepsia, 43*, 855-863.

Golby, A,J., Poldrack, R., Brewer, J.B., Spencer, D., Desmond, J.E., Aron, A.P., Gabrieli, J.D. (2001). Material-specific lateralization in the medial temporal lobe and prefrontal cortex during memory encoding. *Brain, 124*, 1841-1854.

Grossman, M., McMillan, C., Moore, P., Ding, L., Glosser, G., Work, M., Gee, J. (2004) What's a name: voxel-based morphometric analyses of MRI and naming difficulty in Alzheimer's disease, frontotemporal dementia and corticobasal degeneration. *Brain, 127*, 628-649.

Grundman, M., Petersen, R.C., Ferris, S.H., Thomas, R.G., Aisen, P.S., Bennet, D.A., Foster, N.L., Jack, C.R., Galasho, D.R., Dondy, R., Kaye, J., Sano, M., Mohs, R., Gauthier, S., Kim, H.T., Jin, S., Schultz, A.N., Schafer, K., Mulnard, R., van Dyck, C.H., Mintzer, J.,

Zamrini, E.Y., Cahn-Weiner, D., Thal, L.J.; Alzheimer's Disease Cooperative Study. (2004). Mild Cognitive Impairment can be distinguished from Alzheimer disease and normal aging for clinical trials. *Arch Neurol, 61*, 59-66.

Haxby, J.V., Gobbini, M.I., Furey, M.L., Ishai, A., Schouten, J.L., Pietrini, P. (2001). Distributed and overlapping representations of faces and objects in ventral temporal cortex. *Science, 293*, 2425-30.

Hodges, J.R., Salmon, D.P., Butters, N. (1992). Semantic memory impairment in Alzheimer's disease - Failure of access or degraded knowledge. *Neuropsychologia, 30*, 301–314.

Howieson, D.B., Camicioli, R., Quinn, J., Silbert, L.C., Care, B., Moore, M.M., Dame, A., Sexton, G., Kaye, J.A. (2003). Natural history of cognitive decline in the old old. *Neurology, 60*, 1489-1494.

Huettel, S.A., Song, A.W., MCCarthy, G. (2004). *Functional Magnetic Resonante Imaging*. Sinauer Associates Inc., Massachussets, U.S.A.

Iidaka, T., Sadato, N., Yamada, H., Murata, T., Omori, M., Yonekura, Y. (2001). An fMRI study of the functional neuroanatomy of picture encoding in younger and older adults. *Brain Res. Cogn Brain Res, 11*, 1-11.

Jack, C.R. Jr., Petersen, R.C., Xu, Y.C., O'Brien, P.C., Smith, G.E., Ivnik, R.J., Boeve, B.F., Waring, S.C., Tangalos, E.G., Kokmen, E. (1999). Prediction of AD with MRI-based hippocampal volume in mild cognitive impairment. *Neurology, 52*, 1397-1403.

Johnson, S.C., Baxter, L.C., Susskind-Wilder, Connor, D.J., Sabbagh, M.N., Caselli, R.J. (2004), Hippocampal adaptation to face repetition in healthy elderly and mild cognitive impairment. *Neuropsychologia, 42*, 980-989.

Johnson, S.C., Saykin, A.J., Baxter, L.C., Falshman, L.A., Santulli, R.B., McAllister, T.W., Mamourian, A. (2000). The relationship between fMRI activation and cerebral atrophy: comparison of normal aging and Alzheimer disease. *Neuroimage, 11*, 179-187.

Johnson, S.C., Schmitz, T.W., Moritz, C.H., Meyerand, M.E., Rowley, H.A., Alexander, A.L., Hansen, K.W., Gleason, C.E., Carlsson, C.M., Ries, M.L., Asthana, S., Chen, K., Reiman, EM., Alexander, G.E. (2006). Activation of brains regions vulnerable to Alzheimer's disease : The effect of mild cognitivive impairment. *Neurobiology of Aging, 27*, 1604-1612.

Juch, H., Zimine, I., Seghier, M.L., Lazeyras, F., Fsel, J.H. (2005). Anatomical variability of the lateral frontal lobe surface: implications for intersubject variability in language neuroimaging. *NeuroImage, 24*, 504-514.

Kirchhoff, B.A., Wagner, A.D., Maril, A., Stern, C.E. (2000). Prefrontal-temporal circuitry for episodic encoding and subsequent memory. *J Neuroscience, 20*, 6173-6180.

Krishnan, S., Slavin, M.J., Tran, T-TT., Doraiswamy, P.M., Petrella, J.R. (2006). Accuracy of spatial normalization of the hippocampus: Implications for fMRI research in memory disorders. *NeuroImage, 31*, 560-571.

Kuskowski, M.A., Pardo, J.V. (1999). The role of the fusiform gyrus in successful encoding of face stimuli. *Neuroimage, 9*, 599-610.

Laatu, S., Revonsuo, A., Jaykka, H., Portin, R., Rinne, J.O. (2003). Visual object recognition in early Alzheimer's disease: deficits in semantic processing. *Acta Neurol Scand, 108*, 82-9.

Machulda, M.M., Ward, H.A., Borowski, B., Gunter, J.L., Cha, R.H., O'Brien, P.C. (2003). Comparison of memory fMRI response among normal, MCI, and Alzheimer's patients. *Neurology, 61*, 500-506.

Maestu, F., Garcia-Segura, J., Ortiz, T., Montoya, J., Fernandez, A., Gil-Gregorio, P., Campo, P., Fernandez, S., Viano, J., Portera, A. (2005). Evidence of biochemical and biomagnetic interactions in Alzheimer's disease: an MEG and MR spectroscopy study. *Demnt Geriatr Cogn Disord, 20*, 145-152.

Maldjian, J.A., Laurienti, P.J., Burdette, J.B., Kraft, R.A. (2003). An Automated Method for Neuroanatomic and Cytoarchitectonic Atlas-based Interrogation of fMRI Data Sets. *NeuroImage, 19*, 1233-1239.

Maldjian, J.A., Laurienti, P.J., Burdette, J.H. (2004). Precentral Gyrus Discrepancy in Electronic Versions of the Talairach Atlas. *Neuroimage, 21*, 450-455.

Martin, A., Wiggs, C.L., Ungerleider, L.G., & Haxby J.V. (1996). Neural correlates of category-specific knowledge. *Nature*, 1996, 379, 649-652.

Martin, A., Functional Neuroimaging of Semantic Memory. In. R. Cabeza & A. Kingstone (Eds.). *Handbook of Functional Neuroimaging of Cognition.* Cambridge, Massachusetts: The MIT Press; 2000; 153-186.

Brett, M., Antón, J-L., Valabregue, R., Poline J-B. Region of interest analysis using an SPM toolbox [abstract] Presented at the 8th International Conferance on Functional Mapping of the Human Brain, June 2-6, 2002, Sendai, Japam. Available on CD-ROM in NeuroImage, Vol 16, No 2.

McKhann, G., Drachmann, D., Fostein, M., Katzman, R., Price, D., Stadlan, E. (1984). Clinical diagnosis of Alzheimer's disease. Report of the NINCDS-ADRDA Work Group under the auspices of Department of Health and Human Services Task Force on Alzhiemer's disease. *Neurology, 34*, 939-944.

McKhann, G., Drachmann, D., Fostein, M., Katzman, R., Price, D., Stadlan, E. Clinical diagnosis of Alzheimer's disease. Report of the NINCDS-ADRDA Work Group under the auspices of Department of Health and Human Services Task Force on Alzhiemer's disease. *Neurology, 34*, 939-944.

Meyer, J.S., Takshima, S., Terayama, Y., Obara, K., Muramatsu, K., Weathers, S. (1994). CT changes associated with normal aging of the human brain. *J Nerol Sci, 123*, 200-208.

Murtha, S., Chertkow, H., Beauregard, M., Evans, A. (1999). The neural substrate of picture naming. *J Cogn Neurosci, 11*, 399-423.

Oakes, T.R., Fox, S.A., Johnstone, T., Chung, M.K., Kalin, N., Davidson, R.J. (2006). Integrating VBM into the General Linear Model with voxelwise anatomical covariates. *NeuroImage, 34*, 500-508.

Pennanen, C., Kivipelto, M., Tuomainen, S., Hartikainen, T., Laakso, M.P., Hallikainen, M., Bañen, M., Nissinen, A., Helkala, E.L., Vainio, P., Vanninen, R., Partanen, K., Soininen, H. (2004) Hippocampus and entorhinal cortex in mild cognitive impairment and early AD. *Neurobiol Aging, 25*, 303-310.

Petersen, R.C. (2004) Mild cognitive impairment as a diagnostic entity. *J Intern Med, 256*, 183-194.

Petersen, R.C., Smith, G.E., Waring, S.C., Ivnik, R.J., Tangalos, E.G., Kokmen, E. (1999). Mild cognitive impairment: clinical characterization and outcome. *Arch Neurol, 56*, 303-308.

Price, C.J., Devlin, J.T., Moore, C.J., Morton, C., Laird, A.R. (2005). Meta-analyses of object naming: effect of baseline. *Human Brain Mapping, 25*, 70-82.

Rabin, M.L., Narayan, V.M., Kimberg, D.Y., Casasanto, D.J., Glosser, G., Tracy, J.L., French, J.A., Sperling, M.R., Detre, J.A. (2004) Functional MRI predicts post-surgical memory following temporal lobectomy. *Brain, 127*, 2286-2298.

Ranganath, C., Séller, A., Cohen, M.X., Brozinsky, C.J., Rissman, J. (2005) Functional Connectivity with the hippocampus during successful memory formation. *Hippocampus, 15*, 997-1005.

Ries, M.L., Schmitz, T.W., Kawahara, T.N., Torgerson, B.M., Trivedi, M.A., Johnson, S.C. (2006) Task-dependent posterior cingulate activation in mild cognitive impairment. *Neuroimage, 29*, 485-492

Rombouts, S.A.R.B., Barkhof, F., Veltman, D., Machielsen, W., Witter, M., Bierlaagh, M., Lazeron, R., Valk, J., Scheltens, P. (2000) Functional MR imaging in Alzheimer´s disease during memory encoding. *A.J.N.R., 21*, 1869-1875.

Rombouts, S.A.R.B., Scheltens, P., Machielsen, W.C.M., Barkhof, F., Hoogenraad, F.G.C., Veltman, D.J., Valk, J., Witter, M.P. (1999). Parametric FMRI analisis of visual encoding in the human medial temporal lobe. *Hippocampus, 9*, 637-643.

Salat, D.H., Stangl, P.A., Kaye, J.A., Janowsky, J.S. (1999). Sex differences in prefrontal volume with aging and Alzheimer´s disease. *Neurobiol. Aging., 20*, 591-6.

Sanfeliu, M.C., & Fernandez, A. (1996). A set of 254 Snodgrass-Vanderwert pictures standardized for Spanish: Norms for name agreement, image agreement, familiarity, and visual complexity. *Behavior Research Methods, Instruments and Computers, 28*, 537-555.

Sandstrom, C.K., Krishnana, S., Slavin M.M.; Tran, T.-T.T., Doraiswamy P.M., Petrella, J.R. (2006) Hippocampal atrophy confounds template-based functional MR imaging measures of hippocampal activation in patients with mild cognitive impairment. *AJNR, 27*, 1622-1627.

Simons, J.S., Spiers, H.J. (2003) Prefrontal medial temporal lobe interactions in long-term memory. *Nature Rev, 4*, 637-648.

Small, S., Perera, Delapaz, R., Mayeux, R., Stern, Y. (1999) Differential regional dysfunction of the hippocampal formation among elderly with memory decline and Alzheimer´s disease. *Ann Neurol, 45*, 466-472.

Smith, C.D., Andersen, A.H., Kryscio, R.J., Schmitt, F.A., Kindy, M.S. Blonder LX, Avison, M.J. (1999). Altered brain activation in cognitively intact individuals at high risk for Alzheimer´s disease. *Neurology, 53*, 1391-1396.

Snodgrass, J., Vanderwart, M. (1980). Standardized set of 260 pictures: norms of namge agreement, usage agreement, familiarity, and visual complexity. *J Exp Psychol, 6*, 174-215.

Sperling, R., Chua, E., Cocchiarella, A., Rand-Giovannetti, E., Poldrack, R., Schacter, D.L., Albert, M. (2003) Putting names to faces: Successful encoding of associative memories activates the anterior hippocampal formation. *Neuroimage, 20*, 1400-1410.

Sperling, R.A., Bates, J.F., Cocchiarella, A.J., Rentz, D.M., Rosen, B.R., Schacter, D.L., Albert, M.S. (2003). FMRI studies of associative encoding in young and elderly controls and mild Alzheimer´s disease. *J Neurol Neurosurg Psychiatry, 74*, 44-50.

Squire, L.R., Zola-Morgan, S. (1991) The medial temporal lobe memory system. *Science, 253*, 1380-1386.

Talairach, J., Tournoux, P. (1998) *Co-planar stereotaxic atlas of the human brain.* Thieme. Stuttgart.

Tisserand, D.J., Visser, P.J., van Boxel, M.P., Jolles, J. (2000) The relation between gloobal and limbic brain volumes on MRI and cognitive performance in healthy individuals across the age range. *Neurobiology of Aging, 21*, 569-576.

Toga, A.W., Thompson, P.M. (2006). Maps of the brain. *Anat. Rec.265*: 37-53

Ungerleider L, Mishkin M (1982) Object vision and spatial vision: Two cortical pathways. In: *Trends in Neuroscience*. S. 414—417

Wagner, A.D., Schacter, D.L., Rotte, M., Koutstaal, W., Maril, A., Dale, A.M., Rosen, B.R., Buckner, R.L. (1998) Building memories: remembering and forgetting of verbal experiences as predicted by brain activity. *Science, 281*, 1188-1191.

Zakzanis, K.K., Graham, S.J., Campbell, Z. (2003) A meta-analysis of structural and functional brain imaging in dementia of the Alzheimer's type: a neuroimaging profile. *Neuropsychol Rev, 13*, 1-18.

In: Alzheimer's Disease Research Trends
Editor: A.P. Chan, pp. 175-192

ISBN 978-1-60021-712-8

Chapter VIII

PROTECTIVE EFFECT OF VITAMIN C ON OKADAIC ACID-INDUCED OXIDATIVE STRESS AND CYTOSKELETAL ALTERATIONS IN AN *IN VITRO* MODEL SIMILAR TO ALZHEIMER'S DISEASE IN NIE-115 NEUROBLASTOMA CELLS

Isaac Túnez, M. del Carmen Muñoz and Pedro Montilla*

Department of Biochemistry and Biology Molecular, School of Medicine, University of Cordoba, Avda. Menéndez Pidal s/n 10004 – Cordoba, Spain.

ABSTRACT

Oxidative stress (OS) and cytoskeletal changes may be a culprit in neuronal loss in Alzheimer's disease (AD), and that reactive oxygen species (ROS) are involved in the neuronal pathogenesis of this disease, as well as progressive loss of neuronal cytoarchitecture is an event that precedes neural death. Okadaic acid (OA) induces biochemical, physiological and morphological changes similar to AD such as OS, tau hyperphosphorylation, altered cytoskeletal and β-amyloid peptide plaques. Vitamin C is well known as a hydrophilic antioxidant in human cerebrospinal fluid. It is the antioxidant first consumed during the oxidation of plasma and cerebrospinal fluid. In this work we studied the effects of vitamin C on altered cytoskeletal organization and OS induced by OA in N1E-115 neuroblastoma cells. We demonstrated that exposure of cells to 50 nM OA for 2 h induced a reduction in cellular gluthatione transferase (GSH-Tr), glutathione reductase (GSH-Rd) and catalase activities and major axis length. Likewise, this acid prompted an increase in lipid peroxidation products. Treatment of cells with 0.5μg/ml vitamin C partially prevented the effects of OA. The vitamin C effects on

* Correspondence concerning this article should be addressed to Department of Biochemistry and Biology Molecular, School of Medicine, University of Cordoba, Avda. Menéndez Pidal s/n 10004 – Cordoba, Spain. Phone: + 34 957 21 82 68; Fax: + 34 957 21 82 29; E-mail: bb1molop@uco.es; fm2tufii@uco.es.

altered cytoskeletal organization and OS induced by OA were time-dependent, showing its maximum effects when vitamin C was added to the incubation media 2h before OA. These results indicate that OA induces an OS imbalance and cytoskeletal alterations, while vitamin C prevents these changes. Likewise, these data indicate the great importance of OS and the morphological changes in both experimental model and in the development and course of neurodegenerative diseases. These results support the hypothesis that a good level of vitamin C can help to prevent or delay the appearance of neurodegenerative disease; especially AD, as well as they can indicate the participation of vitamin C and micronutrients on oxidative imbalance.

INTRODUCTION

All cells in the body are exposed chronically to oxidants from both endogenous and exogenous sources, but are also equipped with an antioxidant system. The brain tissue is particularly vulnerable to oxidative damage because of a relative lack of antioxidant enzymes like catalase and glutathione peroxidase (GSH-Px) and an abundance of oxidizable substrates such as polyunsaturated fatty acids in neuronal membranes, catecholamines, etc., as well as high oxygen requirements for its metabolism (Halliwell and Gutteridge, 1985; Head et al., 2002; Liu et al., 1996; Floyd and Carney, 1992; Calabrese et al., 2004; Hoyer, 2004; Kang et al., 2004; Montilla et al., 2004; Serrano and Klann, 2004; Túnez et al., 2004a; Túnez et al., 2004b; Warner et al., 2004; Wie and Guo, 2004). Oxidative Stress (OS) has been implicated in various forms of brain damage or altered neuronal functions using in vitro and in vivo models (Morel et al., 1998; Charon et al., 1998; Pocernich et al., 2000; Maier and Chan, 2002; Benítez-King et al., 2003; Túnez et al., 2003). The role played by OS in the genesis of neurodegenerative diseases has been established, and it is widely accepted that OS is an important mechanism of cell death in these disorders including Parkinson's disease (PD), Huntington's disease (HD), Schizophrenia and Alzheimer's disease (AD) (Fariello, 1988; Smith and Perry, 1996; Markesbery, 1997; Christe, 2000; Honda et al., 2004; Mhatre et al., 2004).

AD is the main cause of dementia in elderly people (Luchsinger and Mayeux, 2004). In brain, the pathological signs include deposits of extracellular amyloid-β-peptide (Aβ) in diffuse plaques and in plaques containing elements of degenerating neurons, known as neuritic plaques (Henderson and Finch, 1989; Haass, 1996; Buchet and Pikula, 2000; Dickson et al., 2001; Chauhan, 2003). Intracellular changes include deposits of abnormally hyperphosphorylated tau protein, a microtubule assembly protein, in the form of neurofibrillary tangles, and loss of neurons and synapses is also widespread (Hall et al., 2000; Mukaetova-Ladinska et al., 2000; Mandelkow et al., 2003). Recently, it has been emphasized that OS may be responsible for neuronal loss in AD, and that ROS are involved in the neural pathogenesis of this disease (Olivieri et al., 2000; Pérez et al., 2000; Smith et al., 2000; Zhu et al., 2000). In AD, Aβ has been implicated in OS and free radicals production (Good and Mattson, 1994; McDonald, et al., 1997; Mark et al., 1997; Butterfield et al., 1999; Janciauskiene et al., 1999; Lovell et al., 2003; Smith and Luo, 2003). Furthermore, OS appears to mediate Aβ toxicity by free radicals production, suggesting a pathophysiological link between Aβ, ROS and antioxidative systems (Pappola et al., 1997; Pratico et al., 2001).

Thus, the deposition of Aβ reduces iron and copper concentration in brain tissue, leading to the formation of hydrogen peroxide, OS and neuronal damage (Pappolla et al., 1997).

Under normal conditions, damage by reactive oxygen species (ROS) is kept in check by an efficient array of antioxidant systems that display extensive redundancy. However, in pathological conditions, the oxidants/antioxidant balance is necessarily altered, either primarily or secondarily. Oxidative stress (OS) is the imbalance between oxidants and antioxidants leading to the oxidation of biomolecules including lipids, proteins, carbohydrates and nucleic acids. Several systems operate in a variety of biological compartments to scavenge free radicals and maintain the integrity of lipids, proteins, carbohydrates and nucleic acids. Antioxidants delay or inhibit the oxidation of these molecules (Bastianetto and Quirion, 2004; Schmitt et al., 2004; Willcox et al., 2004). The antioxidant network includes enzymes such as glutathione peroxidase (GSH-Px), superoxide dismutase (SOD) and catalase; and, low molecular weight scavengers such as reduced glutathione (GSH), urate, N-acetyl-5-methoxytryptamine (melatonin) and vitamin C. Water-soluble molecules such as urate, bilirubin, GSH, and vitamin C play greater roles in the aqueous interstitial and intracellular fluid compartments (Reiter et al., 1999; Blokhina et al., 2003).

Vitamin C (ascorbic acid or ascorbate) has been given the name of the antiscorbutic factor, effective against scurvy, a disease that at times reached epidemic proportions in the Middle Ages. In mammals able to synthesize vitamin C, synthesis occurs in the liver from carbohydrates (Chatterjee et al., 1975). In humans, its deficiency is also manifested by body weight loss, general weakness, dyspnoea, heart pain, and palpitations. Following synthesis, vitamin C is distributed in plasma to other tissues where it is transported into cells by sodium dependent uptake.

Ascorbic acid is readily soluble in water, sparingly soluble in ethanol, and practically insoluble in other organic solvents. The structural formulas shown above demonstrate that the most important property of vitamin C is its capacity to be reversibly oxidized to dehydroascorbic acid thereby forming an oxidation-reduction system. Some studies have found that vitamin C is an effective scavenger of reactive oxygen species (ROS) (Rice and Russo-Menna, 1998). Additionally, the evidence indicates vitamin C is the most important antioxidant in plasma (Frei et al., 1989) and it has been shown to minimize ischemic damage in models of cerebral ischemia/reperfusion (Rajan et al., 1993; Henry and Chandy, 1998).

Furthermore, different studies indicate that supplementation with micronutrients (antioxidants) might delay the development of AD. In addition, the brain contains a higher level of vitamin C compared to other tissues (Spector and Eells, 1984). Although generally considered a potent antioxidant, vitamin C in the presence of transition metals can promote oxidative damage to lipids and proteins in purified preparations or crude tissue fractions (Halliwell and Gutteridge, 1989). Data from prospective studies relating intake of antioxidant vitamins with AD are conflicting (Morris et al., 2002; Grodstein et al., 2003).

A recent study carried out by our group shows that vitamin C reduces free radical damage induced by Okadaic acid (OA) in N1E-115 cells, although the reduction was significantly lower than melatonin. Vitamin C treatment significantly reduced the extent of OS. However, vitamin C failed to increase the activity of glutathione transferase (GSH-Tr), and only had a weak effect on catalase activity (Montilla-López et al., 2002).

OA, a diarrhetic shellfish toxin, is a potent promoter of tumours in mouse skin and a specific inhibitor of serine/threonine protein phosphatases 1 (PP1) and 2A (PP2A) (Biolajan and Takai, 1988). This acid has become a useful tool in studying the mechanisms of protein phosphorylation and dephosphorylation. Its administration triggers molecular and structural changes similar to those seen in AD. In PC12 cells (Chiou and Westhead, 1992), neuroblastoma cells (Dupont-Wallois et al., 1995) and primary cultured neurons (Arias et al., 1993) OA induces a cytoskeletal alteration and tau hyperphosphorylation, and when injected into rats, paired helical filaments and Aβ plaques in the hippocampus (Lee et al., 2000). Furthermore, apoptosis and OS have been reported after administration of OA (Chen et al., 2000; Traore et al., 2000).

In the present study, the possible protective effect of vitamin C on OA-induced cytoskeletal alterations and OS in murine neuroblastoma N1E-115 cells was evaluated. The effects of vitamin C on cytoskeletal organization were assessed both by measuring the major axis cell length and by morphology, Coomassie blue staining. OS was determined by levels of lipid peroxidation products, GSH content and enzymatic activities (glutathione transferase, GSH-Tr; glutathione reductase, GSH-Rd and catalase). The results showed that in N1E-115 neuroblastoma, vitamin C partially prevented the changes caused by the phosphatase inhibitor OA. Our data suggest that vitamin C could be a potential therapeutic agent in the treatment of neurodegenerative diseases.

MATERIALS AND METRHODS

Materials

Murine neuroblastoma N1E-115 cells were pruchased from ECACC, the European Collection of Cell Cultures (Porton Down, Salisbury, UK). Culture media, foetal bovine serum, horse serum and antibiotics were purchased from Gibco/BRL (Gaithersburgm MD, USA). Okadaic acid, vitamin C, dimethylsulfoxide (DMSO) and all other chemicals were purchased from Sigma (St. Louis, MO, USA).

Cell Culture

Murine neuroblastoma cells were cultured in Dulbecco's modified Eagle's medium (DMEM) supplemented with 10% foetal bovine serum, 5% horse serum, 100 IU/ml penicillin, 100 mg/ml streptomycin, at 37° C in a 5% CO2 atmosphere for 48 h.

Experimental Design

N1E-115 cells were seed into 35-mm Petri dishes or glass coverslips (18 x 18 mm) at a seeding low density 200,000 cells/mm^2. Forty-four hours after, they were incubated with a final concentation of 50 nM of OA (in 0.1 % DMSO) for 2 h or vehicle. In some experiments, cells were treated with a final concentration of 0.5 μg/ml vitamin C (in saline solution). The vitamin was added (1) 2 h before treating with OA, (2) simultaneously, or (3) 1 h and 45 min after treatment with OA. In all experimental groups, incubation with OA lasted for 2 h.

Light Microscopy

After incubation, cells were washes twice with phosphate buffered saline (PBS: 0.128 M NaCl, 0.010 M Na_2HPO_4, 0.005 M KH_2PO_4, pH 7.2) and fixed for 20 min with methanol at -20° C. Fixed cells were stained with 0.02% Coomassied blue according to Mochizuki and Furukawa (1987). Cells were observed with a Zeiss Axioskop2 microscope equipped with a CCD digital camera. Major cell length axes (as an index of cytoskeletal organization) were measured and cell images processed with the Zeiss Axio Vision software. In all, five cells were measured in for randomized fields per coverslip. Six individual experiments were performed.

Lipid Peroxidation Products

Cells were homogenized with Virtis stirrer in ice cold 20 mM Tris-HCl buffer (pH 7.4). The homogenates were then centrifuged at 10,000 x g for 10 min at 4° C. The supernatant was collected and immediately tested for lipid peroxidation products using the Bioxytech LPO-586 kit (OXIS International, Portland, USA). The kit uses a chromatogenic reagent which reacts with the lipid peroxidation products malondialdehyde and 4-hydroxyalkenals at 45 ± 1°C, yielding a stable chromophore with maximum absorbance 586 nm.

Protein concentration was determined by the Bradford method (1976) using bovine serum albumin as a standard.

Reduced Glutathione Content

Reduced glutathione (gamma-glutamylcysteinglycine or GSH) content was determined in aliquots of cell homogenates. GSH content was carried out using Bioxytech GSH-400 kit (OXIS International, Portland, USA). The method is based on a chemical reaction which proceeds in two steps, obtaining with GSH a chromophoric thione which has a maximal absorbance wavelength at 400 nm.

Protein concentration was determined by the Bradford method (1976) using bovine serum albumin as a standard.

Activity of Antioxidative Enzymes

The activities of glutathione transferase (GSH-Tr) and glutathione reductase (GSH-Rd) were estimated in cell homogenates. The GSH-Tr and GSH-Rd activities were evaluated using the technique described by Jaskot et al. (1983). The glutathione reductase assay cells were homogenized with a Virtis stirrer in ice-cold buffer (0.1M KH_2PO_4/K_2HPO_4, pH 7.0, plus 29.2 mg ethylenediaminetetraacetic acid (EDTA) in 100 ml of distilled water and 10.0 mg digitonin in 100 ml of distilled water, final volume, 2000 ml) to produce a homogenate. The homogenates were then centrifuged at 10,000 x g for 10 min at 4° C. The glutathione transferase assay is based upon the glutathione transferase-catalyzed reaction between CDNB and reduced glutathione, with maximum absorbance at 340 nm, while the glutathione reductase assay is based on the oxidation of NADPH to NAD+, catalyzed by a limiting concentration of glutathione reductase, with maximum absorbance at 340nm.

Catalase was measured in the cell cytosol fraction. Catalase was assayed following Aebi (1984), by the rate of decomposition for H_2O_2 at 240 nm. Cells were homogenized with Virtis stirrer in ice-cold phosphate buffer (6.81 g KH_2PO_4 in water, made up to 1000 ml). The homogenates were then centrifuged at 1,000 x g for 10 min at room temperature. H_2O_2 (10 mM) was used as reagent, with the rate of dismutation of H_2O_2 to water and molecular oxygen being proportional to the concentration of catalase and with maximum absorbance at 240 nm.

Protein concentration was determined by the Bradford method (1976) using bovine serum albumin as a standard.

Statistical Analysis

Data were analyzed using one-way analysis of variance (ANOVA) for repeated measures followed by the Bonferroni correction for multiple comparisons, which was provided by SPSS 11.0 statistical software. Results are expressed as means ± S.E.M. The level of statistical significance was set at $P < 0.05$.

RESULTS

Cellular Morphology and Major Axis Length

In the presence of the vehicle, cytoskeletons stained with Coomassie blue and were observed as a network distributed throughout the cytoplasm (Figure 2A). Also, Coomassiestaining allowed the cellular morphology to be defined as an elongated shape (Figure 2A). Incubation of neuroblastoma N1E-115 cells with OA for 2 h resulted in morphologic changes, characterized by a cytoskeletal retraction toward the nucleus, changing the morphology from an elongated to a rounded shape (Figure 2B), as well as by a reduction in the major axis length of these cells (270.77 ± 14.97 μm in the vehicle group vs. 67.90 ± 3.87 μm in the OA group, $P < 0.001$) (Figure 1).

The effect of OA was partially prevented when N1E-115 cells were treated with vitamin C 2 h before OA incubation (Figure 2C) and the length of major cell axis was of 103.43 ± 10.53 μm (Figure 1). Nevertheless, neither the cellular morphology nor the length of major cell axis were modified when neuroblastoma were incubated with vitamin C simultaneously or after OA addition (Figure 1).

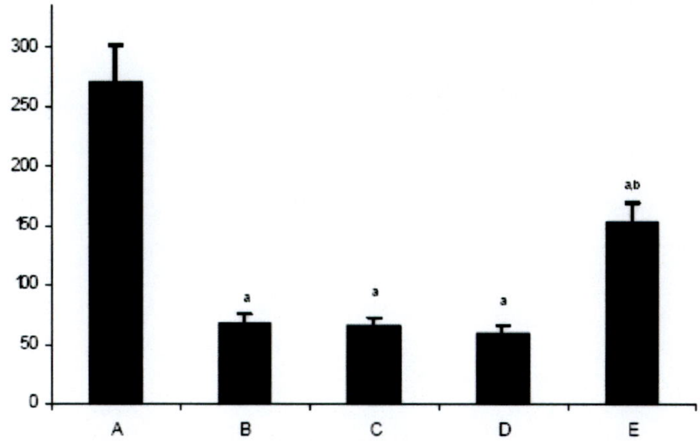

Figure 1. Effects of various time intervals of vitamin C incubation on cytoskeletal changes elicited by OA. N1E-115 neuroblastoma were incubated for various times with 0.5 μg/ml vitamin C and 50 nM OA as follows: vehicle (A), OA for 2 h (B), 50 nM OA for 1 h and 45 min and treated for 15 min with 0.5 μg/ml vitamin C (C), 0.5 μg/mg vitamin C + 50 nM OA for 2 h (D) or 0.5μg/ml vitamin C for 2 h before treatment of 2 h with 50 nM OA (E). Results represent the mean ± S.E.M. of six individual experiments and are expresse as micrometers (μm). [a]P< 0.001 vs vehicle group; [b]P< 0.001 vs OA group.

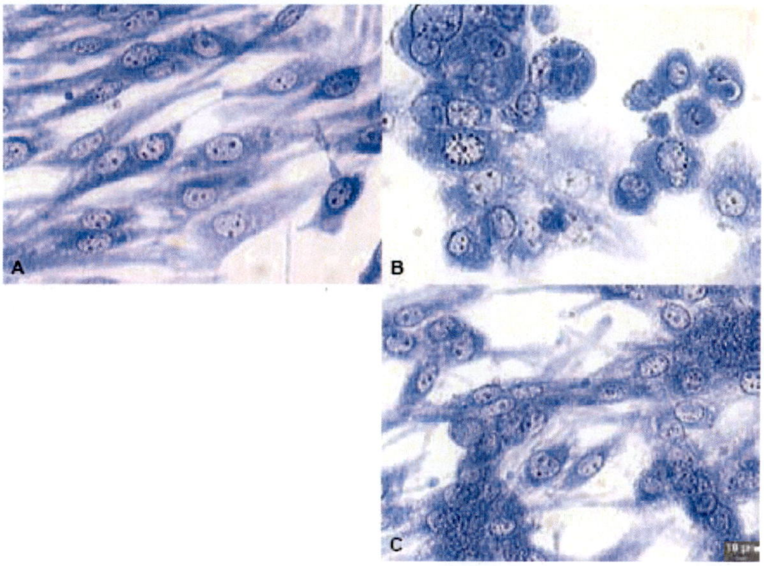

Figure 2. Effect of vitamin C on cytoskeletal rearrangements elicited by OA in N1E-115 cells grown on glass coverslips were treated for 2 h with (A) vehicle, (B) 50 nM OA, and (C) 0.5 mg/ml vitamin C for 2 h before treatment of 2 h with 50 nM. Photomicrographs represents results obtained in six individual experiments. Bar = 10 μm.

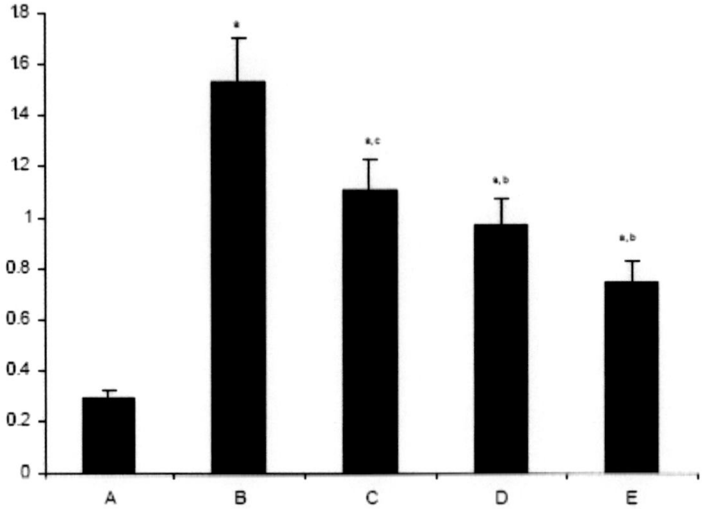

Figure 3. Vitamin C effect on lipid peroxiation products (malondialdehyde + 4-hydroxyalkenals) induced by OA in neuroblatoma. N1E-115 cells were incubated for various times with 0.5 μg/ml vitamin C and 50 nM OA as follows: vehicle (A), OA for 2 h (B), 50 nM OA for 1 h and 45 min and treated for 15 min with 0.5 μg/ml vitamin C (C), 0.5 μg/mg vitamin C + 50 nM OA for 2 h (D) or 0.5μg/ml vitamin C for 2 h before treatment of 2 h with 50 nM OA (E). Results represent the mean ± S.E.M. of six individual experiments and are expresse as nanomoles per milligram of protein (mM/mg protein). $^{a}P < 0.001$ vs vehicle group; $^{b}P < 0.001$ vs OA group; $^{c}P < 0.01$ vs OA group.

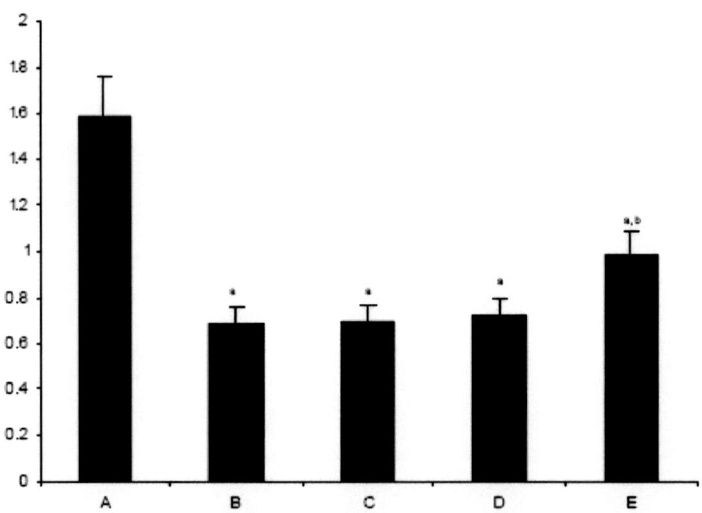

Figure 4. Vitamin C effect on GSH content induced by OA in neuroblatoma. N1E-115 cells were incubated for various times with 0.5 μg/ml vitamin C and 50 nM OA as follows: vehicle (A), OA for 2 h (B), 50 nM OA for 1 h and 45 min and treated for 15 min with 0.5 μg/ml vitamin C (C), 0.5 μg/mg vitamin C + 50 nM OA for 2 h (D) or 0.5μg/ml vitamin C for 2 h before treatment of 2 h with 50 nM OA (E). Results represent the mean ± S.E.M. of six individual experiments and are expresse as nanomoles per milligram of protein (mM/mg protein). $^{a}P < 0.001$ vs vehicle group; $^{b}P < 0.01$ vs OA group.

Lipid Peroxidation Levels and GSH Content

OA induced cytotoxicity at the 50 nM dose. This dose induced consistently a 427.59% increase in lipid peroxidation (MDA+4-HDA) (Figure 3). The effect of OA was partially prevented when N1E-115 cells were treated with vitamin C 2 h before OA incubation (1.53 ± 0.11 nmol/mg protein in the OA group vs 0.75 ± 0.08 nmol/mg protein in the cells treated with vitamin C 2 h before OA incubation; P< 0.01) (Figure 3). Vitamin C added simultaneously or after OA incubation was less effective in diminishing lipid peroxidation levels (Figure 3).

In addition, the GSH measurements showed that OA induced a 57.23% reduction in levels of this molecule (Figure 4). Pre-administration of melatonin protected the cells from the deleterious effect of OA (0.68 ± 0.06 nmol/mg protein in the OA group vs 0.98 ± 0.03 nmol/mg protein in the cells treated with vitamin C 2 h before OA incubation; P< 0.01) (Figure 4), while the changes induced by OA were not reversed when vitamin C was added together with or after OA (Figure 2).

Antioxidative Enzymes Activities

OA caused a reduction in catalase activity (P <0.001 as compared with vehicle) (Table 1). Similarly, GSH-Tr and GSH-Rd activities were reduced in the N1E-115 cells of OA-treated cells (P< 0.01; Table 3). The effect of OA was completely prevented when N1E-115 cells were treated with vitamin C 2 h before OA incubation (P< 0.001) (Table 1). Nevertheless, catalase activity was partially reversed in both cells treated simultaneously with vitamin C and OA (P< 0.01) as well as in cells treated with melatonin after OA (P< 0.05) (Table 1). Furthermore, neither GSG-Rd activity nor GSH-Tr activity were modified when neuroblastoma were incubated with vitamin C before, simultaneously or after OA addition (Table 1).

Discussion

Reactive oxygen species are closely involved in several diseases of the nervous system including Parkinson's disease, Alzheimer's disease, and Schizophrenia (Smythies, 1999). Ascorbic acid is an essential water-soluble antioxidant that has been shown to be an effective scavenger of free radicals and is particularly effective as a plasma antioxidant (Frei et al., 1989).

In this study, we observed that: (i) OA (50 nM) induced a drop in GSH concentration, an increase in lipid peroxidation levels, and reductions in key antioxidative enzymes in neuroblastoma N1E-115 cells; (ii) this cytotoxin triggered cytoskeletal disorganization and morphological changes; (iii) vitamin C had a time-dependent protective effect against the changes induced by OA, so that this micronutrient prevented the OA effects but did not reverse them. Likewise, the collected data indicate the important role of oxidative stress in this experimental model and possibly in the evolution of neurodegenerative diseases and ageing, and supports the hypothesis that vitamin C can act as a scavenger.

Table 1. Effect of various time intervals of vitamin C incubation on enzimatic activities changes elicited by OA. N1E-115 cells were incubated for various times with 0.5 μg/ml vitamin C (Vit C) and 50 nM OA as follows: vehicle, OA for 2 h (OA), 50 nM OA for 1 h and 45 min and treated for 15 min with 0.5 μg/ml vitamin C (OA (105 min)+Vit C (15min), 0.5 μg/mg vitamin C + 50 nM OA for 2 h (OA+Vit C) or 0.5μg/ml vitamin C for 2 h before treatment of 2 h with 50 nM OA (Vit C (- 2h)+OA)

	GSH-Tr (U/mg Protein)	GSH-Rd (U/mg protein)	Catalase (U/mg protein) x 100
Vehícle	0.017 ± 0.002	0.027 ± 0.003	0.025 ± 0.0002
OA	0.013 ± 0.005[b]	0.020 ± 0.004[b]	0.002 ± 0.0001[a]
OA (105 min)+Vit C (15 min)	0.012 ± 0.004	0.002 ± 0.004	0.009 ± 0.0005[d,e]
OA+Vit C	0.012 ± 0.005	0.023 ± 0.004	0.013 ± 0.0004[c,e]
Vit. C (-2h)+OA	0.013 ± 0.004	0.023 ± 0.003	0.024 ± 0.0006[c]

Results represent the mean ± S.E.M. of six individual experiments and are expresse as units per milligram of protein (U/mg protein). [a]*P*< 0.001 vs vehicle group; [b]*P*< 0.01 vs vehicle group; [c]*P*< 0.01 vs OA group; [d]*P*< 0.05 vs OA group; [e]*P*< 0.001 vs Vit. C (-2h)+OA group.

In the present study we found that OA caused oxidative stress and cellular damage similar to other models induced by OA (Arias et al., 1993; Mattson et al., 1997; Arendt et al., 1998; Lee et al., 2000; Creppy et al., 2002; Montilla-López et al., 2002; Pérez et al., 2002; Benítez-King et al., Gong et al., 2003; Túnez et al., 2003). OA is a cell-permeable and specific phosphate 1 and 2A inhibitor (Bialojan and Takai, 1998). This compound has been a useful tool for studying the mechanisms involved in neurodegenerative diseases (Dounay and Forsyth, 2002; Fernández et al., 2002; Holmes et al., 2002; McCluskey et al., 2002). The results presented here support the hypothesis of the suitability of this model to study changes similar to those that occur in neurodegenerative diseases, especially those that involve oxidative stress, morphologic and cytoskeletal alterations, and cellular death, together with the mechanisms of phosphorylation/dephosphorylation (a key mechanism for regulating the biological activity of many human proteins that affect a diverse array of cellular processes, including protein-protein interactions, gene transcription, cell-cycle progression and apoptosis).

So far the evidence indicates that vitamin C prevented free radical damage and partially prevented the changes in cellular morphology and cytoskeletal disorganization. However, vitamin C failed to increase the activity of glutathione transferase and glutathione reductase and only had a significant and time-dependent effect on catalase activity. The increase in this enzyme activity was significantly greater in the group where the vitamin was added 2 h before treating with OA.

These results are in line with other reports from both our group (Montilla-López et al., 2002) and others (van der Loo et al., 2003, Grant et al., 2004; Rodríguez-Martínez et al., 2004), who found that the vitamin C protects against oxidative damage. Thus, van der Loo et al. (2003) demonstrated a drop in vitamin C plasma levels between young and old animals as well as in the heart, liver, kidney, lungs and skeletal muscle. In addition, vitamin C reduction in the heart tissue was associated with increases in lipid peroxidation levels. Furthermore, Grant's group found that ascorbate induces expression of brain-derived neurotrophic factor in SH-SY5Y neuroblastoma after peroxide insult, which is associated with increased survival and decreased oxidative stress; these effects of vitamin C were dose-dependent (Grant et al., 2004). Moreover, Rodríguez-Martínez's group showed that vitamin C partially protected from oxidative damage induced by 3-nitropropionic acid (Rodríguez-Martínez et al., 2004). Additionally, a study of our group showed that vitamin C had a dose-dependent protective effect against the oxidative stress induced by OA in neuroblastoma N1E-115 cells (Montilla-López et al., 2002). This protective effect was characterized by a reduction in the marking parameters of oxidative stress (lipid peroxidation levels and GSH depletion), while vitamin C failed to increase the activity of glutathione transferase and glutathione reductase, and only had a weak effect on catalase activity.

Nevertheless, other authors have shown that the administration of vitamin C may result in increased lipid peroxidation products. Although generally considered a potent antioxidant, ascorbate in the presence of transition metals can promote oxidative damage to lipids and proteins in purified preparations or crude tissue fractions in several different ways (Levine, 1983; Chakraborty et al., 2001). Thus, ascorbate may stimulate lipid peroxidation in brain membrane fractions in combination with iron via the Fenton reaction (Halliwell and Gutteridge, 1989; Buettner and Jurkiewicz, 1996; Dean et al., 1997). Therefore, vitamin C may either enhance oxidative stress or protect against oxidative damage, and the effect depends on the target organ, experimental model, animal strain and age, and the temporal administration regime, as we can deduce from the data in the bibliography.

Moreover, in clinical trials it has been reported that supplementation with antioxidative micronutrients may delay the development of Alzheimer's disease (Sano et al., 1997; Zhang et al., 2002; Luchsinger and Mayeux, 2004). The antioxidative efficacy of α-tocopherol can be considerably increased by co-supplementation with vitamin C (Kontush et al., 2001; Zhang et al., 2002; Zandi et al., 2004). Likewise, different studies show that there is a decrease in vitamin C levels in Alzheimer's disease and Parkinson's disease (Paraskevas et al., 2003; Quinn et al., 2003; Rinaldi et al., 2003). In addition, the results presented by other authors suggested that the use of vitamin C supplements might lower the risk of Alzheimer's disease (Morris et al., 1998; Zaidi and Banu, 2004). Our results are consistent with these data and support the hypothesis that oxygen free radicals and oxidative stress may be the main cause of damage in neurodegenerative disease, especially Alzheimer's disease. The data presented here show that vitamin C provided effective protection but did not reverse the effects induced by OA.

Following on from this, it is possible that different mechanisms are involved in the protective effect of vitamin C against oxidative stress. Thus, we suggest that: (i) vitamin C acts as a free radical scavenger; and (ii) vitamin C enhances the antioxidative efficacy of α-tocopherol and other molecules such as GSH.

In summary, our study proves that: (i) OA induces both oxidative stress, changes in cellular morphologic and cytoskeletal alterations; (ii) vitamin C decreased levels of lipid peroxides and increased the GSH content and catalase activity when N1E-115 cells were treated with vitamin C 2 h before OA incubation. These data indicate that vitamin C has a beneficial effect. However, further investigations are still needed to confirm the role played by vitamin C in neurodegenerative diseases, as well as to clarify its mechanisms.

References

Aebi, H. (1984). Catalase in vitro. *Methods Enzymol, 105*, 121 – 126.

Arias, C., Sharma, N, Davies, P., and Shaftif-Zagardo, B. (1993). Okadaic acid induces early changes in microtubule-associated protein 2 and tau phosphorylation prior to neurodegeneration in cultured cortical neurons. *J Neurochem, 61*, 673 – 683.

Arendt, T., Holzer, M., Brückner, M.K., Janke, C., and Gätner, U. (1998). The use of okadaic acid in vivo and the induction of molecular changes typical for Alzheimer's disease. *Neuroscience, 85*, 1337 – 1340.

Bastianetto, S., and Quirino, R. (2004). Natural antioxidants and neurodegenerative diseases. *Font Biosci, 9*, 3447 – 3452.

Benítez-King, G., Túnez, I., Bellón, A., Ortiz, G.G., and Antón-Tay, F. (2003). Melatonin prevents cytoskeletal alterations and oxidtive stress induced by okadaic acid in N1E-115 cells. *Exp Neurol, 182*, 151 – 159.

Biolajan, C., and Takai, A. (1988). Inhibitory effect of a marine-sponge toxin, okadaic acid, on protein phosphatases: specifity and kinetics. *Biochem J, 256*, 283 – 290.

Blokhina, O., Virolainen, E., and Fagerstedt, K.V. (2003). Antioxidants, oxidative damage and oxygen deprivation stress: a review. *Ann Bot, 91*, 179 – 194.

Bradford, M.M. (1976). A rapid and sensitive method for the quantitation of microgram quantities of protein utilizing the principle of protein-dye binding. *Ann Biochem, 72*, 248 – 254.

Buchet, R., and Pikula, S. (2000). Alzheimer's disease: its origin at the membrane, evidence and questions. *Acta Biochem Pol, 47*, 725 – 733.

Buettner, G.R., and Jurkiewicz, B.A. (1996). Catalytic metals, ascorbate and free radicals: combinations to avoid. *Radiat Res, 145*, 432 – 541.

Butterfield, D.A., Koppal, T., Subramanian, R., and Yatin, S. (1999). Vitamin E as an antioxidant/free radical scavenger against amyloid β-peptide-induced oxidative stress in neocortical synaptosomal membranes and hippocampal neurons in culture: insights into Alzheimer's disease. *Rev Neurosci, 10*, 141 – 149.

Calabrese, V., Boyd-Kimball, D., Scapagnini. G., and Butterfield, D.A. (2004). Nitric oxide and cellular stress response in brain aging and neurodegenerative disorders: the role of vitagens. *In Vivo, 18*, 245 – 267.

Creppy, E.E., Traore, A., Baudrimont, I., Cascante, M., and Carratu, M.R. (2002). Recent advances in the effects induced by phycotoxin okadaic acid. *Toxicology, 181-182*, 433 – 439.

Chakraborty, H., Ray, S.N., and Chakrabarti, S. (2001). Lipid peroxidation associated protein damage in rat brain crude synaptosomal fraction mediated by iron and ascorbate. *Neurochem Int, 39*, 311 – 317.

Charon, I., Zuin-Kornmann, G., Bataille, S., and Schorderet, M. (1998). Protective effect of neutrophic factors, neuropoictic cytokenes and dibutyryl cyclic AMP on hydrogen peroxide induced cytotoxicity on PC12 cells: a possible link sith the state of differentiation. *Neurochem Int*, *33*, 503 – 511.

Chatterjee, I.B., Majumder, A.K., and Nandi, B.K. (1975). Synthesis and some major functions of vitamin C in animals. *Ann N Acad Sci*, *258*, 24 – 47.

Chauhan, N.B. (2003). Membrane dynamics, cholesterol homeostasis, and Alzheimer's disease. *J Lipid Res*, *44*, 2019 – 2029.

Chen, K.D., Lai, M.T., Cho, J.H., Chen, L.Y., and Lai, Y.K. (2000). Activation on p38 mitogen-actived protein kinase and mitochondrial Ca(2+)-mediated oxidative stress are essential for the enhanced expression of grp78 induced by the protein phosphatase inhibitors okadaic acid and calyculin A. *J Cell Biochem*, *76*, 585 – 595.

Chiou. J.Y., and Westhead, E.W. (1992) Okadaic acid, a protein phosphate inhibitor, inhibits never grosth factor-directed neurite outgrowth in PC12 cells. *J Neurochem*, *59*, 1963 – 1966.

Christen, Y. (2000). Oxidtive stress and Alzheimer's disease. *Am J Clin Nutr*, *71*, 621 – S629.

Dean, R.T., Fu, S., Stocker, R., and Davies, M.J. (1997). Biochemistry and pathology of radical-mediated protein oxidation. *Biochem J*, *324*, 1 – 18.

Dickson, T.C., and Vickers J.C. (2001). The morphological phenotype of beta-amyloid plaques and associated neuritic changes in Alzheimer's disease. *Neuroscience*, *105*, 99 – 107.

Dounay, A.B., and Forsyth, C.J. (2002). Okadaic acid: the archetypal serine/threonine protein phosphatase inhibitor. *Curr Med Chem*, *9*, 1939 – 1980.

Dupont-Wallois, L., Sautiere, P.E., Cocquerelle, C., Bailleul, B., Delacourte, A., and Caillet Boudin, M.L. (1995). Shift from fetal-type to Alzheimer-type phosphorylated tau proteins in SKNSH-SY 5Y cells treated with okadaic acid. *FEBS Lett*, *357*, 197 – 201.

Fariello, R.G. (1988). Experimental support for the implication of oxidative stress in the genesis of parkinsonian syndromes. *Funct Neurol*, *3*, 407 – 412.

Fernández, J.J., Candenas, M.L., Souto, M.L., Trujillo, M.M., and Norte, M. (2002). Okadaic acid, useful tool for studying cellular processes. *Curr Med Chem*, *9*, 229 – 262.

Floyd, R.A., and Carney, J.M. (1992). Free radiucal damage to protein and DNA: mechanism involved and relevant observation on brain undergoing oxidative stress. *Ann Neurol*, *32*, S22 – S27.

Frei, B., England, L., and Ames, B.N. (1989). Ascorbate is an outstanding antioxidant in human blood plasma. *Proc Natl Acad Sci USA*, *86*, 6377 – 6381.

Gong, C.X., Wang, J.Z., Iqbal, K., and Grundke-Iqbal, I. (2003) Inhibition of protein phosphatase 2A induced phosphorylation and accumulation of neurfilaments in metabolically active rat brain slices. *Neurosci Lett*, *34*, 107 – 110.

Goodman, Y., and Mattson, M.P. (1994). Secreted forms of beta-amyloid precursor protein protect hippocampal neurons against amyloid beta-peptide-induced oxidative injury. *Exp Neurol*, *128*, 1 – 12.

Grant, M.M., Barber, V.S., and Griffiths, H.R. (2005). The presence of ascorbate induces expression of brain derived neurotrophic factor in SH-SY5Y neuroblastoma cells after peroxide insult, which is associated with increased survival. *Proteomics*, *5*, 534 – 540.

Grodstein, F., Chen, J., and Willet, W.C. (2003). High-dose antioxidant supplements and cognitive function in community.dwelling early women. *Am J Clin Nutr*, *77*, 975 – 984.

Halliwell, B., and Gutteridge, J.M.C. (1985). Oxygen radical and the nervous system. *Trends Neurosci*, *8*, 22 – 26.

Halliwell, B., and Gutteridge, J.M.C. (1989). *Free radicals in biology and medicine*. Clarendon Press, Oxford.

Haass, C. (1996). The molecular significance of amyloid beta-peptide for Alzheimer's disease. *Eur Arch Psychiatry Clin Neurosci*, *24*, 118 – 123.

Hall, G.F., Chu, B., Lee, G., and Yao, J. (2000). Human tau filaments induce microtubule and synapse loss in an in vivo model of neurofibrillary degenerative disease. *J Cell Sci*, *113*, 1373 – 1387.

Halliwell, B., and Gutteridge, J.M.C. (1989). *Free radicals in Biology and Medicine*. Clarendon Press, Oxford.

Head, E., Liu, J., Hagen, T.M., Muggenburg, B.A., Milgram, N.W., Ames, B.N., and Cotman, C.W. (2002). Oxidative damage increases with age in a canine model of human brain aging. *J Neurochem*, *82*, 375 – 381.

Henderson, V.W., and Finch, C.E. (1989). The neurobiology of Alzheimer's disease. *J Neurosurg*, *70*, 335 – 353.

Henry, P.T., and Chandy, M.J. (1998). Effect of ascorbic acid on infarct size in experimental focal cerebral ischaemia and reperfusion in a primate model. *Acta Neurochir*, *140*, 977 – 980.

Holmes, C.F., Maynes, J.T., Perrault, K.R., Dawson, J.F., and James, M.N. (2002). Molecular enzymology underluing regulation of protein phosphatase-1 by natural toxins. *Curr Med Chem*, *9*, 1981 – 1989.

Honda, K., Casadesus, G., Petersen, R.B., Perry, G., and Smith, M.A. (2004). Oxidative stress and redox-active iron in Alzheimer's disease. *Ann N Y Acad Sci*, *1012*, 179 – 182.

Hoyer, S. (2004). Causes and consequences of disturbances of cerebral glucose metabolism in sporadic Alzheimer disease: therapeutic implications. *Adv Exp Med Biol*, *541*, 135 – 152.

Janciauskiene, S., Wright, H.T., and Lindgren, S. (1999). Fibrillar Alzheimer's amyloid peptide Abeta(1-42) stimulates low density lipoprotein binding and cell association, free radical production and cell cytotoxicity in PC12 cells. *Neuropeptides*, *33*, 510 – 516.

Jaskot, R.H., Charlet, E.G., Grose, E.C., Grady, M.A., and Roycroft, J.H. (1983). An automated analysis of glutathione peroxidase, S-transferase and reductase activity in animal tissue. *J Anal Toxicol*, *7,* 86 – 88.

Kang, J.K., Sul, D., Kang, J.K., Nam, S.Y., Kim, H.J., and Lee, E. (2004). Effects of lead exposure on the expression of phospholipid hydroperoxidase glutathione peroxidase mRNA in the rat brain. *Toxicol Sci*, *82*, 228 – 236.

Kontush, A., Mann, U., Arlt, S., Ujeyl, A., Lührs, Ch., Müller-Thamsen, T., and Beisiegel, U. (2001). Influence of vitamin E and C supplementation on lipoprotein oxidation in patients with Alzheimer's disease: noticeable differences in the lipid peroxidation level and in antioxidant defense. *Neurochem Res*, *26*, 353 – 361.

Lee, J., Hong, H., Im, J., Byun, H., and Kim, D. (2000). The formation of PHF-1 and SMI-31 positive dystrophic neurites in rat hippocampues following acute injection of okadaic acid. *Neurosci Lett*, *282*, 49 – 52.

Levine, R.L. (1983). Oxidative modification of glutamine synthase II. Characterisation of the ascorbate model system. *J Biol Chem*, *258*, 11828 – 11833.

Liu, J., Wang, X., Shigenga, M.K., Yoo, H.C., Mori, A., and Ames. B.S. (1996). Immobilization stress causes oxidtive damage to lipid protein and DNA in the brain of rats. *FASEB J*, *10*, 1532 – 1538.

Lovell, M.A., Xie, C., Xiong, S., and Markesbery, W.R. (2003). Protection against amyloid beta peptide and iron/hydrogen peroxide toxicity by alpha lipoic acid. *J Alzheimer Dis*, *5*, 229 – 239.

Luchsinger, J.A., and Mayeux, R., (2004) Dietary factors and Alzheimer's disease. *The Lancet*, *3*, 579 – 587.

Maier, C.M., and Chan, P.H. (2002). Role of superoxide dismutases in oxidative damage and neurodegenerative disorders. *Neuroscientist*, *8*, 323 – 334.

Mandelkow, E.M., Stamer, K., Vogel, R., Thies, E., and Mandelkow, E. (2003). Clogging of axons by tau, inhibition of axonal traffic and starvation of synapses. *Neurobiol Aging*, *24*, 1079 – 1085.

Mark, R.J., Lovell, M.A., Markesbery, W.R., Uchida, K., and Mattson, M.P. (1997). A role for 4-hydroxynonenal, an aldehydic product of lipid peroxidation, in disruption of ion homeostasis and neuronal death induced by amyloid beta-peptide. *J Neurochem*, *68*, 255 – 264.

Mattson, M.P., Fu, W., Waeg, G., and Uchida, K. (1997). 4-Hydroxynonenal, a product of lipid peroxidation, inhibits dephosphorylation of the microtubule-associated protein tau. *Neuroreport*, *8*, 2275 – 2281.

McCluskey, A., Sim, A.T., and Sakoff, J.A. (2002). Serine-threonine protein phosphatase inhibitors: development of potential therapeutic strategies. *J Med Chem*, *45*, 1151 – 1175.

McDonald, D.R., Brunden, K.R., and Landreth, G.E. (1997). Amyloid fibrils activate tyrosine kinase-dependent signaling and superoxide production in microglia. *J Neurosci*, *17*, 2284 – 2294.

Mhatre, M., Floyd, R.A., and Hensley, K. (2004). Oxidative stress and neuroinflammation in Alzheimer's disease and amyotrophic lateral sclerosis: common links and potential therapeutic targets. *J Alzheimer's Dis*, *6*, 147 – 157.

Mochizuki, Y., and Furukawa, F. (1987) Application of Coomassie brilliant blue staining to cultured hepatocytes. *Cell Biol Int Rep*, *11*, 367 – 371.

Montilla-López, P., Muñoz de Águeda, M.C., Feijóo-López, F., Muñoz-Castañeda, J.R., Bujalance-Arenas, I., and Túnez-Fiñana, I. (2002). Comparison of melatonin versus vitamin C on oxidtive stress and antioxidant enzyme activity in Alzheimer's disease induced by okadaic acid in neuroblastoma cells. *Eur J Pharmacol*, *451*, 237 – 243.

Montilla, P., Túnez, I., Muñoz, M.C., Salcedo, M., Feijóo, M., Muñoz-Castañeda, J.R., and Bujalance, I. (2004). Effect of glucocorticoids on 3-nitropropionic acid-induced oxidative stress in synaptosome. *Eur J Pharmacol*, *488*, 19 – 25.

Morel, P., Tallineau, C., Pontcharraud, R., Piriou, A. and Huguet, F. (1998). Effects of 4-hydroxynonenal, a lipid peroxidtion product, on dopamine transport and Na+/K+ ATPase in rat striatal synaptosomes. *Neurochm Int*, *33*, 531 – 540.

Morris, M.C., Beckett, L.A., Scherr, P.A., Hebert, L.E., Bennett, D.A., Field, T.S., and Evans, D.A. (1998). Vitamin E and vitamin C supplement use and risk of incident Alzheimer's disease. *Alzheimer Dis Assoc Disord*, *12*, 121 – 126.

Morris, M.C., Evans, D.A:, Bienias, J.L., Tagney, C.C., and Wilson, R.S. (2002). Vitamin E and cognitive decline in older persons. *Arch Neurol*, *59*, 1125 – 1132.

Mukaetova-Landiska, E.B., García-Siera, F., Hurt, J., Gertz, H.J., Xuereb, J.H., Hills, R., Brayne, C., Huppert, F.A., Paykel, E.S., McGree, M., Jakes, R., Honer, W.G., Harrington, C.R., and Wischik, C.M. (2000). Staging of cytoskeletal and beta-amyloid changes in human isocortex reveals biphasic synaptic protein response during progression of Alzheimer's disease. *Am J Pathol*, *157*, 623 – 636.

Olivieri, G., Brack, C., Muller-Spahn, F., Stahelin, H.B., Herrmann, M., Renard, P., Brockhaus, M., and Hock, C. (2000). Mercury induces cell cytotoxicity and oxidative stress and increases beta-amyloid secretion and tau phosphorylation in SHSY5Y neuroblastoma cells. *J Neurochem*, *74*, 231 – 236.

Pappolla, M.A., Sos, M., Omar, R.A., Bick, R.J., Hickson-Bick, D.L.M., and Reiter, R.J. (1997). Melatonin prevents death of neuroblastoma cells exposed to the Alzheimer's amyloid peptide. *J Neurosci*, *17*, 1683 – 1690.

Paraskevas, G.P., Kapaki, E., Petropoulou, O., Anagnostouli, M., Vagenas, V., and Papageorgiou, C. (2003). Plasma levels of antioxidant vitamins C and E are decreased in vascular parkinsonism. *J Neurol Sci*, *215*, 51 – 55.

Pérez, M., Cuadros, R., Smith, M.A:, Perry, G., and Ávila, J. (2000). Phosphorylated, but not native, tau protein assembles following reaction with the lipid peroxidation product, 4-hydroxy-2-nonenal. *FEBS Lett*, *486*, 270 – 274.

Pérez, M., Hernández, F., Gómez-Ramos, A., Smith, M., Perry, G., and Ávila, J. (2002). Formation of aberrant phosphotay fibrillar polumers in neural. *Eur J Biochem*, *269*, 1484 – 1489.

Pocernich, C.B., La Fontaine, M., and Butterfield, D.A. (2000). In vivo glutathione elevation protects against hydroxyl free radical.induced protein oxidation in rat brain. *Neurochem Int*, *36*, 185 – 191.

Pratico, D., Uryu, K., Leight, S., Trojanoswki, J.Q., and Lee, V.M. (2001). Increased lipid peroxidation precedes amyloid plaque formation in an animal model of Alzheimer amyloidosis. *J Neurosci*, *21*, 4183 – 4188.

Quinn, J., Suh, J., Moore, M.M., Kaye, J., and Frei, B. (2003). Antioxidants in Alzheimer's disease-vitamin C delivery to a demanding brain. *J Alzheimers Dis*, *5*, 309 – 313.

Ranjan, A., Theodore, D., Haran, R.P., and Chandy, M.J. (1993). Ascorbic acid and focal cerebral ischaemia ina primate model. *Acta Neurochir*, *123*, 87 – 91.

Reiter, R.J., Tan, D.X., Cabrera, J., D'Arpa, D., Sainz, R.M., Mayo, J.C., and Ramos, S. (1999). The oxidant/antioxidant network: role of melatonin. *Biol Signals Recept*, *8*, 56 – 63.

Rice, M.E., and Russo-Menna, I. (1998). Differential compartmentalization of brain ascorbate and glutathione between neurons and glia. *Neuroscience*, *82*, 1213 – 1223.

Rinaldi, P., Polidori, M.C., Metastasio, A., Mariani, E., Mattioli, P., Cherubini, A., Catani, M., Cecchetti, R., Senin, U., and Mecocci, P. (2003). Plasma antioxidants are similarly depleted in mild cognitive impairment and in Alzheimer's disease. *Neurobiol Aging, 24*, 915 – 919.

Rodríguez-Martínez, E., Rugerio-Vargas, C., Rodríguez, A.I., Borgonio-Pérez, G., and Rivas-Arancibia, S. (2004). Antioxidant effects of taurine, vitamin C, and vitamin E on oxidtive damage in hippocampus caused by the administration of 3-nitropropionic acid in rats. *Int J Neurosci. 114*, 1133 – 1145.

Sano, M., Ernesto, C., Thomas, R.G., Klauber, M.R., Schafer, K., Grundman, M., Woodbury, P., Growdon, J., and Corman, C.W. (1997). A controlled trial of selegiline, alphatocopherol, or both as treatment for Alzheimer's disease. *N Engl J Med, 336*, 1216 – 1222.

Serrano, F., and Klann, E. (2004). Reactive oxygen species and synaptic in the aging hippocampus. Ageing Res Rev, 3, 431 – 443.Markesbery WR (1997) Oxidative stress hypothesis in Alzheimer's disease. *Free Rad Biol Med, 23*, 134 – 147.

Smith, J.V., and Luo, Y. (2003). Elevation of oxidative free radicals in Alzheimer's disease models can be attenuated by Ginkgo biloba extract EGb 761. *J Alzheimer Dis, 5*, 287 – 300.

Schmitt, B., Bernhardt, T., Moeller, J.J., Heuser, I., and Frolich, L. (2004). Combination therapy in Alzheimer's disease: a review of current evidence. *CNS Drugs, 18*, 827 – 844.

Smith, M.A., and Perry, G. (1996). Alzheimer disease: protein-protein interaction and oxidative stress. *Bol Estatud Med Biol, 44*, 5 – 10.

Smith, M.A., Rottkamp, C.A., Nunomura, A., Raina, A.K., and Perry, G. (2000). Oxidative stress in Alzheimer's disease. *Biochim Biophys Acta, 1502*, 139 – 144.

Spector, R., and Eells, J. (1984). Deoxynucleoside and vitamin transport into the central nervous system. *Fed Proc, 43*, 196 – 200.

Smythies, J. (1999). The neurotoxicity of glutamate, dopamine, iron and reactive oxygen species: functional interrelationship in health and disease. *Neurtox Res, 1*, 27 – 39.

Traore, A., Ruiz, S., Baudrimont, I., Sanni, A., Dano, S.D., Guarigues, J.F., Narbonne, J.F., and Creppy, E.E. (2000). Combined effects of okadaic acid and cadmium on lipid peroxidation and DNA bases modifications (m5dC and8-(OH)-dG) in Caco-2 cells. *Arch Toxicol, 74*, 79 – 84.

Túnez, I., Montilla, P., Muñoz, M.C., and Drucker-Colín, R. (2004a). Effect of nicotine on 3-nitropropionic acid-induced oxidative stress in synaptosomes. *Eur J Pharmacol, 504*, 169 – 174.

Túnez, I., Montilla P., Muñoz, M.C., Feijóo, M., and Salcedo, M. (2004b). Protective effect of melatonin on 3-nitropropionic acid-induced oxidative stress in synaptosomes in an animal model of Huntington's disease. *J Pineal Res, 37*, 252 – 256.

Túnez, I., Muñoz, M.C., Feijóo, M., Muñoz-Castañeda, J.R., Bujalance, I., Valdelvira, M.E., and Montilla, P. (2003). Protective melatonin effect on oxidative stress induced by okadaic acid into rat brain. *J Pineal Res, 34*, 265 – 268.

Van der Loo, B., Bachschmid, M., Spitzer, V., Brey, L., Ullrich, V., and Lüscher, T.F. (2003). Decreased plasma and tissue levels of vitamin C in a rat model of aging: implications for antioxidative defense. *Biochem Biophys Res Commun. 303*, 483 – 487.

Warner, D.S., Sheng, H., and Batinic-Haberle, I. (2004). Oxidants, antioxidants and the ichemic brain. *J Exp Biol*, *207*, 3221 – 3231.

Wie, J., and Guo, G. (2004). AATF protects neural cells against oxidtive dmage induced by amyloid beta-peptide. *Neurobiol Dis*, *16*, 150 – 157.

Willcox, J.K., Ash, S.L., and Catignani, G.L. (2004). Antioxidants and prevention of chronic disease. *Crit Rev Food Sci Nutr*, *44*, 275 – 295.

Zaidi, S.M.K.R., and Banu, N. (2004). Antioxidant potential of vitamins A, E and C in modulating oxidative stress in rat brain. *Clin Chim Acta*, *340*, 229 – 233.

Zandi, P.P., Anthony, J.C., Khachaturian, A.S., Stone, S.V., Gustafson, D., Tschanz, J.T., Norton, M.C., Welsh-Bohmer, K.A., Breitner, J.C.; and Cache County Study Group. (2004). Reduced risk of Alzheimer disease in users of antioxidant vitamin supplements: the Cache County Study. *Arch Neurol*, *61*, 82 -88.

Zhang, S.M., Hernan, M.A., Chen, H., Spiegelman, D., Willett, W.C., and Ascherio, A. (2002). Intakes of vitamins E and C, carotenoids, vitamin supplements, and PD risk. *Neurology*, *59*, 1161 – 1169.

Zhu, X., Rottkamp, C.A., Boux, H., Takeda, A., Perry, G., and Smith, M.A. (2000). Activation of p38 kinase links tau phosphorylation, oxidative stress, and cell cyclerelated events in Alzheimer disease. *J Neuropathol Exp Neurol*, *59*, 880 – 888.

In: Alzheimer's Disease Research Trends
Editor: A.P. Chan, pp. 193-208

ISBN 978-1-60021-712-8

Chapter IX

FOCUS ON DEMENTIA ASSOCIATED WITH PARKINSON'S DISEASE: THE ROLE OF CHOLINESTERASE INHIBITORS

Carmine Fuschillo[1,*], Vincenzo Canonico[2], Silvestro La Pia[1] and Francesca Fortunato[2]

[1]Department of Menthal Health, Neuropsychogeriatric Ward, ASL NA 4, Via Cupa Travi, 30, I-80040 Cercola, Naples, Italy;

[2]Alzheimer Evaluation Unit, Faculty of Medicine, University of Naples "Federico II", Via Pansini, 5, I-80131 Naples, Italy;

ABSTRACT

Parkinson's disease (PD) is a disabling, progressive condition, frequently complicated by a spectrum of cognitive deficits ranging from isolated impairment to severe dementia. The purpose of this paper is to provide an overview of recent findings of dementia associated with PD (PDD), that is increasingly being recognized as a major prognostic factor for progressive disability and nursing home placement. Cholinergic deficits are prominent in PDD and are associated with cognitive slowing, attentional deficiency, memory impairment, and psychotic symptoms, particularly visual hallucinations. The treatment of PDD is challenging. Antipsychotic drugs can precipitate a profound, even fatal worsening in the motor symptoms of patients. On the other hand, dopaminergic agents for parkinsonism frequently cause worsening of hallucinations and cognitive function. The loss of cholinergic functioning suggests a potential utility for cholinesterase inhibitors (ChE-Is) in the treatment of PDD and large studies have been carried out with rivastigmine. This agent appears to moderately improve cognition and to a lesser extent activities of daily living in patients with PDD. Efficacy in other domains

* Correspondence concerning this article should be addressed to Carmine Fuschillo, Via Giovanni da Nola, 60, I-80039 Saviano, Naples, Italy. Phone: +39-081-8203582; Fax: +39-081-5314398; E-mail: c.fuschillo@libero.it.

requires confirmation. Tolerability, in particular nausea, vomiting, and tremor, appears problematic.

Introduction

Parkinson's disease (PD) is a chronic and progressive disorder of the central nervous system estimated to affect 6.3 million people worldwide (Global Declaration on Parkinson's Disease, 2003). It is characterized by a decrease in spontaneous movement, gait difficulty, postural instability, rigidity and tremor. In 1987, when James Parkinson originally described the "shaking palsy", he stated that cognitive decline are not evident until the later stages of the disease. However, the disorder is often complicated by cognitive deficits ranging from isolated cognitive impairment to severe dementia (Merino et al., 2004). Cognitive deficits are common in PD. Frequently, neuropsychiatric symptoms are also present and their profile differs from that exhibited by other forms of dementia (Aarsland et al., 2006).

The prevalence of dementia in PD (PDD) varies widely ranging from 2% in early-onset cases to 81% in an unselected population (Dodel, 2004). A mean of 40% was reported by an analysis of 27 studies (Cummings, 1988). Cross sectional studies suggest a prevalence rate of 30% to 40%, according to Aarsland et al. (2003a), or 37% to 44%, according to Hobson and Meara (1999), and longitudinal studies indicate that the cumulative frequency of dementia in patients with PD varies from 60% to 80% (Aarsland et al., 2003a). The discrepancy in the prevalence rates of dementia in PD is probably due to differences in the cognitive assessment, or in diagnostic criteria of dementia used, as well as it may reflect selection bias or difference in statistical design of the studies. PD patients have approximately a six fold increase in the risk of developing dementia compared with elderly people without PD (Aarsland et al., 2001a; Cummings, 2005). It has been suggested that the prevalence of PDD may be correlated with age and time course of PD (Aarsland et al., 2005).

PDD causes a significant worsening of the quality of life of both patient (Schrag et al., 2000) and caregiver (Aarsland et al., 1999a), inducing a more rapid functional and motor decline (Huber et al., 1988). PDD represents also a cause of nursing home placement of patients (Mayeux et al., 1992; Murat, 2003). Mortality and morbidity is generally higher in patients with PD and dementia than in those without (Merino et al., 2004).

The age at onset of PD appears to be a strong risk factor for the development of subsequent dementia. In fact, dementia occurs rarely in PD patients younger than 50 years of age, but its prevalence increases up to 69% in 80 years patients or older (Mayeux et al., 1992). Others risk factors include: severity of motor symptoms (bradykinesia, especially), presence of psychological and behavioural disturbances (mania, agitation, confusion, depression, psychosis during L-dopa therapy), verbal fluency or executive function impairment, postural and gait disturbance, and low educational level (Ebmeier et al., 1990; Levy et al., 2002; Murat, 2003; Hobson and Meara, 2004). Furthermore, it has been suggested a role of the apolipoprotein E (ApoE) gene alleles (eg, e2, e4) for the development of dementia in PD (Harhangi et al., 2000).

PATHOLOGY AND NEUROCHEMICAL DEFICITS

Pathologic changes occurring in the striatus and substantia nigra, pars compacta, may underlie PD. Tekin and Cummings (2002) described five frontal-subcortcal pathways connecting specific areas of the frontal cortex with the basal ganglia responsible for both motor and behavioural schemata. The neuropathologic basis of dementia in PD is still debated (Dodel, 2004). Deficits in dopaminergic, cholinergic and noradrenergic mechanisms have been proposed. Dopaminergic depletion, i.e., the major cause of the motor impairment of PD, may play even a role in the cognitive deficits (Pillon et al., 2003). Lesional studies found a correlation between PDD and neuronal loss both in the medial part of the substantia nigra (Rinne et al., 1989) and in the mesocortical pathways (Javoy-Agid and Agid, 1980). However, severe damage in other monoaminergic projections (i.e., serotoninergic and noradrenergic) and, more substantially, cholinergic pathways, has been suggested as a cause of cognitive impairment (Pillon et al., 1989; Emre, 2003a). In clinical practice and experimental studies, PDD does not improve with dopaminergic drugs (Apaydin et al., 2002). Reduced fluorodopa uptake in the caudate nucleus and frontal cortex was related to the impairment in neuropsychological tests measuring verbal fluency, working memory, and attentional functioning (Ito et al., 2002). The nucleus basalis of Meynert, which degenerates in AD, is also severely affected in PDD (Whitehouse et al., 1983), indicating the contribution of a cholinergic deficit to the cognitive impairment and dementia (Perry et al., 1993). Extensive reductions of choline acetyltransferase (ChAT), a marker of cortical cholinergic activity, were found in cortical lobes in PD, and the degree of reduction of ChAT in the temporal lobe correlated with the severity of cognitive impairment (Perry et al., 1985). Compared with normal control, the midfrontal ChAT activity was found to be markedly reduced not only in Alzheimer's disease (AD), but also in PD and in Dementia with Lewy bodies (DLB), a condition related to PD, that represents the second most common form of dementia (Neef and Walling, 2006). This reduction was almost twice in PD patients compared with AD subjects (Tiraboschi et al., 2000). Similar findings were found in imaging studies of cortical cholinergic function using positron emission tomography (PET). Compared with controls, mean cortical AChE activity was lower in patients with PDD (-20%) than in those affected by PD without dementia (-13%) and AD patients with comparable severity of dementia (-9%) (Bohnen et al., 2003). In contrast to AD, PDD is associated with neuronal loss in the pedinculopontine cholinergic nuclei that projects to thalamus (Rub et al., 2002). In summary, there is increasing evidence that complex neurotransmitters depletion, other than dopaminergic innervations loss, is crucial for the occurrence of PDD. In particular, cholinergic depletion seems to play a major role in the cognitive and neuropsychiatric symptoms in PDD (Aarsland et al., 2004; Sellal, 2006).

Brain cells loss in PD and DLB seems related to an abnormal aggregation of α-synuclein protein which leads to cytoplasmic inclusions called Lewy bodies (LBs). It has been suggested that the dopaminergic neurons degeneration is due to a mechanism deficit that involves proteins transport from the endoplasmic reticulum to the Golgi apparatus. Moreover, in animal models, certain proteins may reverse this deficit (Parkinson's Disease Mechanism Discovered, 2006). It is now accomplished that cortical LBs are a marker more sensitive and specific neuropathological of dementia than the AD-type pathology, as suggested by a study of 22 PDD patients, compared with 20 PD patients without classical dementia (Hurtig et al, 2000).

Several studies demonstrate a strong correlation between the occurrence of LBs pathology and severity of PDD (Hurtig et al., 2000). PDD and DLB probably represent different points along the synucleinopathies spectrum, sharing some clinical symptoms and similar underlying neuropathological processes. Sellal (2006) questioned whether PPD and DLB should be considered two different syndromes, or represent the same disease. Furthermore, differentiating these conditions may be useful from a clinical point of view, but it may be of a limited value in terms of investigating and treating the underline neurobiology (McKeith and Mosimann, 2004). Although consensus has been reached for DLB diagnosis, an arbitrary 1-year rule has been proposed to distinguish it from PDD. In fact, consensus guidelines for DLB suggest that patients with PD, who develop dementia within 12 months after the initial motor symptoms, should be diagnosed as having DLB; if dementia occurs later in the course of the disease, patients should be diagnosed as PD with dementia rather than DLB (McKeith et al., 1996; McKeith et al., 2004). This approach does not take in account pathologic data, and it is probable than in the next future PDD and DLB will be recognized as the same disease with two different courses (Sellal, 2006).

Clinical Features

Dementia associated with PD has a typical clinical profile. Cognitive impairment manifests itself subtly with slowness of thinking (bradyphrenia) and word finding difficulties (Dodel, 2004), that, at least initially, does not imply a significant impairment in the patient's daily live activities. In the later stages of the disease, the prototypical dementia syndrome associated with PD can be best summarized as a dysexecutive syndrome with prominent impairment of attention, visuo-spatial function, and memory. This clinical picture is often complicated by behavioral symptoms such as apathy and psychosis (Emre, 2003a; Pillon et al., 2001; Aarsland et al., 2003a). Attention deficits occur relatively early in the course of PDD (Emre, 2003a; Ballard et al., 2001) and represent an important treatment target. Impairment in reaction time and vigilance as well as fluctuating attention are present in PDD to an extent comparable to those seen in patients with DLB. Compared with patients with AD, PDD patients are more apathetic and have more cognitive slowing. The magnitude of cognitive slowing is usually exceeding the general level of cognitive performance (Emre, 2005). Changes in different cognitive domains have been extensively assessed in several studies and well described by Pillon et al. (2001). More in detail, the cognitive impairment in PDD may be summarized as follow (Dodel, 2004; Merino et al., 2004):

- Disorders of executive function constitutes the core feature of PDD, and occur early in the course of the disease. Deficits include poor performance in tasks involving rule finding, problem solving, planning, set elaboration, set shifting and set maintenance. Patients have substantial difficulties in developing their own strategies, while performance improves substantially when external cues are provided.

- Visuospatial dysfunction is more severe in PDD than in other form of dementia, including AD. In fact, PDD patients perform worse in all percentual scores, and those with visual hallucinations tend to have worse visual perception than those without. As described by Mosinan et al. (2004), neuropsychological testing reveals a typical pattern of deficits consisting in difficulty with line orientation, block design, and picture arrangement. Patients with severe form of the disease show deficits in non-familiar-face discrimination. Moreover, deficits seem to be, at least in part, independent from motor impairment degree.
- Implicit and explicit memory functions were reported to be impaired in PDD, including working memory and procedural learning. Deficits in working memory could be present even in the early stage of the disease (Emre, 2005). The profile of memory impairment in PDD differs from those seen in AD. In fact, it tends to be less prominent as compared to the overall severity of cognitive impairment in contrast to patients with AD (Emre, 2005). Moreover, it is characterized by a deficit in free recall with preserved recognition, indicating that information is stored, but not adequately accessed. Accordingly, memory performance usually improves when semantic cues or multiple choices are provided.
- Aphasia and ideomotor apraxia don't seem a consistent feature of PDD. The most reported language deficits are anomia and impaired verbal fluency, the latter is more severe than that occurring in AD. As for impairments in other domains, it was suggested that most of the language deficits might not reflect a true involvement of language functions, but it might be rather related to the dysexecutive syndrome.

Recently, Aarsland et al. (2006) have explored the profile of neuropsychiatric symptoms of 537 PDD patients in an international multi-centre clinical trial. Using Neuropsychiatric Inventory (NPI), behavioral and psychological symptoms occurred in 89% of patients, and the most common symptoms were depression (58%), apathy (54%), anxiety (49%), and hallucinations (44%). Moreover, psychotic symptoms could have been precipitated by treatment with dopaminergic agents. In a comparative study, about 83% of PDD patients were found to have a least one psychiatric symptom, as opposed to 95% of those with AD. As individual symptoms were concerned, hallucinations were more severe in PDD, whereas increased psychomotor activity, including aberrant motor behaviour, agitation, disinhibition and irritability, were more common in AD. In the PDD group, apathy was more common in the mild stages, while delusions increased with the progression of the motor and cognitive dysfunctions (Aarsland et al., 2001b).

Patients with PDD usually develop a specific pattern of motor impairment characterized by symmetrical appearance, predominance of bradykinesia, rigidity and postural instability. Patients are also more prone to falls, and they may show a more rapid cognitive decline, whereas tremor dominance has been associated with relative preservation of mental status (Burn et al., 2003). Autonomic symptoms, such as orthostatic and postprandial hypotension, bowel and bladder disturbances and sexual dysfunction are often present in PDD (Kaufmann and Biaggioni, 2003). Furthermore, rapid eye movement (REM) and sleep-behavioral disorder are common in PDD and they can precede clinical symptoms by many years (Boeve et al., 2003).

Diagnostic Methods

Cerebrospinal fluid (CSF) parameters are negative (Holmberg et al., 2003), and electroencephalogram (EEG) shows no specific alterations in PDD (Barber et al., 2000). Using single photon computed tomography (SPECT), Firbank et al. (2003), in 99mcTc-HMPAO-SPECT studies, showed a specific pattern, similar to that observed in DLB, consisting in a perfusion deficit in the precuneus and the inferior lateral parietal regions. By contrast, AD patients revealed a perfusion deficit in the more anterior and inferior regions of parietal cortex, with the involvement of the posterior cingulated cortex as well as of the precuneus. Significant reductions in FP-CIT SPECT binding were reported in the caudate, and anterior and posterior putamen in DLB patients compared with AD subjects and controls (O'Brein et al., 2004). Firbank et al. (2005) measured brain perfusion using Tc99m HMPAO SPECT over one year in 17 PDD, 18 DLB and 34 healthy subjects. They used SPM99 to compare perfusion changes in the two dementia groups, and in the control group. In the DLB, but not in the PDD group, there was a significant increase in putamen perfusion respect to controls. In both DLB and PDD groups, there was a correlation between striatal perfusion increase and worsening of parkinsonism. Perfusion changes were not secondary to changes in antiparkinsonian medication. Compared with the control group, the PDD group showed reduced 18F-dopa PET uptake bilaterally in the striatum, midbrain and anterior cingulated area. Furthermore, a relative difference in 18F-dopa uptake was found between PD and PDD, consisting in a bilateral decline in the anterior cingulated area, in the ventral striatum, and in the right caudate nucleus that was present only in the PDD group (Ito et al., 2002). CT scanning and MRI do not help establish the diagnosis of PDD and no significant differences in whole brain and caudate nucleus volume on MRI between controls, PD and PDD have been reported (Almeida et al., 2003).

Neuropsychological Testing:

Although no specific tests are used in PDD, Dodel (2004) reports that working, episodic, and recall memory is impaired more in AD than in PDD, while semantic memory is equally compromised. In contrast, visuopercetion, visuospatial, and visuoconstruction is impaired more in PDD than in AD. Attentional deficit is predominant in AD, while fluctuating attention is major in PDD and DLB than AD. Executive functions are damaged in both disease.

Treatment

PDD patients may present a combination of motor and non motor symptoms, i.e., cognitive and behavioural symptoms, such as apathy, personality changes and visual hallucinations. These symptoms are often particularly disturbing and represent one of the major determinants of patients' and carers' distress. They also reduce the quality of life leading to institutionalisation (Burn and McKeith, 2003). However, as the disease progresses, the presence of one or more of non motor disorders becomes more likely and physicians should be aware of the need to evaluate and treat these complications. Whereas non motor complications are problematic on their own, they also have multiple effects on the motor complications patients develop (Adler, 2005).

The goal for the clinician in PD therapy is to optimise motor function and cognition, and to minimise depression, hallucinations, delusions, anxiety, daytime hypersomnolence, and orthostatic hypotension. Some time PD therapy can improve motor features, but tolerability is poor because of declines in cognition and behaviour. Levodopa use is hampered by frequent psychotic side-effects. This drug provides only a modest improvement of cognitive functions, probably due to a non-specific effect on arousal or mood (Emre, 2003b). Dopaminergic agents have been shown to produce only limited improvements in cognitive functioning (Kulisevsky et al., 2000). Neuroleptics are typically used in the management of delusions and hallucinations, but even the new generation of atypical neuroleptics can worsen cognition. Furthermore, they aggravate movement disorders, daytime hypersomnolence, and orthostatic hypotension. Discontinuation of any unnecessary medications should be undertaken, including anticholinergics, selegiline, amantadine, tricyclic antidepressants, and sedatives.

Until recently, no specific treatment was recommended for PDD, and treatment options was limited (Sellal, 2006). The observation that these patients have extensive cholinergic deficits suggests a new strategy, after cholinesterase inhibitors (ChE-Is) became available for AD (Emre, 2003a, Emre, 2005). Three ChE-Is are currently available, including donepezil, rivastigmine, and galantamine. They prevent the inactivation of acetylcholine after its release by blocking the acetylcholine esterase. Consequently, they have been proposed for the treatment of cognitive impairment in PDD. The use of these drugs in PDD has shown variable results ranging from general improvement of cognition and psychotic symptoms to no change or even worsening of motor responses. However, increasing cholinergic activity to alleviate cognitive dysfunction may worsen Parkinsonian symptoms (Richard et al., 2002).

The first evidence for a favourable effect of ChE-Is in PDD was carried out with tacrine that improved cognitive and behavioural symptoms, apathy and hallucinations, without no worsening in motor functions (Hutchinson and Fazzini, 1996). Subsequent studies suggested that ChE-Is can improve cognitive and behavioural symptoms in PDD (Aarsland et al., 2002; Marder, 2002; Kurita et al., 2003; Leroi et al., 2004).

In a double-blind, placebo-controlled study, 16 patients treated with donepezil showed an improvement in memory, attention and concentration, and no worsening in motor functions or in the Activity of Dalily Living (ADL) (Leroi et al., 2004). These results are in according to other of previous studies (Aarsland et al., 2002; Fabbrini et al., 2002). An important smaller double-blind, placebo controlled, crossover study with donepezil also showed the beneficial effects of this drug on behaviour and cognition, without worsening parkinsonism (Ravina et al., 2005). Twenty-two patients with PD and dementia were recruited in this study, which consisted of two treatment periods of 10 weeks separated by a 6-week wash out interval. The primary outcome measure was the Alzheimer's Disease Assessment Scale-cognitive subscale (ADAS-cog). The secondary outcome measures included the Mini Mental State Examination (MMSE), the Mattis Dementia Rating Scale (MDRS), the Clinical Global Impression of Change (CGI), and the Brief Psychiatric Rating Scale (BPRS). There was a 1.9-point trend toward better scores on the ADAS-cog on treatment compared with placebo, but this change was not statistically significant. The secondary cognitive measures showed a statistically significant 2-point benefit on the MMSE and a significant 0.37 point improvement on the CGI. No improvements were observed on the MDRS or the BPRS.

In a small open study galantamine was reported to improve cognitive functions, hallucinations, and parkinsonism in some patients, while parkinsonism worsened in others (Aarsland and Hutchinson, 2002). In another study, 16 patients were treated with galantamine for 8 weeks (Aarsland et al., 2003b). Fifty percent of patients improved in test exploring the cognitive functions, such as the Clock Drawing Test, the MMSE, and the Verbal Fluency Test. Some patients reported an improvement in the hallucinations and in parkinsonism, while in 25 percent of subjects no clinical modifications were revealed.

Rivastigmine is the ChE-I agent more used in PDD. In an open study this drug improved cognitive deficit as well as hallucinations, sleep disturbance, and caregiver burden (Reading et al., 2001). In another open-label study, 28 PDD patients were treated with an average of 7.2 mg per day of rivastigmine for 26 weeks (Giladi et al., 2003). Significant improvements were found in the ADAS-cog score, and in the Unified Parkinson's Disease Rating Scales (UPDRS) (including both the total score and the score on the cognitive performance), and no worsening in motor function. The MMSE scores showed improvements, though they remained insignificant. The most frequent undesired effects were hypersalivation, increase in trembling, confusion and hallucinosis.

The first large study assessing the efficacy and safety of rivastigmine in PDD was published by Emre et al. (2004). This study, known as EXPRESS (EXelon in PaRkinson's disEasSe dementia Study), was a 24-week, randomized, multicenter, double-blind, placebo-controlled clinical trial. A total of 541 patients with PDD were enrolled, and 410 completed the study. The mean dose of rivastigmine was 8.6 mg per day (range 3-12 mg per day). At the end of study, 210 patients (55.5 percent) were receiving 9 to 12 mg of drug per day, 76 (21.0 percent) were receiving at least 6 mg but less than 9 per day, 83 (22.9 percent) were receiving at least 3 mg but less than 6 mg per day, and 2 (0.6 percent) were receiving less than 3 mg per day. The primary outcome measures were the ADAS-cog and the Alzheimer's Disease Cooperative Study-Clinician's Global Impression of Change (ADCS-CGIC). Secondary clinical outcomes were the scores of the Alzheimer's Disease Cooperative Study-Activity of Daily Living (ADCS-ADL), the 10-item Neuropsychiatic Inventory (NPI-10), the MMSE, the Cognitive Drug Research (CDR) Computerized Assessment System power of attention tests, the Verbal Fluency test, and the Ten Point Clock-Drawing test. Statistically significant benefit was seen for both primary measures in favour of rivastigmine. As compared with placebo group, patients treated with this drug had improvements in ADAS-cog scores at week 24 (mean improvement of 2.1 points, as compared with a worsening of 0.7 point in the placebo group; $p<0.001$). On the ADCS-CGIC more patients on rivastigmine showed an improvement (40.8% vs. 29.7% on placebo; $p=0.02$) and more patients on placebo deteriorated (42.5% on placebo vs. 33.7% on rivastigmine; $p=0.007$). Likewise on all secondary efficacy parameters there were statistically significant differences in favour of rivastigmine including neuropsychiatric symptoms, computerized tests of attention, Clock Drawing test, Verbal Fluency test, MMSE and the ADL scale. A comparable beneficial effect on behavioral disorders was demonstrated. In particular, this improvement was marked for hallucinations and sleep disturbances, and moderate for cognitive functions. Adverse events were significantly more frequent in patients treated with rivastigmine. The most frequent side-effects were nausea (affecting 29.0 percent of patients in the rivastigmine group and 11.2 percent of those in the placebo group, $p<0.001$), vomiting (16.6 and 1.7 percent, $p<0.001$), and tremor (10.2 and 3.9 percent, respectively; $p=0.01$). The objective measures of motor symptoms, however, as assessed by UPDRS part III, did not reveal any significant differences between the two treatments. This important clinical trial has induced, in February 2006, the European Commission to grant a marketing authorization for rivastigmine for the symptomatic treatment of mild to moderately severe PDD.

An interesting study directly compared DLB and PDD patients and found similar treatment effects in both disorders (Minett et al., 2003). However, when withdrawn from the drug, patients with PDD deteriorated markedly, suggesting that DLB and PDD patients, who benefit from ChE-Is, should be treated long-term and the treatment discontinuation might have detrimental effects.

In a review of studies describing the use of ChE-Is in PDD, Maidment and co-workers (2005) showed that ChE-Is have a moderate effect against cognitive symptoms, and no clear evidence of a noticeable clinical effect against neuropsychiatric symptoms. Moreover, due to the exacerbation of tremor, the tolerability was poor, and this might limit the utility of ChE-Is.

Psychotic symptoms, such as hallucinations and delusions, may also benefit by the use of antipsychotic drugs. Typical antipsychotics (first generation antipsychotics) are contra-indicated because they can induce a worsening of motor function. There have been several studies with atypical neuroleptics (second generation antipsychotics) to treat psychosis in PD (Fuschillo et al., 2006). There are robust evidences concerning clozapine in the treatment of psychosis in PD (Friedman and Fernandez, 2002; Factor et al., 1994; Wagner et al., 1996). Evidence from randomized, placebo controlled studies demonstrating significant improvement of psychosis without worsening of motor symptoms exist for clozapine (The Parkinson Study Group, 1999; Factor et al., 2001), and low doses of this drug (<50 mg/day) appear effective in PDD, with an acceptable tolerability. In several open label studies, quetiapine induced an improvement in psychotic symptoms of PD (Fernandez et al, 2000; Friedman et al, 1999; Menza et al., 1999). Roberts et al., (2001), in a 24-week trial, showed a significant improvement in 29 PD patients treated with quetiapine in both behavioural and cognitive domains, compared with those receiving placebo. Similar findings were found by Juncos et al. (2004). In the Ondo et al.'s trial (2005) no significant change was reported in patients treated with quetiapine compared to placebo-group. Although in some studies risperidone and olanzapine has been shown effective and well tolerated (Mohr et al., 2000; Aarsland et al., 1999b; Wolters, 1999), other reports indicated that many patients are unable to tolerate these drugs due to deterioration of motor function (Molho and Factor, 1999; Graham et al., 1998).

Recently, in a report the Quality Standards Subcommittee of the American Academy of Neurology indicated relevant practice parameters to make evidence-based treatment recommendations for PD patients with dementia, depression, and psychosis (Miyasaki et al., 2006). The results showed that amitriptyline might be considered to treat depression in PD without dementia (Level C); for psychosis in PD, clozapine should be considered (Level B), quetiapine might be considered (Level C), but olanzapine should not be considered (Level

B). Regarding ChE-Is treatment in PDD, donepezil or rivastigmine should be considered (Level B) and rivastigmine should be considered for DLB (Level B), but improvement is modest and motor side effects might occur.

Conclusion

Although no drug treatments can provide a cure for PPD, its pharmacologic management can be challenging. Drug treatments could temporarily slow down the progression of cognitive symptoms in patients with this form of dementia. In patients with acute psychotic symptoms, other causes of symptoms, such as pain, intercurrent infection, subdural haematoma, or adverse drug reaction must be excluded. Medications capable of causing confusion should be discontinued. Antiparkinsonian medication should be reviewed and a gradual, graded withdrawal undertaken in the order of anticholinergics, amantadine, selegiline, and dopamine agonists (Dodel, 2004). If there is no improvement in psychotic features, an antipsychotic agent may be used (e.g. clozapine, quetiapine) (Friedman and Factor, 2000).

Recently, according to several studies showing the presence of a cortical cholinergic deficit in PDD, it has suggested that the treatment with ChE-Is may be beneficial (Aarsland et al., 2004; Cummings, 2005), and may be helpful in improving cognitive function and reducing neuropsychiatric symptoms. Tolerability, and in particular nausea, vomiting, and tremor, appears poor and problematic. Additional researches are needed to determine whether all ChE-Is are of equal efficacy in this setting, the duration of benefit to be expected, and the interaction with dopaminergic agents and psychotropic drugs commonly used in this patient population.

References

Aarsland, D; Andersen, K; Larsen, JP, Lolk, A; Krag-Sorensen, P. Prevalence and characteristics of dementia in Parkinson disease: an 8-year prospective study. *Arch Neurol*, 2003a 60, 387-392.

Aarsland, D; Andersen, K; Larsen, JP; Lolk, A; Nielsen, H; Kragh-Sorensen, P. Risk of dementia in Parkinson's disease: a community-based, prospective study. *Neurology*, 2001a 56, 730-736.

Aarsland, D; Laake, K; Larsen, JP; Janvin, C. Donepezil for cognitive impairment in Parkinson's disease: a randomised controlled study. *J Neurol Neurosurg Psychiatry*, 2002 72, 708-712.

Aarsland, D; Bronnick, K; Ehrt, U; De Deyn, PP; Tekin, S; Emre, M; Cummings, JL. Neuropsychiatric symptoms in patients with PD and dementia: frequency, profile and associated caregiver stress. *J Neurol Neurosurg Psychiatry*, 2006 4 July, [Epub ahead of print]. doi:10.1136/jnnp.2005.083113.

Aarsland, D; Cummings, JL; Larsen, JP. Neuropsychiatric differences between Parkinson's disease with dementia and Alzheimer's disease. *Int J Geriatr Psychiatry*, 2001b 16, 184-191.

Aarsland, D; Hutchinson, M. Galantamine for Parkinson's disease with dementia. *Eur Neuropsychopharm*, 2002 12(suppl 12), S378-79.

Aarsland, D; Hutchinson, M; Larsen, JP. Cognitive, psychiatric and motor response to galantamine in Parkinson's disease with dementia. *Int J Geriatr Psychiatry,* 2003b 18, 937-941.

Aarsland, D; Larsen, JP; Karlsen, K; Lim, NG; Tandberg, E. Mental symptoms in Parkinson's disease are important contributors to caregiver distress. *Int J Geriatr Psychiatry*, 1999a 14, 866-874.

Aarsland, D; Larsen, GP; Lim, NG; Tandberg, E. Olanzapine for psychosis in patients with Parkinson's disease with and without dementia. *J Neuropsychiatry Clin Neurosci,* 1999b 11, 392-394.

Aarsland, D; Mosimann, UP; McKeith, IG. Role of cholinesterase inhibitors in Parkinson's disease and dementia with Lewy bodies. *J Geriatr Psichiatry Neurol,* 2004 17, 164-171.

Aarsland, D; Zaccai, J; Brayne, C. A systematic review of prevalence studies of dementia in Parkinson's disease. *Mov Disord*, 2005 20, 1255-1263.

Adler, CH. Nonmotor complications in Parkinson's Disease. *Mov Disord,* 2005 20(suppl.11), S23-S29.

Almeida, OP; Burton, EJ; McKeith, I; Gholkar, A; Burn, D; O'Brien, JT. MRI study of caudate nucleus volume in Parkinson's disease with and without dementia with Lewy bodies and Alzheimer's disease. *Dement Geriatr Cogn Disord*, 2003 16, 57-63.

Apaydin, H; Ahlskog, E; Parisi, JE; Boeve, BF; Dickson, DW. Parkinson disease neuropathology. Later-developing dementia and loss of the levodopa response. *Arch Neurol,* 2002 59, 102-112.

Ballard, C; O'Brein, J; Grey, A; Cormack, F; Ayre, G; Rowan, E; Thompson, P; Bucks, R; McKeith, I; Walker, M; Tovee, M. Attention and fluctuating attention in patients with dementia with Lewy bodies and Alzheimer disease. *Arch Neurol,* 2001 58, 977-982.

Barber, PA; Varma, AR; Lloyd, JJ; Haworth, B; Snowden, JS; Neary, D. The electroencephalogram in dementia with Lewy bodies. *Acta Neurol Scand*, 2000 101, 53-56.

Boeve, BF; Silber, MH; Parisi, JE; Dickson, DW; Ferman, TJ; Benarroch, EE; Schmeichel, AM; Smith, GE; Petersen, RC; Ahlskog, JE; Matsumoto, JY; Knopman, DS; Schenck, CH; Mahowald, MW. Synucleinopathy pathology and REM sleep behavior disorder plus dementia or parkinsonism. *Neurology*, 2003 61, 40-45.

Bohnen, NI; Kaufer, DI; Ivanco, LS; Lopresti, B; Koeppe, RA; Davis, JG; Mathis, CA; Moore, RY; DeKosky, ST. Cortical cholinergic function in more severely affected in parkinsonian dementia than in Alzheimer disease: an in vivo positron tomographic study. *Arch Neurol*, 2003 60, 1745-1748.

Burn, DJ; McKeith, IG. Current treatment of dementia with Lewy Bodies and Dementia associated with Parkinson's Disease. *Mov Disord,* 2003 18, S72-S79.

Burn, DJ; Rowan, EN; Minett, T; Sanders, J; Myint, P; Richardson, J; Thomas, A; Newby, J; Reid, J; O'Brein, JT; McKeith, IG. Extrapiramidal features in Parkinson's disease with and without dementia and dementia with Lewy bodies: a cross-sectional comparative study. *Mov Disord*, 2003 18, 884-889.

Cummings, JL. Intellectual impairment in Parkinson's disease: clinical, pathologic, and biochemical correlates. *J Geriatr Psychiatry Neurol*, 1988 1, 24-36.

Cummings, JL. Cholinesterase inhibitors for treatmemnt of dementia associated with Parkinson's disease. *J Neurol Neurosurg Psychiatry*, 2005 76, 903-904.

Dodel, R. Dementia in Parkinson' disease. Orphanet Encyclopedia, November 2004. http://www.orpha.net/data/patho/GB/uk-PDD.pdf

Ebmeier, KP; Calder, SA; Crawford, JR; Stewart, L; Besson, JA; Mutch WJ. Clinical features predicting dementia in idiopathic Parkinson's disease: a follow-up study. *Neurology*, 1990 40, 1222-1224.

Emre, M. Dementia associated with Parkinson's disease. *Lancet Neurol,* 2003a 2, 229-237.

Emre, M. What causes mental dysfunction in Parkinson's disease? *Mov Disord*, 2003b 18(suppl 6), S63-S71.

Emre, M; Aarsland, D; Albanese, A; Byrne, EJ; Psych, FRC; Deuschl G., De Deyn, Durif, F; Kulisevsky, J; van Laar, T; Lees, A; Poewe, W; Robillard, A; Rosa, MM; Wolters, E; Quarg, P; Tekin, S; Lane, R. Rivastigmine for Dementia Associated with Parkinson's Disease. *N Engl J Med*, 2004 351, 2509-2518.

Emre, M. Expert review: dementia associated with Parkinson's disease- features, cause and treatment. Published on CNSforum, 27 Sep 2005. http://www.cnsforum.com/magazine/asktheexpert/pd/

Fabbrini, G; Barbanti, P; Aurilia, C; Pauletti, C; Lenzi, GL; Meco, G. Donepezil in the treatment of hallucinations and delusions in Parkinson's disease. *Neurol Sci*, 2002 23, 41-43.

Factor, SA; Brown, D; Molho, ES; Podskalny, GD. Clozapine. A 2-year open trial in Parkinson's disease patients with psychosis. *Neurology,* 1994 44, 544-546.

Factor, SA; Friedman, JH; Lannon, MC; Oakes, D; Bourgeois, K; Parkinson Study Group. Clozapine for the treatment of drug-induced psychosis in Parkinson's disease: results of the 12 week open label extension in the PSYCLOPS trial. *Mov Disord,* 2001 16, 135-139.

Fernandez, HH; Lannon, MC; Friedman, JH; Abbott, BP. Clozapine replacement by quetiapine for the treatment of drug-induced psychosis in Parkinso's disease. *Mov Disord,* 2000 15, 579-581.

Firbank, MJ; Colloby, D.J; Burn, D.J; McKeith, I.G; O'Brien, J.T. Regional cerebral blood flow in Parkinson's disease with and without dementia. *Neuroimage*, 2003 20, 1309-1319.

Firbank, MJ; Burn, DJ; McKeith, IG; O'Brein, JT. Longitudinal study of cerebral blood flow SPECT in Parkinson's disease with dementia, and dementia with Lewy bodies. *Int J Geriatr Psychiatry*, 2005 20, 776-782.

Friedman, JH; Factor, SA. Atypical antipsychotics in the treatment of drug-induced psychosis in Parkinson's disease. *Mov Disord*, 2000 15, 201-211.

Friedman, JH; Fernandez, HH. Atypical antipsychotics in Parkinson-sensitive population. *J Geriatr Psychiatry Neurol,* 2002 14, 156-170.

Friedman, JH; Fernandez, HH; Jacques, C. Quetiapine for the treatmnent of dopamimetic psychosis in Parkinson's disease. Presented at the 152nd annual meeting of the American Psychiatric Association; May 15-20, 1999, Washington, DC.

Fuschillo, C; La Pia, S; Canonico, V. Prescribing psychotropic drugs in the elderly: treatment controversies in the management of behavioral and psychological symptoms of dementia (BPSD). In: Welsh EM (editor). *Trends in Alzheimer's disease research.* New York, Nova Science Publishers 2006, 1-52.

Giladi, N; Shabtai, H; Gurevich, T; Benbunan, B; Anca, M; Korczyn, AD. Rivastigmine (Exelon) for dementia in patients with Parkinson's disease. *Acta Neurol Scand,* 2003 108, 368-373.

Global Declaration on Parkinson's Disease launched by the Working Group on PD at the World PD International Symposium, 7th December 2003 in Mumbai, India. http://www.epda.eu.com/globaldeclaration-about.shtm.

Graham, JM; Sussman, JD; Ford, KS; Sagar, HJ. Olanzapine in the treatment of hallucinosis in idiopatic Parkinson's disease: a cautionary note. *J Neurol Neurosurg Psychiatry,* 1998 65, 774-777.

Harhangi, BS; de Rijk, MC; van Duijn, CM; Van Broeckhoven, C; Hofman, A; Breteler, MM. APOE and risk of PD with or without dementia in a population-based study. *Neurology*, 2000 54, 1272-1276.

Hobson, P; Meara, J. The detection of dementia and cognitive impairment in a community of elderly people with Parkinson's disease by use of the CAMCOG neuropsychological test. *Age Ageing*, 1999 28, 39-43.

Hobson, P; Meara, J. Risk and incidence of dementia in a cohort of older subjects with Parkinson's disease in the United Kingdom. *Mov Disord,* 2004 19, 1043-1049.

Holmberg, B; Johnels, B; Blennow, K; Rosengren, L. Cerebrospinal fluid Abeta42 is reduced in multiple system atrophy but normal in Parkinson's disease and progressive supranuclear palsy. *Mov Disord*, 2003 18, 186-190.

Huber, SJ; Paulson, GW; Shuttleworth, EC. Relationship of motor symptoms, intellectual impairment, and depression in Parkinson's disease. *J Neurol Neurosurg Psychiatry*, 1988 51, 855-858.

Hurtig, H; Trojanowski, JQ, Galvin, J; Ewbank, D; Schmidt, ML; Lee, VM; Clark, CM; Glosser, G; Stern, MB; Gollomp, SM; Arnold, SE. Alpha-synuclein cortical Lewy bodies correlate with dementia in Parkinson's disease. *Neurology*, 2000 54, 1916-1921.

Hutchinson, M; Fazzini, E. Cholinesterase inhibition in Parkinson's disease. *J Neurol Neurosurg Psychiatry*, 1996 61, 324-325.

Ito, K; Nagano-Saito, A; Kato, T; Arahata, Y; Nakamura, A; Kawasumi, Y; Hatano, K; Abe, Y; Yamada, T; Kachi, T; Brooks, DJ. Striatal and extrastriatal dysfunction in Parkinson's disease with dementia: a 6-[18F]fluoro-L-dopa PET study. *Brain*, 2002 125(Pt 6), 1358-1365.

Javoy-Agid, F; Agid, Y. Is the mesocortical dopaminergic system involved in Parkinson's disease? *Neurology*, 1980 30, 1326-1330.

Juncos, JL; Roberts, VJ; Evatt, ML; Jewart, RD; Wood, CD; Potter, LS; Jou, HC; Yeung, PP. Quetiapine improves psychotic symptoms and cognition in Parkinson's disease. *Mov Disord,* 2004 19, 29-35.

Kaufmann, H; Biaggioni, I. Autonomic failure in neurodegenerative disorders. *Semin Neurol,* 2003 23, 351-363.

Kulisevsky, J; Garcia-Sanchez, C; Berthier, ML; Barbanoj, M; Pascual-Sedano, B; Gironell, A; Estevez-Gonzalez, A. Chronic effects of dopaminergic replacement on cognitive function in Parkinson's Disease: a two-year follow-up study of previously untreated patients. *Mov Disord,* 2000 15, 613-626.

Kurita, A; Ochiai, Y; Kono, Y; Suzuki, M; Inoue, K. The beneficial effect of donepezil on visual hallucinations in three patients with Parkinson's disease. *J Geriatr Psychiatry Neurol,* 2003 16, 184-188.

Leroi, I; Brandt, J; Reich, SG; Lyketsos, CG; Grill, S; Thompson, R; Marsh, L. Randomized placebo-controlled trial of donepezil in cognitive impairment in Parkinson's disease. *Int J Geriatr Psychiatry,* 2004 19, 1-8.

Levy, G; Jacobs, DM; Tang, MX; Cote, LJ; Louis, ED; Alfaro, B; Mejia, H; Stern, Y; Marder, K. Memory and executive function impairment predict dementia in Parkinson's disease. *Mov Disord,* 2002 17, 1221-1226.

Maidment, ID; Fox, C; Boustani, M. A review of studies describing the use of acetyl cholinesterase inhibitors in Parkinson's disease dementia. *Acta Psychiatr Scand,* 2005 111, 403-409.

Marder, K. Donepezil for cognitive impairment in Parkinson's disease: a randomized controlled trial. *Curr Neurol Neurosci Rep,* 2002 2, 390-391.

Mayeux, R; Denaro, J; Hemenelgildo, N. A population-based investigation of Parkinson's disease with and without dementia: relationship to age and gender. *Arch Neurol,* 1992 49, 492-497.

McKeith, IG; Galasko, D; Kosaka, K; Perry, EK; Dickson, DW; Hansen, LA; Salmon, DP; Lowe, J; Mirra, SS; Byrne, EJ; Lennox, G; Quinn, NP; Edwardson, JA; Ince, PG; Bergeron, C; Burns, A; Miller, BL; Lovestone, S; Collerton, D; Jansen, EN; Ballard, C; de Vos, RA; Wilcock, GK; Jellinger, KA; Perry, RH. Consensus guidelines for the clinical and pathological diagnosis of dementia with Lewy bodies (DLB): Report of the consortium on DLB international workshop. *Neurology,* 1996 47, 1113-1124.

McKeith, IG; Mintzer, J; Aarsland, D; Burn, D; Chiu, H; Cohen-Mansfield, J; Dickson, D; Dubois, B; Duda, JE; Feldman, H; Gauthier, S; Halliday, G; Lawlor, B; Lippa, C; Lopez, OL; Carlos Machado, J; O'Brien, J; Playfer, J; Reid, W; International Psychogeriatric Association Expert Meeting on DLB. Dementia with Lewy bodies. *Lancet Neurol,* 2004 3, 19-28.

McKeith, IG; Mosimann, UP. Dementia with Lewy bodies and Parkinson's disease. *Parkinsonism Relat Disord,* 2004 10(suppl 1), S15-18

Menza, MM; Palermo, B; Mark, M. Quetiapine as an alternative to clozapine in the treatment of dopamimetic psychosis in patients with Parkinson's disease. *Ann Clin Psychiatry,* 1999 11, 141-144.

Merino, JG; Luchsinger, J; Zhigao, H; Schmetzer, AD; Talavera, F; Ahmed, I; Harsch, HH; Soreff, S. Parkinson disease dementia. *WebMD,* October 13, 2004. www.emedicine.com7med7topic3110.htm

Minett, TS; Thomas, A; Wilkinson, LM; Daniel, SL; Sanders, J; Richardson, J; Littlewood, E; Myint, P; Newby, J; McKeith, IG. What happens when donepezil is suddenly withdrawn? An open label trial in dementia with Lewy bodies and Parkinson's diseases with dementia. *Int J Geriatr Psychiatry*, 2003 18, 988-993.

Miyasaki, JM; Shannon, K; Voon, V; Ravina, B; Kleiner-Fisman, G; Anderson, K; Shulman, LM; Gronseth, G; Weiner, WJ; Quality Standards Subcommittee of the American Academy of Neurology. Practice Parameter: Evaluation and treatment of depression, psychosis, and dementia in Parkinson disease (an evidence-based review): report of the Quality Standards Subcommittee of the American Academy of Neurology. *Neurology,* 2006 66, 996-1002.

Mohr, E; Mendis, T; Hildebrand, K; De Deyn, PP. Risperidone in the treatment of dopamine-induced psychosis in Parkinson's disease: an open pilot trial. *Mov Disord,* 2000 15, 1230-1237.

Molho, ES; Factor, SA. Worsening of motor features of parkinsonism with olanzapine. *Mov Disord,* 1999 14, 1014-1016.

Mosinan, UP; Mather, G; Wesnes, KA; O'Brein, JT; Burn, DJ; McKeith, IG. Visual percetion in Parkinson's disease dementia and dementia with Lewy bodies. *Neuroloy,* 2004 63, 2091-2096.

Murat, E. Dementia associated with Parkinson disease. *Lancet Neurol,* 2003 2, 229-237.

Neef, D; Walling, AD. Dementia with Lewy bodies: an emerging disease. *Am Fam Physician*, 2006 73, 1223-1229.

O'Brein, JT; Colloby, S; Fenwick, J; Williams, ED; Firbank, M; Burn, D; Aarsland, D; McKeith, IG. Dopamine transporter loss visualized with FP-CIT SPECT in the differential diagnosis of dementia with Lewy bodies. *Arch Neurol*, 2004 61, 919-925.

Ondo, WG; Tintner, R; Dat Voung, K; Lai, D; Ringholz, G. Double-blind, placebo-controlled, unforced titration parallel trial of quetiapine for dopaminergic-induced hallucinations in Parkinson's Disease. *Mov Disord,* 2005 20, 989-994.

Parkinson's Disease Mechanism Discovered, HHMI Research News. 2006. http://www.hhmi.org/news/lindquist20060622.html. June 22

Perry, EK; Irving, D; Kerwin, JM. Cholinergic transmitter and neurotrophic activities in Lewy body dementia: similarity to Parkinson's and distinction from Alzheimer disease. *Alzheimer Dis Assoc Disord,* 1993 7, 69-79.

Pillon, B; Boller, F; Levy, R; Dubois, B. Cognitive deficits and dementia in Parkinson's disease. In: Boller F and Cappa S (editors). *Handbook of Neuropsychology. 2 ed.* Amsterdam, Elsevier Sciences 2001, 311-371.

Pillon, B; Czernecki, V; Bubois, B. Dopamine and cognitive function. *Curr Opin Neurol,* 2003 16(suppl 2), S17-22.

Pillon, B; Dubois, B; Cusimano, G; Bonnet, AM; Lhermitte, F; Agid Y. Does cognitive impairment in cognitive disease result from non-dopaminergic lesion? *J Neurol Neurosurg Psychiatry,* 1989 52, 201-6.

Ravina, B; Putt, M; Siderowf, A; Farrar, JT; Gillespie, M; Crawley, A; Fernandez, HH; Trieschmann, MM; Reichwein, S; Simuni, T. Donepezil for dementia in Parkinson's disease: a randomised, double blind, placebo controlled, crossover study. *J Neurol Neurosurg Psychiatry*, 2005 76, 934-939.

Reading, PJ; Luce, AK; McKeith, IG. Rivastigmine in the treatment of parkinsonian psychosis and cognitive impairment: preliminary findings from an open trial. *Mov Disord,* 2001 16, 1171–74.

Richard, IH; Justus, AW; Greig, NH; Marshall, F; Kurlan, R. Worsening of motor function and mood in a patient with Parkinson's disease after pharmacologic challenge with oral rivastigmine. *Clin Neuropharmcol,* 2002 25, 296-299.

Rinne, JO; Rummukainen, J; Paljarvi, L, Rinne, UK. Dementia in Parkinson's disease is related to neuronal loss in the medial substantia nigra. *Ann Neurol,* 1989 26, 47-50.

Roberts, HE; Juncos, JL; Wood, CD; et al. Quetiapine for psychosis in patients with Parkinson's disease. Presented at the 32nd annual meeting of the American Society of Consultant Pharmacists Senior Care, Nov 7-10, 2001, Chicago, Ill.

Rub, U; Del Tredici, K; Schultz, C; Ghebremedhin, E; de Vos, RA; Jansen Steur, E; Braak, H. Parkinson's disease: the thalamic components of the limbic loop are severely impaired by alpha-synuclein immunopositive inclusion body pathology. *Neurobiol Aging,* 2002 23, 245-254.

Schrag, A; Jahanshahi, M; Quinn, N. What contributes to quality of life in patients with Parkinson's disease? *J Neurol Neurosurg Psychiatry,* 2000 69, 308-312.

Sellal, F. Parkinson's disease with dementia and dementia with Lewy body disease: two syndromes, the same disease? *Psychogeriatrics,* 2006 6, S30. doi:10.1111/j.1479-8301.2006.00132.x.

Tekin, S; Cummings, JL. Frontal-subcortical neuronal circuits and clinical neuropsychiatry: an update. *Psychosom Res,* 2002 53, 647-54.

The Parkinson Study Group. Low-dose clozapine for the treatment of drug-induced psychosis in Parkinson's disease. *N Engl J Med,* 1999 349, 757-763.

Tiraboschi, P; Hansen, LA; Alford, M; Sabbagh, MN; Schoos, B; Masliah, E; Thal, LJ; Corey-Bloom, J. Cholinergic dysfunction in diseases with Lewy Bodies. Neurology, 2000 54, 407-411.

Wagner, ML; Defilippi, IL; Menza, MA; Sage, IL. Clozapine for the treatment of psychosis in Parkinson's disease: chart review of 49 patients. *J Neuropsychiatry Clin Neurosci,* 1996 8, 276-280.

Whitehouse, PJ; Hedreen, JC; White, CL 3rd; Price, DL. Basal forebrain neurons in the dementia of Parkinson's disease. *Ann Neurol,* 1983 13, 243-248.

Wolters, EC. Dopaminomimetic psychosis in Parkinson's disease patients: diagnosis and treatment. *Neurology,* 1999 52(suppl 3), S10-S13.

In: Alzheimer's Disease Research Trends
Editor: A.P. Chan, pp. 209-223
ISBN 978-1-60021-712-8

Chapter X

Writing Errors Induced in Normal Subjects: A Comparison with Writing Alterations in Alzheimer's Patients

Rita Moretti*, Paola Torre and Rodolfo M. Antonello
Dipartimento di Medicina Clinica e Neurologia, U.C.O. di Clinica Neurologica,
Università degli Studi di Trieste, Italy.

Abstract

Writing is a complex process requiring visual memory, attention, phonological and semantic operations and motor performance. For that reason, it can easily be disturbed by interfering with attention, memory, by interfering subvocalization, and so on. Using 23 female third-year students (23.4 ± 0.78 years old) from the University of Trieste, we investigated the production of errors in three experimental conditions (control, articulatory suppression and tapping). In the articulatory suppression condition, the participants produced significantly more linguistic impairments (such as agrammatism, unrelated substitutions, sentence omissions, and semantically deviant sentences), which are similar to linguistic impairments found in aphasia. On the tapping condition there were more perseverations, deletions, and substitutions, both of letters and of words. We then have considered 50 patients suffering from Alzheimer's Disease (CDR average' score=1.76±0.56): we evaluated their writing production, in the spontaneous, under dictation and on copy tasks. We collected the samples and analysed their production, with the same schema of mistake' classification score. We compared the results, and try to find a correlation with specific items of the AD population.

These data suggest that writing is not an automatic skill. Only after many years of experience and practice of processing information (through cortical subcortical channels) can writing be considered an automatic skill. Limited experimental conditions can disrupt

* Correspondence concerning this article should be addressed to Rita Moretti M.D., Dipartimento di Medicina Clinica e Neurologia, U.C.O. di Clinica Neurologica, Università degli Studi di Trieste, Ospedale di Cattinara 34149 Trieste, Italy or e-mail (moretti@univ.trieste.it).

the writing system in normal subjects, probably interfering with the cortical subcortical loops, and link normality to pathology. In neurodegeneration, such as in Alzheimer' Disease, writing is precociously impaired and the disruption is early macroscopically evident.

Writing is an expression of language. However, even the most prolific authors speak more than they write, and for the bulk of the population, writing is far and away the least used of their language skills. Traditional neuropsychologists seem to have thought about writing as a skill, and appear to assume it to be closely dependent upon speech skills. Within cognitive neuropsychology, the study of writing processes has tended to concentrate on the writing in aphasic writers.

Writing is a cognitive system with a complex architecture consisting of many functionally independent procedural and memory components. It involves central and peripheral processes, where the central process integrates the output modalities involved in the spelling of familiar and unfamiliar words (Beauvois, and Derousne, 1981; Shallice, 1981; Alexander, Fischer, and Friedman, 1982; Bub, and Kertesz, 1982; Alexander, Friedman, Loverso, and Fischer, 1992). The peripheral processes realize the motor output of spelled words, with their allographic variants (Papagno, 1992). A popular view in the classical literature on dysgraphia states that writing requires the mediation of "inner speech" (Luria, 1970). More specifically, writing takes place through the acoustic analysis of the input, the recoding of each phoneme of the stimulus into a grapheme, and the recoding of graphemes in motor schemes (Luria, 1970). Children who were asked to open their mouths and keep them open while writing something produced more letter omissions, mis-spellings, and repetitions than the control group. In recent years, this phonological mediation hypothesis has been modified. For example, the dissociation between poor writing of familiar words and good writing of novel words in specific clinical cases (Beauvois, and Derousne, 1981; Ellis and Young, 1988) had been interpreted as evidence for the existence of two functionally independent routines: a lexical mechanism, which does not require phonological mediation and is used for spelling known words, and a phonological mechanism, which requires phonological mediation and is used for spelling words not previously encountered.

Many years have underwent since it was noted that the ability to write depende critically on both linguistic and motoric functions and that agraphia might be related to apraxia and visuospatial impairment. However, till that moment, some Authors have demonstrated that apractic agraphia were not intimately bound to apraxia of the limbs (Roeltgen, and Heilman, 1983). We report a clinical case of a 71-year-old man, with an eighth-grade education, in his usual state of health until two days before admission, when he noted difficulty in writing and a slight clumsiness of his right hand. At examination, he was right-handed (+22 at Briggs and Nebes Test) (Briggs, and Nebes, 1975); the medical history was remarkable for mild congestive heart failure and atrial fibrillation; he was alert and oriented. Calculations, right/left discrimination, stereognosis, graphestesia and memory appeared normal. He had no neglect, nor extinction. He exhibited a moderate right central facial weakness but no clear weakness or sensory loss in his extremities. Reflexes were symmetric. A CT of the head shoed a small area of presumed infarction involving the left-superior temporo-parietal cortex. Neuropsychological exams noted a slight dysprosodia, without a slow rate of speech. No aphasia was noted with the Aachner Aphasia Test (Luzzati, Wilmes, and DeBleser, 1992). Reading aloud and for comprehension was normal, as well preserved were his denomination, oral spelling, and his praxis (Christensen, 1975). The patient's writing was assessed under different conditions: he was asked to copy, write to dictation and spontaneously letters, words and sentences. He exhibited a profound impairment in grapheme production under all conditions and when writing single letters as well as entire sentences. Morphological, lexical and semantic aspects were not influenced by his writing impairment, which seems to interest only the motor sub-system, and in particular, its spatial realization. When he was asked to write with anagram letters, he did well, both with his right and left hand, and moreover, writing was not influenced by closing his eyes. He did not ameliorate when asked to write larger letters, and moreover, he noted that writing into a specific spatial pattern was very difficult. For example, he could not complete crossword puzzle anymore. His coordination pattern was equally disrupted when he intended to write following the horizontal line of a paper. He was tested three times during hospitalization, and he gradually began to improve, after the first week: firstly, we assisted to a better motor execution of the graphemic pattern, and lastly, to an improvement of spatial realization of his writing production.

Attention is also involved in writing. Writing was found to be impaired in a large number of acutely confused patients (Chedru, and Geschwind, 1972) without focal brain lesions. These impairments involved the motor and spatial aspects of writing as well as spelling and syntax, with a high error rate in terms of omissions and substitutions of consonants and of grammatical morphemes. Any visual scene contains multiple objects, where each object is composed of multiple features such as colour, shape, motion and location. Writing process needs the selection of the objects of interest (letters) based on any feature or combination of features. Such sort of spatial cueing enhances visual performance in a large variety of visual tasks, including threshold and supra-threshold detection of luminance increments and discriminations involving shape and colour (Eriksen, and Hoffman, 1972). Two locations are also selected in the context of a large class of vasomotor behaviours including orienting to peripheral stimuli; overt orienting refers to a set of processes by which stimuli of interest in a visual scene are detected in the periphery of the visual field and rapidly brought into the fovea by means of rapid saccadic eye movements. On the contrary, covert orienting is relevant for the fact that the behaviourally relevant stimuli can be attended to in the absence of exploratory saccadic eye movements. It is a well-known fact that we can move our attention around in visual space without moving our eyes; yet when the eyes do move, there appears to be an obligatory shift of attention. Therefore, cover orienting and overt orienting implicate oculomotor programming in the generation of attentional shifts. Both the systems are involved in writing, where higher vision is fundamental for its realization (Corbetta, 2001). Ullman (1984) proposed that the computation of various spatial relations between objects requires the application of visual routines to selected stimulus locations. However, because of computational limitations visual routines can be applied only to one or two locations. The analysis of the visual scene therefore requires a mechanism for selecting and switching the focus of processing from one location to another. Writing, as a cognitive system under lied by many functionally independent procedural and memory components, tightly relies on visuo-spatial attention. A recent work (Olive, and Kellogg, 2002) used interference reaction time for detecting auditory probes to measure attentional demands of copying, and composing a text in children and adults. With motor execution being relatively automatic, adults were able to attend fully to the high-level processes required in mature, effective composition. One reason that children fail to engage in such high-level processes is that motor processes deplete available attention.

Importantly, writing errors are not exclusive to aphasic patients as normal individuals also make errors in writing (Ellis, 1979). The errors referred here to are not spelling errors, but unintentional "slips of the pen", which can be perceived to be incorrect as soon as one becomes aware of them. One of the insights gleaned from studies of normal errors has to do with the planning of writing. If an error involves the intrusion of an element (e.g. a letter or a word) due later in a sequence, then the intruding element mostly likely must already have been selected from memory (Lashley, 1951; Miceli, Silveri and Caramazza, 1988). The orthographic representation is stored in the graphemic output buffer (Wing, and Baddeley, 1980; Miceli, et al. 1988), which seems to be part of the working memory. Information apparently decays in this buffer very rapidly (Wing, and Baddeley, 1980), and has to be refreshed for normal writing. The stored graphemic representations specify the identity and order of the component letters and their status as consonants or vowels. Different methods were proposed for classifying errors by collecting samples of spontaneous writing from Broca's, Wernicke's, and conduction aphasics (Sgaramella, Ellis, and Semenza, 1991), or by collecting a corpus of mistakes produced by normal persons (Ellis, 1979). We used a modified classification of mistakes, which gave good results in the study of the writing production in different neurological population (Moretti, Torre, Antonello, Carraro, Zambito-Marsala, Ukmar, Capus, Gioulis, Cazzato, and Bava, 2002). Spelling mistakes were not considered for this study. The remaining errors were classified into word-level (movement and selection) and letter-level (movement and selection) types of mistakes.

This study was conducted, at the beginning, precisely to evaluate various experimental manipulations of writing, in three conditions (spontaneous, copying, and dictation) in normal subjects: normal standard state, articulatory suppression and tapping. The articulatory suppression may interfere with phonological control, or reduce the number of the so-called parasitic thoughts, by activating the articulatory loop from the working memory. The tapping condition might interfere with motor development of intended act. Four questions have arisen in our minds, when we began the study:

1. do normal subjects produce movement or selection mistakes?
2. do normal subjects produce more mistakes in different experimental conditions?
3. could we distinguish specific types of mistakes in different experimental conditions, specific to the condition?
4. which type of writing modality (spontaneous, dictation or summary) is more sensitive to external stimuli?

The null hypothesis form is that there will be no significant differences in the number of errors between the conditions. What we found suggest that there are different and specific errors in the two experimental conditions (articulatory suppression and tapping), when compared to normal standard situation. The number of mistakes are significantly different, allowing us to reject the null hypothesis and claim support to the possibility to get in the way of writing procedure with two given stimuli, by altering the articulatory loop of the working memory, or by interfering with motor execution of the act.

But then, we decided to test 30 patients, suffering from Alzheimer's Disease (AD), at the very beginning of their clinical history, and to evaluate their writing production, in three conditions (spontaneous, copying, and dictation). We have detected their mistakes, evaluate them with the same criteria proposed for the normal subject group, and then compared them with the corpus collected from the samples of normal subjects.

We discuss the results, trying to examine the possible brain correlates with graphemic output realisation.

METHOD

Subjects

30 female third-year students (22.15 ± 0.54 years old) from the Faculty of Medicine at the University of Trieste. We chose a group of female students due to the probable minor hemispheric lateralization of linguistic areas (see data and literature in: Fabbro, and Bava, 1990). The participants have been enrolled randomly from an original group of 67 volunteers. We decided to limit the number of participants due to the duration of the tests (trials before test, instructions, explanations, and effective time for the test amount for more than four hours for each subjects), but have expanded their number, starting from a previous experience (Moretti, Torre, Antonello, Fabbro, Cazzato, and Bava, 2003). All the students were right handed according to the Briggs and Nebes test (Briggs, and Nebes, 1975). None of the subjects had ever suffered from language impairment, of learning disability or other neurological or auditory impairments.

30 patients, diagnosed as suffering from probable AD, in accordance with NINCDS-ADRDA (McKahnn, Drachman, Folstein, Katzmann, Price, and Stadlan, 1984), (73,84 ± 7,14 years old), right handed according to the Briggs and Nebes test (Briggs, and Nebes, 1975), at the very beginning of their clinical history, according to the Clinical Dementia Rating (CDR) (mean score= 1.765 ± 0,14) (Hughes, Berg, Danizger, Coben, and Martin, 1982), have been examined.

Materials and Procedures

The normal subjects' tasks were to write on set topics, to take dictation, to copy, and to summarize. The students were asked to write 3 compositions, given the following instructions: "Describe a trip near Trieste"; "Describe Your favourite topic at University"; "Describe your best friend". Then the subjects were asked to write a dictation of 90 words and non-words (see Appendix 1A) and 30 sentences, chosen from the Bilingual Aphasia Test (Paradis, 1987; Paradis, and Canzanella, 1990) (see Appendix 1B). Subjects were told that it might be possible that some phonemes, put together, could be presented to them, and in that case, it was part of the experiment, so they should write the same sounds they have heard. No specific mention has been made to the presence of non – words in the test. All the words, non-words and sentences were recorded and were allowed 5 seconds between words and 10 seconds between sentences. The students were then asked to summarize three tales recorded on audio tape (see Appendix 1C), given a maximum time of ten minutes each, and to copy three written passages, each of which contained 87 words (see Appendix 1D), given a maximum time of five minutes each.

The subjects had to carry out the trials under the following conditions: normal control; articulatory suppression (the subject must pronounce indefinite sounds such as "bla-bla" aloud; this causes an articulatory suppression of the subvocalizing enhancement of the memory process); tapping (the subject must tap with the forefinger of the left hand while writing with the right hand).

The order of the various conditions was counterbalanced across the subjects.

They were requested to execute their task on different pieces of paper (white sheets, without lines). No preference was indicated by the examiner whether to write in cursive or in print.

The AD patients were asked to write five sentences, spontaneously; then they were asked to write a dictation of 30 words and 30 non-words, and 5 sentences. They were asked to summarize a short story they have heard extracted from the Bilingual Aphasia Test (Paradis, 1987; Paradis, and Canzanella, 1990) and to copy five sentences from the same test. They were requested to execute their task on different pieces of paper (white sheets, without lines). No preference was indicated by the examiner whether to write in cursive or in print.

All the material was classified and corrected independently by two trained neurologists (with a good inter-rater reliability, kappa=0.79) and then the results were compared: spelling mistakes were not taken into account, nor were doubtful strokes, or inaccurate or imprecisely written letters. For disagreements between-raters, after comparison, there was a discussion and a final decision derived from a mutual consensus.

Spelling mistakes were not considered: "aqua" for "acqua", or "a" instead of "ha", or "artilio" for "artiglio", "perche" for "perché". The remaining significant errors were classified into word-level (movement and selection) and letter-level (movement and selection) types of mistakes. Letter Movement mistakes comprised adjacent and nonadjacent letter reversals (such as "catrolina" for "cartolina" or "fanira" "farina") and perseverations of single letters (such as "lamponee" for "lampone") (Kirk, Blonder, Wertman, and Heilman, 1991). Letter Selection mistakes comprised insertions (such as "penotola" for "pentola"), substitutions (such as "penta" for "penna") and deletions (such as "penola" for "pentola") (Kirk et al., 1991). Word Movement errors comprised perseverations (such as "andammo al al mare" for "andammo al mare") and regularizations of non-words (such as "catrame" for "catrumo") (Sgaramella, et al., 1991). Word Selection errors comprised omissions (such as "andammo mare" for "andammo al mare"), additions (such as "partirono per di Torino" for "partirono per Torino"), verbal substitutions (such as "cantina" for "catino"), and unrelated substitutions (such as "catrumpo" for "catrame") (Sgaramella, et al., 1991) of single words (data and Literature have been reported in: Moretti, Torre, Antonello, Fabbro, Cazzato, and Bava, 2003).

Statistical analysis was performed using the Statistical Package for the Social Sciences (SPSS-PC, version 10.0). In the comparison between groups, paired samples t-test, and analysis of variance (ANOVA) were used, as appropriate.

RESULTS

All the 30 students completed all the trials. We try to proceed accordingly to the four preliminary questions, presented in the introduction:

1. Do normal subjects produce movement or selection mistakes?The total number of errors was 943. The subjects produced 169 mistakes (19% of the total errors) under the control condition; in particular, they produced 19 letter-movement, 121 letter selection, 20 word-movement and 9 word-selection mistakes.
2. Do normal subjects produce more mistakes in different experimental conditions?

The total number of errors was 932. The subjects produced 169 mistakes (19% of the total errors) under the control condition, 330 (35%) under the tapping condition, and 433 (46%) under the articulatory suppression condition. In particular, they produced 20 letter-movement, 109 letter selection, 21 word-movement and 19 word-selection mistakes in normal condition; they produced 43 letter-movement, 235 letter selection, 17 word-movement and 35 word-selection mistakes in tapping condition; finally, they produced 44 letter-movement, 302 letter selection, 42 word-movement and 45 word-selection mistakes in articulatory suppression condition (Table 1).

Table 1. Summary of mistakes in the three experimental conditions

	NORMAL	TAPPING	ARTICULATORY SUPPRESSION
Letter movement mistakes	**20**	**43**	**44**
Letter selection mistakes	**109**	**235**	**302**
Word movement mistakes	**21**	**17**	**42**
Word selection mistakes	**19**	**35**	**45**
TOTAL	**169**	**330**	**433**

3. Could we distinguish specific types of mistakes in different experimental conditions, specific to the condition?

All the individual results were analyzed with an analysis of variance (condition: control, articulatory suppression and tapping; type of error: letter-level, word-level). The factor condition was significant ($F(2, 30) = 21.45$; $p<.001$). Type of error was also found to be significant ($F (1,15) = 59.91$; $p<.001$). The interaction condition/error type was significant ($F (2,30) = 8.67$; $p<.001$). Therefore, according to the Bonferroni test, the subjects produced significantly fewer errors under the control condition than under the tapping and articulatory suppression conditions. Moreover, the subjects produced significantly more errors in the articulatory suppression condition (Table 2).

4. Which type of writing modality (spontaneous, dictation or summary) is more sensitive to external stimuli?

Considering the single task proposed, subjects'errors could be divided as follows: 110 were found among dictated words; 183 were found among dictated non-words; 104 were found among dictated sentences; 166 were made in the summary task; 220 were made in the copy task; 149 were found in the composition task (Table 3). Paired samples t-tests (2-tailed) were done within tasks, considering letter-level and movement-level. In the word dictation task, the number of errors in the control condition was significantly different from articulatory suppression condition ($p<0.01$). No difference could be detected at the word level. In the non word dictation task, no significant difference emerged among the three different conditions, as far as letter level is concerned; the number of mistakes is significantly different in the articulatory suppression condition ($p<0.01$) in the word-level.

Table 2. Synopsis of qualitative analysis of total number of mistakes on different writing tasks

	TYPES OF MISTAKES	CONTROL	TAPPING	ARTICULATORY SUPPRESSION
Letter movement errors	**Adjacent letter reversals**	**10**	**6**	**15**
	Perseverations	**10**	**31**	**15**
	Non adjacent letters Reversals	**0**	**6**	**14**
Letter selection errors	**Insertions**	**7**	**20**	**34**
	Substitutions	**76**	**124**	**143**
	Deletions	**26**	**91**	**125**
Word movement errors	**Perseverations**	**0**	**2**	**13**
	Regularizations	**21**	**15**	**29**
Word selection	**Omissions**	**11**	**12**	**22**
	Additions	**0**	**8**	**0**
	Verbal substitutions	**4**	**6**	**11**
	Unrelated substitutions	**4**	**9**	**12**

Table 3. Synopsis of mistakes in three experimental conditions

	CONTROL				TAPPING				ART. SUPPRESSION				TOTAL
	Letter		**Word**		**Letter**		**Word**		**Letter**		**Word**		
	Sel	**Mov**	**Sel**	**Mov**	**Sel**	**Mov**	**Sel**	**Mov**	**Sel**	**Mov**	**Sel**	**Mov**	
Word-dictation	4	6	2	8	28	2	0	0	42	12	6	0	110
Non Word-dictation	27	0	8	8	38	0	4	14	32	4	18	30	183
Sentences dictation	16	0	0	0	14	8	0	0	54	2	10	0	104
Summary	16	10	2	0	45	8	8	0	50	8	9	10	166
Copy	27	0	4	5	69	16	11	3	74	8	1	2	220
Composition	19	4	3	0	41	9	12	0	50	10	1	0	149
Total	**109**	**20**	**19**	**21**	**235**	**43**	**35**	**17**	**302**	**44**	**45**	**42**	**932**

In the sentence task, paired sample t-tests suggested a significant difference among the number of mistakes in control versus articulatory suppression condition ($p<0.01$) at letter level. No difference was demonstrated at the word-level. In the copy task, paired sample t-tests suggested a significant difference in the number of letter-level mistakes in control versus tapping ($p<0.001$) and versus articulatory suppression ($p<0.001$). When compared to word level mistakes, only the control versus tapping conditions were significantly different ($p<0.001$).

In the summary task, paired sample t-tests suggested a significant difference in the number of letter level mistakes in the control versus the tapping ($p<0.05$) and versus the articulatory suppression conditions ($p<0.001$). When compared to word level mistakes, the control versus tapping conditions were significantly different ($p<0.01$), as were the control versus articulatory suppression ($p<0.001$). Lastly, in the composition task, paired sample t-tests put in evidence a significant difference in the number of letter-level mistakes in control versus tapping ($p<0.01$) and versus articulatory suppression ($p<0.001$). When compared word-level mistakes, control versus tapping condition is significantly different ($p<0.01$), as well as control versus articulatory suppression ($p<0.001$).

Table 4. Summary of mistakes in the AD group

	NORMAL	AD
Letter movement mistakes	20	309
Letter selection mistakes	109	247
Word movement mistakes	21	125
Word selection mistakes	19	104
TOTAL	**169**	**785**

Table 5. Synopsis of mistakes in AD patients

	AD				TOTAL
	Letter		**Word**		
	Sel	**Mov**	**Sel**	**Mov**	
Word-dictation	40	49	25	21	135
Non Word-dictation	56	45	31	35	167
Sentences dictation	34	34	24	5	97
Summary	49	56	21	15	141
Copy	27	56	6	11	100
Composition	41	69	18	17	145
Total	**247**	**309**	**125**	**104**	**785**

The AD patients were asked to write five sentences, spontaneously; then they were asked to write a dictation of 30 words and 30 non words, and 5 sentences. They were asked to summarize a short story they have heard extracted from the Bilingual Aphasia Test and to copy five sentences from the same test. Now, considering the corpus of mistakes made by the AD patients, it must be said that it is more consistent than that of the normal subjects, even in the articulatory suppression condition (Table 4). Considering the obvious reduction of given stimuli to the AD group (inferior to 54%, when comparing to the normal subjects stimuli), there is a larger corpus of mistakes in AD condition. AD patients made 785 mistakes in the only normal condition, which is significantly superior to the number of mistakes made by the normal subjects in all the condition (169; $p<0.001$), but even superior to the whole number of mistakes made by the normal subjects in the three conditions, if hypothesized that the number of stimuli is the same of the AD patients ($p<0.001$). Copy is the most preserved task, considering the ratio mistakes/given items (100/145=0.68). The other are the following: word dictation ratio mistakes/given items is 135/30=4.5; non word dictation ratio mistakes/given items is 167/30=5.66; sentences dictation ratio mistakes/given items is 97/45=2.15; summary ratio mistakes/given items (considering an average number of words produced of 45.3) is 141/45.3=3.11; composition ratio mistakes/given items (considering an average number of words produced of 40.23) is 145/40.23=3.604 (Table 5).

There is a significant number of mistakes in the letter-movement corpus of mistakes, when considering the letter level ($p<0.05$); no difference can be detected in the word-level groups.

Discussion

The analysis of a group of subjects studied under standardized conditions represents, first of all, a contribution to the description of writing errors in normal subjects, characteristically described as slips of the pen. New corpora of slips of the pen and of forced errors in normal spellers seem to be of interest, to the extent that they allow further insight into theoretical issues germane to the development of theories of spelling.

Even if the theoretical background of writing is not completely understood, the idea of looking at the disrupting effect of interfering tasks on writing might offer explanations for errors; on the contrary, the results can only be taken to show that normal subjects write more accurately if their attention is unperturbed, which is hardly surprising. To answer the four questions established in the introduction, our results demonstrate that normal subjects produced, in normal conditions, movement and selection mistakes. In normal conditions, letter – level mistakes were more frequent than word-level mistakes. When imposed experimental conditions, they interfere with writing production, heavier the articulatory suppression than the tapping condition, but both of them deeper than control condition. Moreover, during articulatory suppression condition, one can observe the doubling up of "paraphasic" mistakes, such as verbal or unrelated substitutions; the number of types of errors is clearly and significantly reduced, as well as the number of words produced. They were not analyzed parametrically, though there were a higher number of omissions of free grammatical morphemes, associated with a more conspicuous number of semantically deviant sentences, in the articulatory suppression condition. In the tapping condition, on the other hand, high percentage of perseverations of letters and omissions of words was found. Finally, tapping and articulatory suppression interfere with all the writing tasks executed by our volunteers, heavier and differently considering the larger amount of word-level mistakes produced.

Then, it might be hypothesized that articulatory suppression and tapping work somehow to interfere writing process. Once, it might be supposed that articulatory suppression interferes with the phonological mediated linguistic control. The writing process can be divided into different parts (Luria, 1970): words can be divided into phonemes, phonemes are converted into graphemes, and only then writing is possible. The importance of phonetic analysis in writing had been demonstrated in children; when learning to write, they are more likely to anticipate stressed than atonics syllables. In cases reported of sensory alalia (Luria, 1970), patients lose the ability to do phonetic analysis and are only able to copy written language. Stuttering children or children with uranoschisis, develop writing impairments, once interpreted due to the inaccuracy of their phonetic analysis. However, the phonological mediation hypothesis of writing is no longer tenable, especially in the light of recent evidence from adult aphasia (Ellis and Young, 1988). Thus, a "surface dysgraphic" patient may lose the capacity to retrieve once-familiar spellings from some form of lexical store, without losing the capacity to retrieve spoken word-forms; similarly, a "phonological dysgraphic" patient may lose the capacity for phoneme-grapheme conversion required to generate plausible spellings for unfamiliar words or non words without losing the capacity for grapheme-phoneme conversion in reading (Beauvois and Derousne, 1981). As clearly pointed out by Ellis and Young (1988), the cognitive neuropsychology of spelling and writing is not built solely upon patients in whom spelling and writing are impaired. For example, patients who can spell words correctly despite not having access to their correct spoken forms show that spelling of familiar words is not done by phoneme-grapheme conversion (Shallice, 1981). Baddeley (1982; Baddeley, Lewis, and Vallar, 1984; Baddeley, Papagno, and Vallar, 1988) proposed that articulatory suppression may reduce the number of the so-called parasitic thoughts, by activating the articulatory loop from the working memory. He determined that during tests of articulatory suppression, the number of spontaneous thoughts were significantly fewer compared to those registered during the quiet state. More recent experimental designs (Hanley, 1997) confirm that vision, and supplement it. A more precise study design (Calvo, and Eysenck, 1996) demonstrates that articulatory suppression interferes with the articulatory loop, which has been considered by those authors as a sort ancillary mechanism enhanced in the reading operational system when other strategies, such as regressive fixations and control of speed cannot be used. As far as has been demonstrated in a previous work (Moretti, Torre, Antonello, Carraro, Zambito-Marsala, Ukmar, Capus, Gioulis, Cazzato, and Bava, 2002) that reading and writing strongly depend on the integrity of oculomotor regressive fixation and attention, one might suppose that articulatory suppression might interfere with the attention system and above all, disrupting the articulatory loop, eliminates the possible auxiliary control system which guarantees correct execution of writing.

Tapping, considered as a movement itself, interferes both with attention input and with motor development of actions. When tapping is done with the left hand, functional imaging has put in evidence a bilateral activation of motor and supplementary motor areas(Moretti, Torre, Antonello, Ukmar, Longo, and Bava, 2002). Nobody described tapping as interference stimulus in writing process. Bilateral activation of motor and supplementary motor areas might interfere with motor control exerted by the right hand, dedicated at the same moment to a complex distal motor act. When tapping with the left hand, our volunteers persevered and repeat the last letter, or syllables, of the words or delete the last portions of words. There is an interesting analogy between the tapping condition and writing disturbances in acute confusional states (Chedru, and Geschwind, 1972), where an increase in substitution and perseveration of the last letter of words is found. This fact leaves us the possibility that tapping might interfere somehow in attention control of complex motor act, perhaps limiting the bimanual coordination requested in the specific task.

What can be created, as an experimental model, with the results of the tapping and articulatory suppression conditions might be considered a pseudo-agraphic situation (Sgaramella, et al., 1991). When the type of errors is considered, it must be emphasized that, under the articulatory suppression condition, subjects produced "unrelated word substitution," an increased number of semantically deviant sentences, an increase in the number of omissions of free grammatical morphemes, a reduction of total number of words, and an increase in types of errors specific which stand out as a variety typical only among pathological conditions. On the contrary, when tapping is activated, there is an higher number of perseveration in letters and syllables.

On the contrary, in the AD patients, the corpus of mistakes is higher than normal subjects, in all the three experimental conditions. The study is rather new, as far as we know of another one, systematic study, on writing in AD patients, but the latter did not consider different writing conditions (such as dictation, spontaneous writing, summary and copying) (LaBarge, Smith, Dick, and Storandt, 1992).

The study described graphic errors made in writing a simple sentence in 368 healthy older adults and individuals in different stages of dementia of the Alzheimer type. Errors of agraphia were present in both healthy and demented people and, in general, increased with the severity of dementia. The errors of agraphia were not correlated with measures of aphasia or psychometric measures of language and motor performance. Writing skill may represent procedural memory, and agraphia errors indicate alterations in long-term memory in dementia of the Alzheimer type (LaBarge, Smith, Dick, and Storandt, 1992).

What we have seen in our AD patients corresponds to an increase of mistakes, in all the tasks, with a relative preservation of copy. Thus, it seems that in AD condition, writing, an overlearned skill is disrupted in several parts, in the graphemic motor control, in phonological and in semantic procedure. Graphemic area has been postulated for distinguishing grapheme motor control and other motor skills coordination (Rothi and Heilman, 1981): however, nothing is known about the parietal role (real or putative) in spatial execution of graphemic patterns. We hypothesize that parietal lobe mediate visual input and high-definition control for specific-motor engrams (and among them, graphemes). As far as writing is concerned, parietal lobe may be involved in regularization of visuokinesthesic engrams (Liepmann and Maas, 1907), which realize the selection, timing and spatial relationships of learned motor skills, such as graphemes. Sitting at the junction of the temporal, parietal, and occipital lobes, the inferior region of the parietal area, particulary vulnerable to AD (which includes the angular and supramarginal gyri) has no strict anatomical boundaries, is partly coextensive with the posterior-superior temporal gyrus, and includes part of area 7 as well as area 37. It maintains rich interconnections with the visual, auditory, and somesthetic associations areas including the middle (basal) temporal lobe, the superior colliculus via the pulvinar, the lateral geniculate nucleus of the thalamus, and massive interconnections with the frontal lobes, inferior temporal region, and other higher order assimilation areas throughout the neocortex. Hence, the inferior parietal lobule has auditory and thus (in the left hemisphere) language capabilities. Given its location at the border regions of the somesthetic, auditory, and visual neocortices, and containing neurons and receiving input from these modalities, as the inferior parietal lobule evolved it became increasingly multimodally responsive; a single neuron simultaneously receiving highly processed somesthetic, visual, auditory and movement related input from the various association areas. Hence, many of the neurons in this area are multi-specialized for simultaneously analyzing auditory, somesthetic, and spatial-visual associations, and have visual receptive properties which encompass almost the entire visual field, with some cells responding to visual stimuli of almost any size, shape, or form (Moretti et al., 2005, in press). It has been argued that the sensory motor engrams necessary for the production and perception of written language are stored within the parietal lobule of the left hemisphere. In fact, given that the parietal lobes are concerned with the hands and lower visual fields, they not only guide and observe hand movements, but learn and memorize these actions, including those involved in writing. Hence, when lesioned, patients sometimes have difficulty writing and forming letters due to an inability to access these engrams. Writing samples may be characterized by mispellings, letter ommissions, distortions, temporal-sequential misplacements, and inversions. Sometimes agraphia is accompanied by alexia (Data and literature in: Rhawn, 2000).

Writing could be easily disrupted: it is an overlearned, extra-sophisticated skill, which requires fine and highly precise movements, depending on acquired rules. It is drammatically different from the other motor sequences, almost automatic of acts of real life: that is probably only a part of the truth and much more must be said on this topic.

In conclusion, it can be seen that writing is actually fragile and it is possible to disturb it because it depends on many components. Moreover, writing is not, or is only very rarely, an automatic skill. Limited experimental conditions can produce errors which somehow make normal subjects performance mimic those of subjects with specific pahologies.

REFERENCES

Alexander, M., Fischer, R., and Friedman, R. (1982) Lesion localization in apractic agraphia. *Archives of Neurology*, *49*, 246-251.

Alexander, M., Friedman, R., Loverso, F., and Fischer, R. (1992) Lesion localization of phonological agraphia. *Brain and language*, *43*, 83-95.

Baddeley, A. D, Lewis, V., And Vallar, G. (1984) Exploring the articulatory loop. *Quarterly Journal of Experimental Psychology*, *36A*, 233-252.

Baddeley, A. D, Papagno, C., and Vallar, G. (1988) When long-term learning depends on short-term storage. *Journal of Memory and Language*, *27*, 586-595.

Baddeley, A. D. (1982) Amnesia: a minimal model and interpretation. In L. S. Cermak (Ed.), *Human memory and amnesia.* Hillsdale, NJ: Erlbaum. Pp. 305-336.

Beauvois, M. F., and Derousne, J. (1981) Lexical or orthographic agraphia. *Brain*, 104, 21-49.

Briggs, G., and Nebes, R. (1975) Patterns of hand preference in a student population. *Cortex*, *11*, 230-23

Bub, D., and Kertesz, A. (1982) Deep agraphia. *Brain and Language*, *17*, 146-165.

Calvo, M. G., and Eysenck, M. W. (1996) Phonological working memory and reading in test anxiety. *Memory, 4(3)*, 289-305.

Chedru, F., and Geschwind, N. (1972) Writing disturbances in acute confusional states. *Neurpsychologia, 10*, 343-353.

Corbetta, M. (2001) *A neuroimaging exploration of human attention.* American Academy of Neurology (AAN), Phildelphia, 7FC.006, 98-108.

Ellis, A. (1979) Slips of the pen. *Visible language, XIII (3)*, 265-282.

Ellis, A., and Young, A. (1988) Spelling and writing. In: A. Ellis, and A. Joung, (Eds.), *Human cognitive neuropsychology*. Hillsdale , NJ: Erlbaum. Pp. 163-191.

Eriksen, C. W., and Hoffman, J. E. (1972) Temporal and spatial characterisitcs of selectinve encoding from visual displays. *Perception and Psychophysics, 12*, 210-204.

Fabbro, F., and Bava, A. (1990) *Asimmetrie dell'encefalo umano: filogenesi ed ontogenesi.* Firenze: Editrice Il Sedicesimo.

Hanley, J. R. (1997) Does articulatory suppression remove the irrelevant speech effect? *Memory, 5(3)*, 423-431.

Hughes C., Berg L., Danizger W., Coben L., and Martin R. (1982) A new clinical scale for the staging of dementia. *Brit. J. Psychiatry, 140*: 566-572.

Kirk, A., Blonder, L. X., Wertman, E., and Heilman, K. M. (1991) Phonolexical agraphia: superimposition of acquired lexical agraphia on developmental phonological dysgraphia. *Brain, 114/4*, 1977-1996.

Labarge E., Smith D. S., Dick L., and Storandt M. (1992) Agraphia in dementia of the Alzheimer type, *Archives of Neurology, 49*; 11: 121-134.

Lashley, K. (1951) The problem of serial order in behavior. In: L. A. Jeffress (Ed.), *Cerebral mechanism in behavior: the Hixon Symposium*, New York: J. Wiley. Pp. 112-136.

Liepman H., and Maas O. (1907) Einfall von linksseitiger Agraphie und Apraxie bei Rechtseitiger Lahmung. Translated by C. Wirsig and RT Watson *Monatschrift fur Psychologie und Neurologie, 10*, 214-227.

Lurjia, A. R. (1970) *Neuropsicologia del linguaggio grafico.* Padova: Editore Messaggero.

McKahnn G., Drachman D., Folstein M., Katzmann R., Price D., and Stadlan E.M. (1984) Clinical diagnosis of AD: report of the NINCDS-ADRDA work group under auspices of the Department of health and human services task forces on AD. *Neurology, 34*: 939-944.

Miceli, G., Silveri, M., and Caramazza, A. (1988) The role of the phoneme to grapheme conversion system and of the graphemic output buffer in writing. In: R. Coltheart, G. Sartori (Eds.), *The cognitive Neuropsychology of the language.* Hillsdale, NJ: Erlbaum. Pp. 235-251.

Moretti R., Torre P., Antonello R.M., Fabbro F., Cazzato G., Bava A. (2003). Writing errors by normal subjects. *Perceptual and Motor Skills*; *97*: 215-229.

Moretti, R., Torre, P., Antonello, R. M., Carraro, N., Zambito-Marsala, S., Ukmar, M., Capus, L., Gioulis, M., Cazzato, G., and Bava, A. (2002) Peculiar aspects of reading and writing performances in patients with olivopontocerebellar atrophy. *Perceptual and Motor Skills, 94*, 677-694.

Moretti, R., Torre, P., Antonello, R. M., Ukmar, M., Longo, R., and Bava, A. (2002) Learned movements in a left-handed pianist: an f-MRI evaluation. *Journal of Clinical Neuroscience, 9 (6)*, 680-684.

Olive, T., and Kellogg, R. T. (2002) Concurrent activation of high- and low-level production processes in written composition. *Mem. Cognit., 30 (4)*, 594-600.

Papagno, C. (1992) A case of peripheral dysgraphia. *Cognitive Neuropsychology, 9(3)*, 259-270.

Paradis, M. (1987) *The assessment of bilingual aphasia*. Hillsdale, NJ: Erlbaum.

Paradis, M., And Canzanella, M. (1990) *Test per l'afasia in un bilingue: versione italiana*. Hillsdale, NJ: Erlbaum.

Rhawn J. (2000) *The inferior parietal lobe. Neuropsychiatry, Neuropsychology, Clinical Neuroscience*. Academic Press, New York.

Rothi L.J., and Heilman K.M. (1981) Alexia and agraphia with spared spelling and letter recognition abilities. *Brain and Language*, *12*, 1-13.

Sgaramella, T., Ellis, A., and Semenza, C. (1991) Analysis of the spontaneous writing errors of normal and aphasic writers. *Cortex*, *27*, 29-35.

Shallice, T. (1981) Phonological agraphia and the lexical route in writing. *Brain*, *104*, 413-431.

Ullman, S. (1984) Visual routines. *Cognition*, *18*, 97-159.

Wing, A., and Baddeley, A.D. (1980) Spelling errors in handwriting: a corpus and a distributional analysis, In U. Frith (Ed.), *Cognitive Processes in Spelling*. New York: Academic Press. Pp. 252-285.

In: Alzheimer's Disease Research Trends
Editor: A.P. Chan, pp. 225-239

ISBN 978-1-60021-712-8

Chapter XI

THE ROLE OF ALLELES 4 AND 2 OF THE APOE GENE AND COGNITIVE TESTS IN THE EARLY CONVERSION OF MILD COGNITIVE IMPAIRMENT TO ALZHEIMER DEMENTIA

Ana Barabash[1], Alberto Marcos[2], Inés Ancin[1], Blanca M. Vazquez[1], Pedro Gil[3], Cristina Fernández[4], Juan José López-Ibor[1] and José Antonio Cabranes[1,]*

[1]Department of Psychiatry, [2]Department of Neurology, [3]Department of Geriatrics, [4]Epidemiological Unit, Hospital Clínico San Carlos, Madrid, Spain.

ABSTRACT

Late onset Alzheimer's disease (AD) is considered as a polygenic disorder resulting from the coincidence of a moderate number of genetic functional variants, located in candidate genes and others, each contributing small effects. Many studies focused mainly on identifying common risk alleles make it possible to predict the conversion from normal cognitive individual to Mild Cognitive Impairment (MCI), and from MCI to neurodegenerative dementia. We review the increasing literature about the genetics of AD under the light of our experience. We report a prospective study of apolipoprotein E (APOE) genotype in 89 patients diagnosed as MCI based on the Petersen criteria and supported by the MMSE, GDS scale and neuropsychological tests. After a median follow up of 49.6 months, 27 subjects remained with MCI and 62 subjects developed AD. This latest group was stratified again into two subgroups considering whether they converted to AD before (n=40) or after (n=22) 20 months of evolution. In order to assess the risk associated to each genotype, a control group (n=90) matched for age and sex and without

* Correspondence concerning this article should be addressed to Jose Antonio Cabranes, Psychiatry Department, Hospital Clínico San Carlos, C/ Martín Lagos s/n. 28040, Madrid, Spain. Tel: 0034913303808; Email: jcabranes.hcsc@madrid.salud.org.

memory impairment (MMSE≥28) was included. Patients who developed AD showed significantly lower values than MCI subjects in the CAMCOG (76% sensitivity and 67% specificity), for prompt detecting the onset of AD, with a 4.65-fold times increased risk of converting to AD (p<0.001). The presence of at least one APOE 4 allele was associated with risk of developing MCI (OR: 6,04; 95%CI: 2,76–13,23; p<0,001) but did not have an effect on the predictive cumulative hazard ratio (HR: 1.2; 95%CI: 0.73-2.1; p:0.32) of developing AD. Though it did not reach a statistically significant level, the presence of at least one APOE 2 allele showed a protective effect for the risk of developing MCI (OR: 0,57; 95%CI: 0,14–2.26). No patient was homozygous for 2/2 and no patient with rapidly progressive disease carried the 2 allele either (HR: 0.4; 95%CI: 0.05-2.7; p: 0.25). Our data demonstrated a strong association of APOE 4 carrier status by itself with MCI, predicting a higher risk to suffer MCI. APOE 2 variant showed an interesting protective effect to MCI. Notwithstanding, the presence of at least an allele 4 when the patient is suffering MCI did not change the probability of progression to AD.

Introduction

Mild Cognitive Impairment (MCI) is considered a transitory clinical entity toward dementia. MCI is characterized by memory complains with normal global cognitive function [1,2]. However there is epidemiological evidence that a lot of MCI diagnosed subjects do not deteriorate over time and even some of them can return to a normal state, being the initial impairment a consequence of concomitant depression, stress situation or metabolic alterations. These reasons and the lack of consensuated criteria for their classification have induced some authors to consider the MCI as a non-homogeneous clinical syndrome [3].

Different diagnostic criteria, time of evolution and source of derivation of the patients between the reported studies are the probable cause of the dispersion of the results about the outcome and heterogeneity of the patients included in this syndrome [1,2,4-11]. A recent report [12] recommended the development of proper and sensible functional and neuropsychological measures, sure methods to assess the clinical outcome and sensible epidemiologically oriented instruments across different cultures.

In spite of the fact that we can assess that amnestic MCI subjects frequently progress to Alzheimer's disease (AD) and we can depend on reported criteria and global consensus for the diagnosis of MCI [1,13-15], including clinical subtypes and probable aetiologies, there is a fairly high degree of heterogeneity about the clinical outcome within this group of patients. So, new classifications based on neuropsychological and genetical profiles are needed.

In one hand, clinical prediction methods as the Clinical Dementia Rating (CDR) criteria could not predict group membership, having poor sensitivity in healthy older people for detecting memory decline [16]. Standard neuropsychological evaluations are sensitive and specific for distinct types of impairments described in preclinical stages of AD, they are inexpensive and useful for the identification of changes in brain function, and have the advantage of not requiring sophisticated instrumental methods [17-27]. MCI subjects declined faster on daily life advance activities, episodic, semantic and logical memory, perceptual speed and attention compared with normal age-matched people. As well as among AD there are also frontally-mediated behaviours, consist of apathy and executive dysfunction. In normal ageing there are mild impairment in episodic memory function involving retrieval strategy, but it affects also and preferentially encoding in both AD and MCI. The selective amnesia of the MCI patient was joined next by semantic and other linguistic disorders and emerging difficulties with visuospatial skills and since the impairment progressed, they had problems with response inhibition and speed of attentional switching. In a previous study [28], we report that a broad neuropsychological battery together with clinical scales and activities of daily living assessment can differentiate MCI from AD patients on the first evaluation. Lawton and Reisberg Scale for Global Deterioration (GDS), Mini-Mental State Examination of Folstein et al (MMSE), Blessed scale, global CAMCOG (Global Cognitive subscale of the Cambridge Mental Disorders in the elderly Examination Assessment schedule) and some of its subtests scoring showed differences between the individuals that progress or do not to dementia. Also, the global score of the CAMCOG joined to Calculus, Orientation, Memory, Attention and Perception subtest had the highest sensitivity and specificity for distinguishing patients who develop AD, three of them (CAMCOG, Memory and Perception) being able to predict the risk of progression from MCI to AD with high sensitivity. Although these neuropsychological parameters could help in the clinical differentiation of MCI and prognostic purposes its value applied to particular individuals outside epidemiological studies is still controversial.

In the other hand, the possibility to identify genes participating in the etiology of MCI could open great opportunities to improve their diagnosis and outcome, even allowing initiating early treatments before the degenerative process was established. Considering that the distinct entities that probably form the MCI diagnosis concept (AD, vascular dementia, neuropsychiatric diseases) could had a genetical origin, different genes can be implicated. The four genes currently related to AD are the amyloid precursor protein [29], presenilin-1 [29-31] and presenilin-2 [32], all of them included in the unusual autosomical dominant forms of AD and the Apolipoprotein E (APOE) which is a common genetic risk factor to AD.

Having in mind the previous reports that find an association between the APOE gene and the cognitive decline and MCI, we decide to study the polymorphisms of this glycoprotein to establish if the presence of the allele 4 and/or the 2 allele changed the risk to develop AD.

METHODS

We performed a longitudinal prospective study on 89 individuals (59 female, 30 male) who consecutively attended the Memory Units within the Neurology and Geriatrics Departments of the Hospital Clínico San Carlos, Madrid, Spain. All of them complained of memory problems with no difficulties on daily life activities, and fulfilled the MCI established diagnostic criteria by Petersen et al [14]: 1) The presence of a subjective memory complain, 2) preserved general intellectual functioning as estimated by performance on a vocabulary test, 3) demonstration of a memory impairment by cognitive testing, 4) intact ability to perform activities of daily living, and 5) absence of dementia criteria. The study was performed in accordance with both the international ethical recommendations regarding research and human clinical trials as set out in the Helsinki Declaration (1964) and the guidelines for good clinical research practice (WHO, 1995). The procedure of the research project was explained to the patients participating in the study. All subjects signed an informed consent form. A clinical interview with a close relative was done. We analysed age, gender, educational level, social support and professional status. Appropriate classification of MCI was based on the MMSE [33] and GDS, supported by functional assessment and neuropsychological tests (Table I). To assess the risk associated to each genotype a case control study was carried out. For this purpose a control group of 90 subjects matched in age and sex (56 female, 34 male) recruited from day Care units, without mental disturbances and without memory impairment (MMSE score $\geq$ 28) was included. We excluded subjects who met dementia criteria as per DSM-IV or ICD-10, with functional or social disabilities, with a GDS score higher than 3, with more than 4 points in the Hachinski Ischaemia Scale, with history of stroke, toxic abuse, metabolic, endocrine, inflammatory, infectious, terminal, renal, hepatic or current psychiatric diseases, with uncertain development or very low educational level. On every subject we performed complementary explorations (Class II evidence level) recommended by the American Neurology Association [34], blood and urine test, basic biochemical with Gamma-Glutaril-Transpeptidase, B_{12}, folate and thyroid analysis and luetic serology, and Cranial Tomography (CT) or Magnetic Resonance Imaging (MRI).

Table I. Neuropsychological evaluations performed to the 89 subjects of the study

Cognitive domain:

- Minimental State Examination of Folstein et al (MMSE)
- Global Cognitive subscale (CAMCOG) of the Cambridge Mental Disorders in the elderly Examination Assessment schedule, and the items:
  - Orientation
  - Praxis
  - Language
  - Calculus
  - Memory
  - Abstract thinking
  - Attention
  - Perception
- Rivermead Barrage Memory Test (RBMT)
- Benton visual memory test
- Wechsler Adult Intelligence Scale (WAIS) with the items:
  - Vocabulary
  - Digits
  - Number codes
  - Incomplete figures
  - Puzzles

Functional domain:

- Blessed Dementia scale
- Lawton and Brody activities scale

Affective domain:

- Yesavage Geriatric Depression scale.

Genetic Study

Genomic DNA was extracted from EDTA-anticoagulated whole blood samples using standard DNA isolation methods. APOE genotyping was performed using polymerase chain reaction-restriction length polymorphism (PCR-RFLP) assays. Detection of APOE genotype was done using a method adapted from Zivelin et al. [35] but using forward primer from method described by Hixton and Vernier [36] that yields a 227 bp DNA fragment. Double digestion of this fragment with *Afl*III and *Hae*II yields on 4% agarose metaphor electrophoresis three specific fragments: 195 bp for APOE E4 allele, 177 bp for E2 allele and 145 bp for E3 allele respectively.

The median time of follow-up was 49.6 months. Our final patient's population emanate from a group of amnestic MCI individuals and the individuals were followed up with symptomatic and cognitive assessment. After this follow-up period some patients developed AD while others retained the initial diagnosis of MCI, being then divided into two groups:

1/ Group I, 62 patients were diagnosed with probable AD according to the DSM-IV criteria supported by neuropsychological tests. They can be considered as Progressive Mild Cognitive Impairment Patients (PMCI). The appropriate classification of dementia as AD was based on the National Institute of Neurological and Communicative Disorders and Stroke and the Alzheimer's disease and Related Disorders Association (NINCDS-ADRDA) criteria, a score in the Hachinski Ischaemia Scale lower than 5, with no evidence of cerebral cortical

infarcts and no more than a subcortical lacunar infarct lower than 1.5 cm on CT or MRI. PMCI were in the 4 to 7 stages of the GDS;

2/ Group II, 27 subjects who did not develop dementia and retained the initial of MCI.

They can be considered as Stable Mild Cognitive Impairment Patients (SMCI). SMCI individuals were in the 1 to 3 stages of the GDS.

Statistical Analysis

Qualitative variables are shown with their frequency distribution together with their 95% confidence interval. Quantitative variables are represented by their mean and standard deviation or median and its IQR. Their association was assessed by means of the chi-squared or *t* -test. The effect size was estimated by absolute differences between the study groups and their 95% confidence interval. Areas below the curve and cut-off points with the highest predictive values (maximum sensitivity and specificity) were estimated. The significance of the area below the curve was established by the fact that 0.5 was not included within the 95% confidence interval. Neuropsychological validity parameters were calculated with sensitivity and specificity. Hardy-Weinberg (H-W) equilibrium was determined by χ^2 exact test. Comparisons of genotype frequencies were performed according to the χ^2 analysis. Odds Ratios (OR) were estimated to assess the risk of developing MCI. Kaplan-Meier survival-analysis method and Cox proportional hazard analyses with dementia diagnosis used as an event were done to study the effect of each genotype in the MCI progression to dementia. Adjusted Hazard Ratio (HR) was calculated. In all hypothesis contrasts the null hypothesis was rejected with a type 1 or α error of less than 0.05. In all cases 95% confidence intervals were calculated. Data were analysed with SPSS 12.0 for Windows® and Epidat 2.01.

RESULTS

Sociodemographic data for groups PMCI and SMCI are shown on Table II. The PMCI group was older (p=0.008) than the SMCI group at inclusion. Although more females than males progress to dementia, there were no significant differences between them in sex distribution, in length of disease evolution, years of schooling, professional status or social support. Sixty-two patients met clinical criteria for dementia over four years from an initial population of 89 subjects, with a rate of progression to dementia of 69.7% in our population.

Table II. Sociodemographical data for the study groups

VARIABLE	PMCI n=62	SMCI n=27	p
Age (years)*	77 (74-80,2)	74 (65-77)	0,008
Age range (years)	53-92	53-80	
Male (%) **	22 (35,5)	8 (29,6)	0.58
Duration of disease evolution (months)*	24 (18-36)	22 (12-36)	0,45
Length of schooling ** ≤10 years (%)	54 (87,1)	22(81,5)	0,49
Professional status ** (% unqualified)	43 (72,9)	19 (70,4)	0,81
Social support ** (% with low rating)	11 (19,6)	5 (20,8)	0.90

* Median (IQR); ** Absolute number (%); PMCI: Progressive Mild Cognitive Impairment Patients; SMCI: Stable Mild Cognitive Impairment Patients.

With regard to the cognitive variables, PMCI patients showed significantly lower values (p=0.01-0.001) than SMCI subjects on Lawton and GDS basal scoring, MMSE, Blessed scale, Vocabulary, Puzzles and Number Codes subtest of the WAIS, global CAMCOG scoring, including its Orientation, Language, Memory, Perception, Calculus, Attention and Abstract thinking subtests and the Rivermead score (Table III).

The best tools for separating both SMCI and PMCI groups were the MMSE and Blessed scale score, the global CAMCOG score with its subtest Orientation and Memory and the Rivermead score (Table IV). All of them have ROC areas near or higher than 80%, with sensitivities from 76 to 87 and specificities from 67 to 71. We calculated the Hazard Ratio (HR) with the optimum sensitivity and specificity data (Table V). The survival curve of the global study group is showed in Figure 1. We can appreciate an inflexion point at 20 months, meaning the moment on evolution that divide the patients with quick from slow progression. The global and after 20 months of follow-up survival curves from the CAMCOG score are showed in Figures 2 and 3. Considering the SMCI subjects face to the PMCI patients, we can appreciate a cumulative probability to develop an AD until 4.65 times (95%CI: 2.5-8.7; p<

0.001) if the scoring is lower than 82.5 points. With regard to the patients with quick evolution face to the slow or no evolution patients, we can appreciate a cumulative probability to develop an AD until 9.10 times (95%CI: 3.4-23.4; p<0.001) if the scoring is lower than 78.5 points.

Table III. Neuropsychological data of the 89 studied subjects

GROUP	Group I (PMCI) (n =62)	Group II (SMCI) (n =27)	p
Lawton	6.7 (1.3)	7.3 (0.8)	0.009
MMSE	26.4 (3.6)	30.4 (3.4)	<0.001
GDS	2.4 (0.6)	1.9 (0.5)	0.004
Blessed	4.0 (2.4)	2.0 (1.5)	0.01
Hachinski	1.0 (0.9)	0.01 (0.6)	0.191
Yesavage	3.0 (2.3)	2.0 (1.4)	0.177
Vocabulary*	11.5 (12.9)	16.0 (22.5)	0.004
Digits*	8.0 (1.7)	7.9 (2.2)	0.92
Figures*	8.3 (3.0)	9.5 (3.9)	0.281
Number Codes*	5.0 (6.7)	11.0 (15.1)	0.001
Puzzles*	6.5 (5.9)	11.5 (10.3)	0.003
CAMCOG Score	76.0 (8.5)	89.8 (10.3)	<0.001
Orientation**	8.4 (1.2)	9.5 (0.8)	<0.001
Language**	23.7 (2.4)	26.2 (2.7)	<0.001
Praxis**	8.6 (2.9)	9.8 (3.1)	0.063
Memory**	16.4 (3.5)	20.8 (4.1)	<0.001
Attention**	4.5 (2.1)	6.1 (2.8)	0.005
Calculus**	1.5 (0.5)	1.8 (0.4)	0.007
Perception**	6.8 (1.4)	7.8 (1.1)	0.001
Abstract Thinking**	6.1 (1.5)	7.2 (1.9)	0.007
Benton	3.5 (1.8)	3.2 (0.5)	0.814
RBMT	6.0 (2.6)	9.2 (1.9)	0.001

Data shown are mean (and standard deviation) or #median (and 25-75 IQR); PMCI: Progressive Mild Cognitive Impairment Patients; SMCI: Stable Mild Cognitive Impairment Patients; MMSE: Mini-Mental Examination of Folstein et al; GDS: Reisberg Scale for Global Deterioration; CAMCOG: Global Cognitive subscale of the Cambridge Mental Disorders in the elderly Examination Assessment schedule;*: WAIS' subtest; **: CAMCOG's subtest; RBMT: Rivermead Barrage Memory Test.

Considering the genetic variables, as has been done by other authors, APOE genotypes were divided either into E4 positive (E4E4, E4E3, E4E2), E2 positive (E2E3 and E2E2) and E3 homozygote (E3E3). There were no subjects in the group of patients presenting the E2E2 genotype. As some evidence suggests that E2 may be protective, two control subjects with the E2E4 genotype were included in the E4 positive group, after analyzing that the deleterious effect of E4 was higher than the protective effect of E2 when E2E4 subjects were alternatively included or excluded in any of the groups. Possession of at least one APOE 4 allele was associated with the risk of developing MCI (OR: 6, 04; 95%CI: 2, 76–13, 23; p<0,001) but did not have an effect on the predictive cumulative hazard ratio (HR: 1.2; 95%CI: 0.73-2.1; p: 0.32) of developing AD. Though it did not reach a statistically significant level, the possession of at least one E2 allele showed a protective effect for the risk to develop MCI (OR: 0, 57; 95%CI: 0, 14–2.26). No patient was homozygous for E2E2 and no patient with rapidly progressive disease carried the E2 allele neither (HR: 0.4; 95%CI: 0.05-2.7; p: 0.25) (Table VI and Figures 4 and 5).

Table IV. Validity of the neuropsychological data for the detection of clinical progression from SMCI to PMCI of the 89 studied patients

Data	ROC (95% CI) Cut-off Point (%)	Se	Sp
MMSE	0.79 (0.7-0.9) 29.5	79	71
GDS	0.70 (0.6-0.8) 2.5	40	92
Blessed	0.79 (0.7-0.9) 2.25	76	70
Vocabulary**	0.56 (0.4-0.8) 18.5	71	50
Puzzles**	0.72 (0.6-0.9) 8.5	58	56
Number codes**	0.65 (0.5-0.8) 11.5	79	50
CAMCOG	0.85 (0.8-0.9) 82.5	76	67
Orientation*	0.78 (0.7-0.89) 9.5	81	70
Language*	0.75 (0.6-0.8) 25.5	77	56
Memory*	0.80 (0.7-0.9) 19.5	79	70
Attention*	0.68 (0.6-0.8) 4.5	53	70
Calculus*	0.63 (0.5-0.7) 1.5	45	71
Perception*	0.71 (0.6-0.8) 7.5	71	63
Abstract Thinking*	0.68 (0.6-0.8) 7.5	74	51
RBMT	0.85 (0.7-0.9) 8.5	87	70

PMCI: Progressive Mild Cognitive Impairment Patients; SMCI: Stable Mild Cognitive Impairment Patients; ROC: ROC area; 95% CI: 95% Confidence Interval; Se: Sensitivity; Sp: Specificity; MMSE: Mini-Mental Examination of Folstein et al; GDS: Reisberg Scale for Global Deterioration; CAMCOG: Global Cognitive subscale of the Cambridge Mental Disorders in the elderly Examination Assessment schedule; *: CAMCOG's subtest; **: WAIS's subtest; RBMT: Rivermead Barrage Memory Test.

CONCLUSION

Since the introduction of prescription drugs against dementia, which may soon be indicated on MCI subjects, its early detection has become a vast issue. The prompt prediction of cognitive impairment will be essential to delay the progression of the disease.

Table V. Likelihood of progression to AD from 89 MCI subjects by the neuropsychological data

SUBTEST	Cut-off Point	HR (95 % CI)	p
MMSE	< 29.5	4.22 (2.22-8.02)	< 0.001
	> 29.5	1	
Blessed	< 2.25	0.34 (0.18-0.62)	< 0.001
	> 2.25	1	
CAMCOG	< 82.5	4.65 (2.50-8.65)	< 0.001
	> 82.5	1	
Orientation*	< 9.5	3.81 (2.01-7.24)	< 0.001
	> 9.5	1	
Memory*	< 19.5	3.59 (1.93-6.70)	< 0.001
	> 19.5	1	
RBMT	< 8.5	4.45 (1.3-4.45)	0.005
	> 8.5	1	

HR: Hazard Ratio; *: CAMCOG subtest; 95% CI: 95% Confidence interval; MMSE: Mini-Mental Examination of Folstein et al.; RBMT: Rivermead Barrage Memory Test.

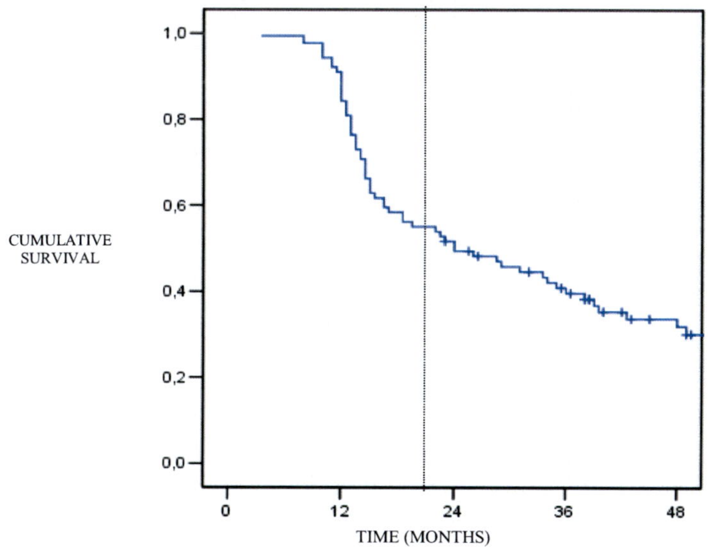

Figure 1. Survival curve of the global group of study.

The APOE is a 299 aa glycoprotein codified by a gene localized in the 19q 13.2, founded in the neuritic plaques and the neurofibrilary tangles which promote the amyloid formation. Given its role in early as well as late-onset forms of AD, the APOE gene may be a more useful model for studies aiming to improve diagnostic criteria for MCI and as evolution marker. Despite the studies reported about the APOE role in MCI have not produced consistent features, it may be due to the use of small and heterogeneous samples of individuals, short following-up periods and without controlled confusion variables.

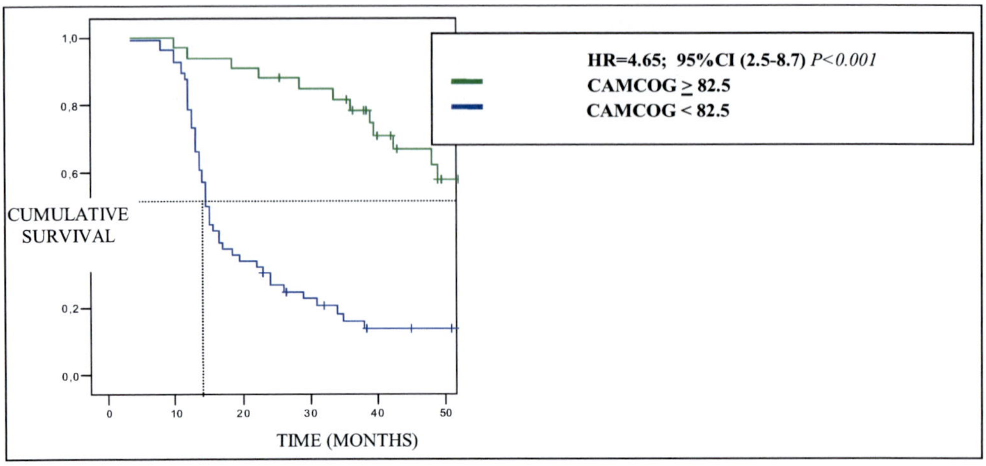

Figure 2. Cumulative probability to develop AD in the follow-up according to the CAMCOG scoring between PMCI and SMCI patients.

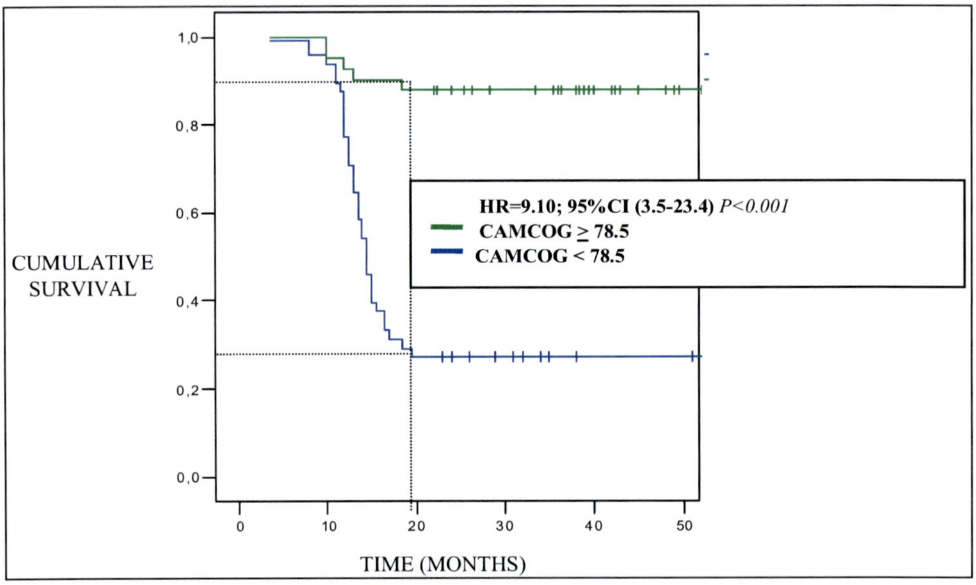

Figure 3. Cumulative probability to develop AD at 20 month of the follow-up according to the CAMCOG scoring between quickly or slowly progressive dementia groups.

Some authors have reported that the presence of the E4 allele is associated with different degrees of memory decline on elderly subjects, being more frequent among lately developing dementia individuals [37-39]. But there are few longitudinal prospective studies reported, which are also controversial. Petersen et al. [4] and Tierney et al. [5] after at least a two year follow-up have showed that the presence of the E4 allele is a good predictor to dementia in the evolution. However other authors [40-42] do not find this association.

We studied a group of control individuals and amnestic MCI subjects, emanating from specialized neurological and geriatric clinics, and after the exclusion of the subjects that in the sucesive follow-up normalized the neuropsychological and memory scores or a psychiatric disease emerged. So, our final subject's population were in the probable AD group on evolution. Our findings prove that the APOE gene is a risk gene to developing MCI, that the risk depends on the presence of the E4 allele and that the E4 carriers have a six-fold higher risk to have a MCI than the non-carriers individuals. On the contrary we have found that the E2 carriers have a protection factor as the risk to developing MCI is decreased by half. After a wide follow-up period we have observed that the presence of the E4 allele does not increase the risk of developing AD, so we think that the evolution from MCI to dementia does not seem related to the APOE 4 allele status. Notwithstanding the APOE 2 allele presence seems to be a protective character, as if the subject carries the 2 allele he has a median disease-free time of 24 months, much superior than the non carriers, and in front of the 33 or 4 allele carriers. This argument is reinforced by the fact that none of the PMCI patients has the homozygous character to 22, but it was present in the control group. In addition if we divide the MCI group according to the velocity of the progression none of the E2 allele carriers develops dementia in less than 20 months, as the statistically significant HR shows.

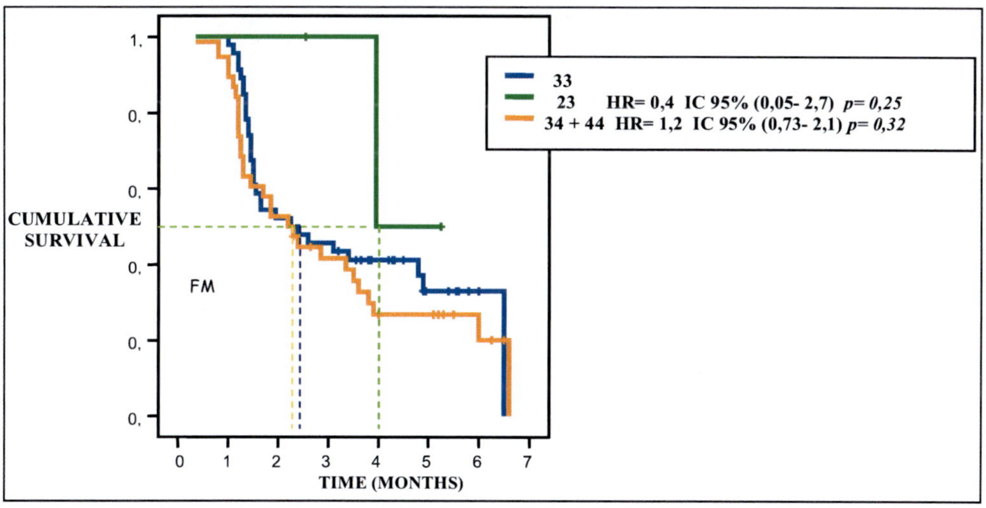

Figure 4. Cumulative probability to develop AD in the follow-up according to the APOE genotype between PMCI and SMCI groups.

From the neuropsychological study we can conclude that some cognitive variables (Lawton and GDS, MMSE, Blessed scale, Vocabulary, Number Codes and Puzzles subtests of the WAIS, the global CAMCOG and its Orientation, Language, Memory, Perception, Calculus, Attention and Abstract thinking subtests and the Rivermead memory test) were different between the individuals that progress or not to dementia. Some of them (MMSE, Blessed scale, global score of the CAMCOG joined to Orientation and Memory subtest and the Rivermead memory test) have high sensitivity and specificity for distinguishing patients who develop AD. Patients that score lower than 82.5 points in the CAMCOG score have an accumulated likelihood to develop an AD up to 4.65 times, the accumulated likelihood to develop an AD in the first 20 months being up to 9.10. These neuropsychological variables classified the patients according to the deterioration process, differentiated and predicted if a patient affected with memory complains was suffering a cognitive impairment in its early stage and could inform about the risk of culminating in dementia. Punctuations higher than the established cut-off points can identify with high probability the risk to developing dementia among the MCI group of subjects, and were an useful tool for clinical practice, easily available in the majority of Memory Units for cognitive assessment.

Our results confirm the discriminative power for distinguishing MCI from AD patients of some cognitive variables obtained even from the first neuropsychological evaluation. From the genetic study we can infer that the presence of the APOE E4 allele confers a risk to develop MCI, but if the MCI is established it does not modify the evolution to AD. And finally the presence of the 2 allele seems to generate a protective effect both to develop MCI and/or AD. The combination of neuropsychological and genetic variables classified the patients according to the deterioration process, differentiated and predicted if a patient affected with memory complains have high risk of developing dementia.

Table VI. Genotypic frequencies and risk to develop MCI associated to the APOE genotype

		Controls*		Cases				
APOE	Genotype	N	%	N	%	OR	CI 95%	P
	33	70	77.8	46	52.9	1		< 0,001
	22 + 23	8	8.9	3	3.4	0.57	0.14 – 2. 26	
	24+ 34 + 44	12	13.3	38	43.7	6. 04	2.76 – 13. 23	

OR: Odds Ratio; 95% CI: 95% Confidence interval; * The distribution of the genotypes was in Hardy-Weinberg equilibrium.

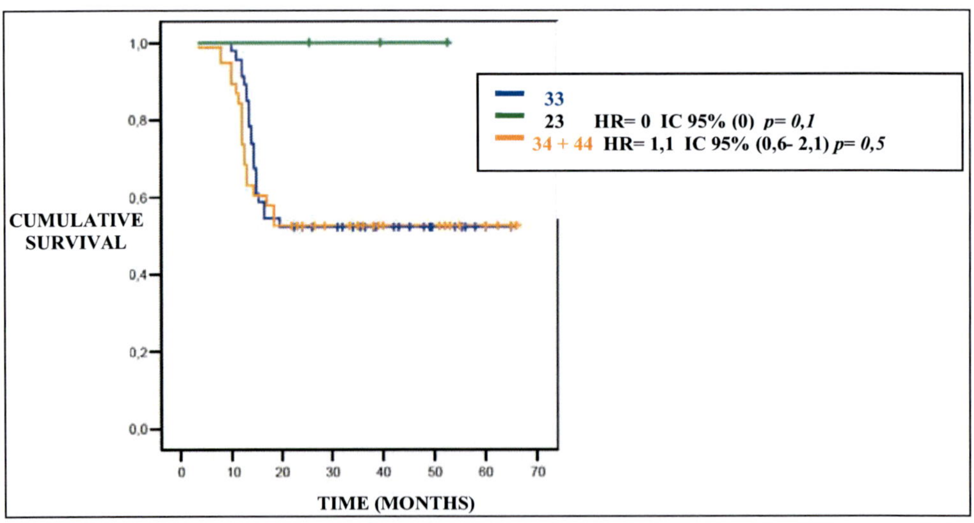

Figure 5. Cumulative probability to develop AD at 20 month of the follow-up according to the APOE genotype between quickly or slowly progressive dementia groups.

REFERENCES

[1] Petersen RC, Morris JC. Clinical features. In: Petersen RC, ed. *Mild Cognitive Impairment: aging to Alzheimer's disease*. New York: Oxford University Press, Inc, 2003c: 15-40.

[2] Flicker C, Ferris SH, Reisberg B. Mild Cognitive Impairment in the elderly: predictors of dementia. *Neurology* 1991; 41: 1006-1009.

[3] Gauthier S, Touchon J. Mild cognitive impairment is not a clinical entity and should not be treated. *Arch Neurol* 2005; 62, 7: 1164-6.

[4] Petersen RC, Smith GE, Ivnik RJ, et al. ApoE status as a predictor of the development of Alzheimer's disease in memory-impairment individuals. *JAMA* 1995; 273: 1274-1278.

[5] Tierney MC, Szalai JP, Snow WG, et al. A prospective study of the clinical utility of ApoE genotype in the prediction of outcome in patients with memory impairment. *Neurology* 1996; 46: 149-154.

[6] Ritchie K, Artero S, Touchon J. Classification criteria for mild cognitive impairment. A population-based validation study. *Neurology*, 2001; 56: 37-42.

[7] Larrieu S, Letenneur L, Orgogozo JM, et al. Incidence and outcome of mild cognitive impairment in a population-based prospective cohort. *Neurology* 2002; 59: 1594-1599.

[8] Palmer K, Wang H, Backman L, et al. Differential evolution of cognitive impairment in nondemented older persons: results from the Kungsholmen Project. *Am J Psychiatry* 2002; 59: 436-442.

[9] Encinas M, de Juan R, Marcos A, Gil P, Barabash A, Frenéndez C, de Ugarte C, Cabranes JA. Regional cerebral blood flow assessed with 99mTc-ECD SPET as a marker of progression of mild cognitive impairment to Alzheimer´s disease. *Eur J Nucl Med Mol Imaging* 2003; 30: 1473-1480.

[10] Cabranes JA, De Juan R, Encinas M, Marcos A, Gil P, Fernandez C, De Ugarte C, Barabash A. Relevance of functional neuroimaging in the progression of mild cognitive impairment. *Neurol Res*. 2004; 26: 496-501.

[11] Marcos A, Barabash A, Gil P, Encinas M, de Juan R, Payno M, Ancín I, Vázquez B, Cabranes JA. The role of functional neuroimaging in mild cognitive impairment. *Current Medical Imaging Reviews* 2006; 2: 237-243.

[12] Luis CA, Loewenstein DA, Acevedo A, Barker WW, Duara R. Mild Cognitive Impairment. Directions for future research. *Neurology* 2003; 61: 438-444.

[13] Petersen RC. Mild Cognitive Impairment as a diagnostic entity. *J Intern Med* 2004; 256: 183-194.

[14] Petersen RC, Stevens JC, Ganguli M, et al. Early detection of dementia: mild cognitive impairment (an evidence based review). Report of the Quality Standards Subcommitte of the American Academy of Neurology. *Neurology* 2001b; 56: 1133-1142.

[15] Petersen RC, Morris JC. Mild cognitive impairment as a clinical entity and treatment target. *Arch Neurol* 2005; 62, 7: 1160-3.

[16] Tuokko H, Frerichs R, Graham J, et al. Five-year follow-up of Cognitive Impairment with no dementia. *Arch Neurol* 2003, Apr; 60 (4): 577-582.

[17] Bennett DA, Wilson RS, Schneider JA, et al. Natural history of mild cognitive impairment in older persons. *Neurology* 2002; 59: 198-205.

[18] Palmer K, Wang H, Backman L, et al. Differential evolution of cognitive impairment in nondemented older persons: results from the Kungsholmen Project. *Am J Psychiatry* 2002; 59: 436-442.

[19] Marquis S, Moore M, Howieson DB, et al. Independent predictors of cognitive decline in healthy elderly persons. *Arch Neurol.* 2002; 59: 601-606.

[20] Collie A, Maruff P, Shafiq-Antonacci R et al. Memory decline in healthy older people. Implications for identifying mild cognitive impairment. *Neurol* 2001; 56: 1533-1538.

[21] Luis CA, Barker W, Loewenstein DA, et al. Conversion to dementia among two groups with cognitive impairment. *Dement Geriatr Cogn Disord* 2004; 18: 307-313.

[22] Visser PJ, Verhey FR, Scheltens P, et al. Diagnostic accuracy of the Preclinical AD scale (PAS) in cognitively mildly impaired subjects. *J Neurol* 2002 Mar; 249 (3): 312-319.

[23] Visser PJ, Verhey FR, Ponds RW, Jolles J. Diagnosis of preclinical Alzheimer's disease in a clinical setting. *Int Psychogeriatr* 2001 Dec; 13 (4): 411-423.

[24] Perry RJ, Watson P, Hodges JR. The nature and staging of attention dysfunction in early (minimal and mild) Alzheimer's disease: relationship to episodic and semantic memory impairment. *Neuropsychologia* 2000; 38 (3): 252-271.

[25] Arnaiz E, Almkvist O. Neuropsychological features of mild cognitive impairment and preclinical Alzheimer's disease. *Acta Neurol Scand* 2003 Suppl Feb; 179: 34-41.

[26] Cullum C, Huppert FA, McGee M, et al. Decline across different domains of cognitive functioning in normal ageing: results of a longitudinal population-based study using CAMCOG. *Int Geriatr Psychiatry* 2000; 15: 853-862.

[27] De Jager CA, Hogervorst E, Combrinck M, Budge MM. Sensitivity and specificity of neuropsychological tests for mild cognitive impairment, vascular cognitive impairment and Alzheimer's disease. *Psychol Med* 2003; 33(6): 1039-1050.

[28] Marcos A, Gil P, Barabash A, Rodríguez R, Encinas M, Fernández C and Cabranes JA. Neuropsychological markers of progression from Mild Cognitive Impairment to Alzheimer´s Disease. *American Journal of Alzheimer's disease and other Dementias* 2006; 21: 189-196.

[29] van Broekhoven CL. Molecular genetics of Alzheimer's diseases: identification of genes and gene mutations. *Eur Neurol* 1995; 35: 8-19.

[30] Schellenberg GD, Bird TD, Wijsman EM, et al. Genetic linkage evidence for a familiar Alzheimer's disease locus on chromosome 14. *Science* 1992; 258: 668-671.

[31] van Broekhoven CL, Backhovens H, Guts M, et al. Mapping of a gene predisposing to early-onset Alzheimer's disease to chromosome 14 q 24.3. *Nat Genet* 1992; 2: 335-339.

[32] Rogaer EI, Sherrington R, Rogaeva EA, et al. Familiar Alzheimer's disease in kindreds with missense mutations in a gene on crhomosome 1 related to the Alzhimer's disease type 3 gene. *Nature* 1995; 376: 775-798.

[33] Folstein MF, Folstein SE, McHugh PR. Mini-Mental State. A practical method for grading the cognitive state of patients for the clinician. J Pschyatr Res 1975; 12: 189-98.

[34] Report of the Quality Standards Subcommittee of the American Academy of Neurology. Practice parameters for diagnosis and evaluation of dementia (Summary Statement). *Neurology* 1994; 44: 2203-2206.

[35] Zivelin A, Rosenberg N, Peretz H et al. Improved method for genotyping apolipoprotein E polymorphisms by a PCR-based assay simultaneously utilizing two distinct restriction enzymes. *Clin Chem* 1997; 43: 1657-1659.

[36] Hixson JE, Vernier DT. Restriction isotyping of human apolipoprotein E by gene amplification and cleavage with Hhal. *J Lipid Res* 1990; 31: 545-548.

[37] Coria FRI, Bayon C, SantaEngracia N, rodriguez-Artalejo F. Apoprotein E allelic variants predict dementia in elderly patients with memory impairment. *Eur J Neurol* 1995; 2: 1-3.

[38] Dik MG, Jonker C, Bouter LM, Geerlings MI, van Kamp GJ, Deeg DJ. APOE-epsilon4 is associated with memory decline in cognitively impaired elderly. *Neurology* 2000; 54: 1492-1497.

[39] Rosich-Estrago M, Figuera-Terre L, Mulet-Perez B, et al. Dementia and cognitive impairment pattern: its association with epsilon$ allele of apolipoprotein E gene. *Rev Neurol* 2004; 38: 801-807.

[40] Jack CR, Petersen RC, Xu YC, et al. Prediction of AD with MRI-based hippocampal volume in mild cognitive impairment. *Neurology* 1999; 52: 1397-1403.

[41] Johnson Ka, Jones K, Holman BL, et al. Preclinical prediction of Alzheimer's disease using SPECT. *Neurology* 1998; 50: 1563-1571.

[42] Visser PJ, Verhey FR, Ponds RW, Cruts M, van Broeckhoven CL, Jolles J. Course of objective memory impairment in non-demented subjects attending a memory clinic and predictors of outcome. *Int J Geriatr Psychiatry* 2000; 15: 363-372.

In: Alzheimer's Disease Research Trends
Editor: A.P. Chan, pp. 241-251
ISBN 978-1-60021-712-8

Chapter XII

NEUROINFLAMMATORY ONSET DYNAMICS AND PROGRESSION IN ALZHEIMER DISEASE

Lawrence M. Agius*
Department of Pathology, St Luke's Hospital Gwardamangia University of Malta Medical School, Msida, Malta Europe.

ABSTRACT

Nitric oxide and free oxygen molecular species would constitute integral system components in the realization of a neuroinflammatory series of events damaging cerebral cortical neurons in the Alzheimer brain. The impact of such processes of reactive injury would be manifested particularly in the development of injury to cerebral endothelial cells as progressive amyloid deposition and amyloid angiopathy in these patients. The blood-brain barrier and the distribution of neuritic plaques would attest to the evolving onset dynamics of a process of cell injury culminating in death of neurons. Nitric oxide as a primarily locally diffusible agent in the progression of neuritic and neuronal injury would implicate microglia as active participants in the progression of the Alzheimer brain process. Recognition of the various pathways that would contribute to neuroinflammation in Alzheimer disease would attest to a multiplicity of events in onset and progression culminating in ischemia/reperfusion injury and of excitotoxity of both neurons and endothelial cells. Thus a coupled series of parallel pathways would evolve implicating a neuronal and endothelial cell series of interactive pathologic lesions in the Alzheimer disease onset and progression of injury.

* Correspondence concerning this article should be addressed to Lawrence M. Agius 27 "Ballarat" Guzeppi Caruana Street, Tal-Virtu, Rabat, RBT09 Malta Europe. Tel.: 356-21451752; (Work): 356-2595-1663; E-mail: lawrence.agius@um.edu.mt, lawrence.agius@gov.mt.

Nitric Oxide Modulates Smooth Muscle Relaxation

The neuroinflammaory cycle has been proposed as a potential therapeutic target to alter progression of Alzheimer disease [20]. Nitric oxide would constitute a generic modulator system superimposed on essential networks of functional neurotransmitter effects and of smooth muscle relaxation. It appears to represent, in a partly hierarchical sense, another level of modulation that operates on a fully functional system of networks central to both neurotransmission and smooth muscle relaxation; these would interrelate with each other and also as individual operative systems in their own right. Characterization of neuronal nitric oxide as an inhibitory neurotransmitter does represent a system of modulation of the effects of vasoactive intestinal polypeptide release at neuromuscular or of acetylcholine release at cholinergic nerve terminals beyond simple systems of innervation of smooth muscle at only one primary level of operability. Neuroinflammation in particular would implicate neuronal type nicotinic acetylcholine receptors and peroxisomal proliferators-activated receptors in Alzheimer disease [25].

The endothelial nitric oxide isoform as a local vasodilator on vascular smooth muscle would represent another system of modulation exerted by the effects of nitric oxide beyond even strict operability of innervation systems.

cDNA array evidence shows selectively altered synaptic plasticity in cases at high risk for Alzheimer disease, including in particular the expression of a-type synapsins [23].

Endothelial nitric oxide operates at a level of modulation that influences considerably relaxation effects as exerted on smooth muscle contractility of the vascular wall. Hence, particularly with regard to inducible nitric oxide generated by macrophages, this would operate as an essential, locally diffusible, system as innervation and neurotransmission in terms of inflammatory reactive mediators and of endothelial reactivity constituting a single integral system. Oxidative damage to lipids, nucleic acids and proteins progresses as neuroinflammation and with accumulation of reactive astrocytes and microglia [19].

Nitric oxide would represent an integrated system that modulates and coordinates effects regarding smooth muscle relaxation that might develop as a consequence to a wide variety of possible stimulatory systems.

The local mode of operative nitric oxide would represent a system that transcends at a higher level variable degrees of smooth muscle relaxation as observable in the lower esophageal sphincter region, stomach, ileocolon and also in the vascular wall.

Within the nervous system, nitric oxide would, in terms of locally diffusible effects, operate in a retrograde manner and contribute to the essential phenomenon of latent presynaptic potentiation as proposed for systems such as learning and memory.

Nitric oxide would constitute a general biologic principle whereby local diffusible mediators might actually represent the final pathway by which multiple systems influence a target they converge on. In addition, there is currently intense debate on the potential use of nonsteroidal anti-inflammatory drugs in Alzheimer disease [22].

Smooth muscle, whether in the gastrointestinal tract, or vascular wall, might act as a single final target for complex systems including neural and neurotransmitter mediators, inflammatory cytokines, and as templates for endothelial cells; a whole series of agonists might ultimately be finely modulated by the locally diffusible nitric oxide. In fact, the different nitric oxide synthase isoforms might represent a system adapted to implicate various pathobiologic systems in an overall scheme that converges on smooth muscle fibers or neurons in particular.

INFLAMMATORY RESPONSES AND INTERACTIONS BETWWEN FREE OXYGEN RADICALS AND NITRIC OXIDE

Free super-radical –induced injury has been proposed as a central phenomenon akin to the very nature of the inflammation-induced injury, whether this ultimately is protective for the organism or else is self-progressive in the generation of either septic shock or chronic neuro-inflammatory states. Neuroinflammation can be both a cause and a result of oxidative stress [29]. Even chronic relapsing inflammation as represented by inflammatory bowel disease, arthritis and osteomyelitis, does belie a distinction between acute and chronic inflammation in conditions as characterized in many cases of pancreatitis. Many normal aging inflammatory processes are linked not only to Alzheimer disease but also to cancer, diabetes and cardiovascular disease [2].

A chronic relapsing course for an inflammatory condition would function as agents such as nitrosylating and free oxygen radical reactivity. Such reactivity would implicate a specific etiologic agent that gives rise to the onset of the inflammatory or neuroinflammatory state in the first instance. The metallothionein family of proteins, particularly MT-I and MT-II are upregulated in neuroinflammation of Alzheimer brains together with oxidative stress associated with amyloid plaques [3].

It is this intrinsic susceptibility of an inflammatory reaction to either become chronic or to follow a recurrent cycle of remissions and relapses that would help characterize the nature and scope of operability of an inflammatory state per se. Within such a concept, one might consider the essentially ambivalent nature of nitric oxide as either a cytoprotective or as a cytoinjurious agent in various disorders such as Alzheimer's disease. Early stages of Alzheimer disease show upregulated cell cycle protein, adhesion and inflammatory factors [12]. The essential modulatory role of nitric oxide as a locally diffusible agent would be operative within a setting of local production also of free oxygen radicals. Such a situation would classically be represented by the inflammatory state that induces much of the central aspects of possible interactions of nitric oxide with free oxygen radicals. Neuroinflammation would interact with systems of proteolysis, protein misfolding and oxidative stress in multiple pathogenic pathways of beta amyloidosis and tau phosphorylation in the Alzheimer brain [9].

Inflammatory reactions would be largely translatable in terms of reactivity subsequent to interactions between nitric oxide and free oxygen radicals. In the case of ischemia/reperfusion, a set of conditions would arise that are associated with serious cellular injury due to the presence of excess production locally of free oxygen radicals.

The endothelially-derived nitric oxide would be implicated as another participant in the induction of cell/tissue injury in cases of ischemia/reperfusion of tissues including the cerebral hemispheres.

Various reactive products are possibly produced by interactions of nitric oxide and oxygen free radicals with various residues such as thiols, metallo-compounds such a hemoglobin, myoglobin and cytochrome oxidase. A process particularly conducive to the production of direct damage to subcellular components would also operate in the generation or activation of various enzymatic reactions including, for example, cyclooxygenase [11]. Inhibition of cyclooxygenase would prevent programmed cell death of neurons in familial Alzheimer disease [14]. It might be particularly relevant to consider the essential interactions between nitric oxide and free oxygen radicals in the formation, centrally, of the inflammatory reaction. A generic mechanism of amyloid aggregation appears to operate that interacts with various component systems of cholinergic neurotransmission in Alzheimer disease [4].

The inflammatory response would be characterized constitutively by the generation and also progression of its component systems [7,16].

The very nature of inflammatory states would constitute induced cell/tissue damage in terms that would specifically relate to modes of generation of bouts of inflammatory response or reactivity. This would relate particularly in terms of specific interactions between nitric oxide and free oxygen radicals.

In this sense, a chronic relapsing inflammatory reaction, even a chronic inflammatory state per se, would necessarily implicate an endless series of the generative steps as interactive phenomena between nitric oxide and free oxygen radicals. Expression of MAPK-associated protein kinase 2 correlates with beta amyloidosis, microgliosis and upregulation of tumor necrosis factor alpha and macrophage inflammatory protein 1 alpha in a transgenic model of Alzheimer disease [5]. In this context, especially, endothelial nitric oxide and inducible nitric oxide of macrophage origin would constitute the specific self-generators of a successive series of inflammatory responses in terms of increased nitrosylation and oxygen super-radical formation as these specifically interact with each other. Complement mediated neuroinflammation in Alzheimer disease may implicate activated microglia, secretion of proinflammatory cytokines and generation of oxidative products [8].

Nitric Oxide from Endothelial Cells and Renin Synthesis

Vascular pathology would appear to play a crucial pathogenic role in neurodegenerative dementia. Nitric oxide dysregulation due to microvasculopathy would result in regional metabolic dysfunction. Increased nitric oxide upregulates neuroinflammation due to its free radical properties, impairing mitochondria [28].

The question of nitric oxide-induced secretion and synthesis of renin by juxtaglomerular granular cells appears to revolve around the identity of such JGG cells as modified smooth muscle cells. Such a concept would implicate a mutually dual system of operability whereby nitric oxide release from endothelial cells would involve feedback mechanisms with nitric oxide synthesis and release from juxtaglomerular granular cells in the afferent arteriolar wall of the glomerulus.

It would appear that nitric oxide is a generic product of endothelial cells that preferentially act on vascular smooth myofibers in the vascular wall. This would be in keeping with the local diffusion properties of nitric oxide in its paracrine mode of operation.

Such a basic system would adapt to a system of synthesis and release of renin from the juxtaglomerular granular cells in a mode that in some way would be analogous to relaxation of smooth vascular smooth myofibers as seen commonly in the action of nitric oxide.

Relaxation of smooth muscle fibers of the vascular wall would involve an active process of induction of the modified cells of the JGG cell type resulting in the synthesis and release of renin. One might understand the nature of the metaplastic type transformation that smooth muscle fibers of the afferent glomerular arteriole undergo to form JGG cells in trying to clarify the role of production and action of nitric oxide in terms of renin production.

Renin is a protease directly implicated in the production of angiotensin II, the most powerful natural vasoactive substance circulating in the blood. As such, renin would appear to represent an intermediate metabolite acting as a protease within the same system of vasoactive and vasodilator regulation including nitric oxide.

It is perhaps in this sense that through the intermediary production of renin, the generally vasodilatory action of nitric oxide is converted to a powerful vasoconstrictor mode of action.

The variability of action in terms of stimulation or inhibition by nitric oxide on renin secretion would operate as either acute or subchronic infusion and as chronic availability of nitric oxide over a number of weeks. These would represent a summation complex of effects resulting from primary stimulation of synthesis and release of renin. Secondary effects are also induced by nitric oxide directly on vascular smooth muscle cells as found in the cerebrum.

In cases of chronically raised levels of circulating nitric oxide, the direct vasodilatory effect of this on the vascular smooth muscle in general would result in a secondary effect of inhibition of renin release from the JGG cells. These could counterbalance any direct stimulatory effect of nitric oxide on the specialized smooth myofibers as juxtaglomerular granular cells of the afferent arteriole of the glomerulus.

Maturation of Alzheimer neuropathology and ischemic lesions in the central nervous system evolve in terms of an important role for neuroinflammation. Activation of glial cells and upregulation of inflammatory mediators induce an increased neuronal susceptibility to ischemia [24].

Nitric Oxide-Induced Tissue Injury

How is it that nitric oxide both causes and protects against tissue injury in states of inflammation, septic shock and ischemia/reperfusion of the brain? Does such a dually contrasting mode of action intrinsically arise from the mode of action of nitric oxide itself? Multiple gene transcription pathways in Alzheimer neuroinflammation induce secretion of cytokines and chemokines and matrix metalloproteinases; also chronic activation of many potentially toxic products would develop [13]. It might perhaps be relevant to consider the nitric oxide that proves contradictory in its modes of action in terms specifically of vascular phenomena as they relate to inflammatory response. The vascular blood flow with its concurrent tendency to increased endothelial/leukocyte adherence at slow rates of blood perfusion might lie close to the central mode of effect of nitric oxide in terms of protective action against cell injury in persistent inflammatory states such as inflammatory bowel disease or neuroinflammation.

Nitric oxide would prove particularly significant in the perpetuation of the inflammatory response in terms of vascular slowing of blood flow. Cerebral microvascular amyloid deposition rather than parenchymal amyloid correlates often with dementia [18]. There would evolve consequent increased tendency for endothelial/leukocyte adherence.

Such a scheme would necessarily appear to lead to increased chemotactic attraction of successive further waves of inflow of neutrophils from the blood stream into the already inflamed tissues, and consequently would tend to effectively result in perpetuation of the already established neuroinflammatory state.

Inflammation contributes to Alzheimer type neurodegeneration primarily as a significant source of pathology rather than simply as a secondary phenomenon [30].

Such considerations, when applied to ischemia/reperfusion of the brain, might implicate slowing of blood flow with generation of free oxygen radicals at the level of the endothelial cell. It is in the presence of large amounts of oxygen carried by the reperfusing stream of blood into a cerebral cortical region that is initially ischemic that the essential role of nitric oxide would derive from presumably partly damaged endothelial cells. This is particularly implicated in the generation of large amounts of free oxygen radicals.

It is an essential property of endothelially derived nitric oxide in the presence of a damaged endothelial cell bed that would generate cerebral tissue injury due to reactive free oxygen radical production.

The ischemic state of the tissues that are suddenly exposed to large amounts of liberated oxygen molecular species might constitute an important aspect of the mode of cell injury in cases of cerebral ischemia/reperfusion.

A phenomenon of excessive oxygen delivery that is of an abnormal distributive pattern of delivery would, within the setting of regional groups of cells, promote an anaerobic adaptation in cases of tissue ischemia. This would further accentuate the sudden release of excessive amounts of nitric oxide as a consequence of injury to endothelial cells of vessels within the ischemic cerebral cortical region.

Inflammatory Self-Progression

Both the progressiveness and the persistence of neuroinflammatory reactions would characterize reactive changes as a fundamental series of mechanisms contributing integrally to the basic pathobiology of Alzheimer disease. The purinergic receptor subtype P2X7R, a nonselective cationic channel activated by high levels of adenosine triphosphate, mediates microglial inflammatory responses in Alzheimer disease [1]. The self-amplifying aspect of such inflammatory reactive changes would be based at least partly on cyclooxygenase catalytic function that underlies a fundamental susceptibility of reactive processes to self-perpetuation of the disease impact on cerebral tissues.

Inflammatory reactions would constitute mechanisms prone to self-progression rather than to self-limitation in terms particularly related to dynamics of genesis of the disease process. Glial cells appear activated by beta-amyloid accumulation in Alzheimer brains and involve reactive oxygen molecular species and the release of inflammatory cytokines [10].

MICROGLIA IN NEURONAL INJURY ARISING IN PATIENTS WITH NEUROINFLAMMATION

The microglia and macrophage cell populations [21] appear initial sites of involvement leading to neurodegeneration in cases of viral encephalitis as seen particularly in patients with HIV infection of the central nervous system. Herpes simplex virus type 1 has been implicated in the etiology of Alzheimer disease and also Down syndrome [34]. Much of the damage inflicted during the course of a viral encephalitis would start primarily as a microglial reactivity. Much of the clinical impact of the subsequent disease course would be dependent on a central participation as mediators of various cytokines, complement components and interferon gamma besides nitric oxide.

The formation of active microglial nodules in cases of neuroinflammation would represent not only a response to neuronal injury but also an initiator of the neuronal injury subsequent to stimulation by a putative primary agent.

An overall process of combined integral effect in the development of neuronal damage in many cases of viral encephalitis would originate as a result of involvement of reactive microglial progression. Such a cell population would be particularly significant in terms of induced and maintained progression of the neuronal injury in view of the vast repertoire of cytokine secretory potential of the microglia. Such an essential attribute would correlate with the exquisite responsiveness to aggregate as distinctly defined microglial nodules throughout much of the central nervous system in cases of active neuroinflammation.

REACTIVE MICROGLIAL ACTIVATION AND BETA-AMYLOID DEPOSITION IN NEURITIC PLAQUES

Glial and particularly microglial reactivity is an emerging morphologic feature of many states of neurodegeneration. There appears to be some correlation between microglial and astrocytic activation in conditions such as Alzheimer's disease in a strictly focal or multifocal distribution pattern. Neuroinflammation would link beta-amyloid deposition to neuronal damage and clinical disease [31]. Such focal sites of glial activation would seem to directly localize the distribution of the dystrophic neurites as senile or neuritic plaques in Alzheimer's disease.

The nature of the glial activation process is unclear but would incorporate an important element of phagocytosis, on the part of the microglial cells. This is particularly significant in the light of the morphologic evolution of the neuritic plaque as a phenomenon eventually resulting in a burnt out plaque with dense central deposits of beta-amyloid. Interleukin (IL)-1,

IL-6, Tumor Necrosis Factor-alpha and Transforming Growth Factor-beta are probable key players in progression of the Alzheimer disease process [27].

It is this association of initial demonstration of microglial activation pathways that would progressively decrease and burn out in apparently strong inverse relationship to the accumulation of beta-amyloid. This would emphasize much of the dynamic evolution of the neuritic plaque. Iron in particular might be important in neuroinflammation and progression of Alzheimer disease [15].

Beta-amyloid production in the central nervous system might represent an important and fairly common pathobiologic event, one that appears to be safeguarded against mainly by microglial activation and phagocytic activity in general. The dystrophic neurites that develop and progress in the neuritic plaque would be significant in that they surround the central deposit of densely accumulated beta-amyloid.

As such, beta-amyloid could well represent an integral morphologic lesion as a product of combined activation/phagocytic activity on the part of microglia and also an element of neuritic degeneration. Although beta-amyloid peptide vaccination effectively reduces Abeta burden in Alzheimer model mice, meningoencephalitis developed in some patients [6]. The beta-amyloid deposits would progress in terms of an ongoing microglial activation process.

Hence, beta-amyloid deposits might, in fact, result from reactive phenomena associated with the activated microglia, in strict relation to the development of dystrophic neurites. Hence, with the subsequent association of reactive and phagocytic activities, as exhibited by microglia in the neuritic plaques, there might remain a dense central deposit of amyloid in these plaques. S100B activation of glia would appear to contribute to the generation of oxidative stress in the Alzheimer brain; S100B would stimulate inducible nitric oxide synthase with activation of Nuclear Factor kappaB [33].

Beta-amyloid deposits appear a direct result of reactive breakdown and processing by microglia with a possibly strong immune component as well. Such a phenomenon would presumably directly develop as a process of active agent participation incorporated in the production of the dystrophic neurites.

Cyclooxygenase-2 would influence amyloid precursor protein processing and promote cerebral amyloidosis [32].

Such activated immune response, with an important phagocytic component, would conceptually constitute a mechanism of phagocytosis with localization of the pathobiologic agent promoting development of the dystrophic neurites. The central localization of the beta-amyloid deposits within the neuritic plaques would represent the nature of evolution of the final endproduct series of mechanisms in the eventual production of the inactive and burnt out plaques.

Oxidative stress, Ca(2+) and metal ion dysregulation, dysfunction of endoplasmic reticulum and mitochondria, impaired homeostasis of cholesterol and of neurotransmission appear implicated in the production of cognitive deficit [17].

Endothelial Cell Viability and the Blood-Brain Barrier

A central point of interest is the degree of viability or nonviability of endothelial cells in cases of disruption of the blood brain barrier [26]. In cases of neuroinflammation, the viability of the immediately adjoining endothelial cells constituting the blood-brain barrier would depend on the integrity of the intercellular tight junctions.

This structural organization of the endothelial cell lining of a vessel would specifically be directed at strict maintenance of control of tight intercellular junctions. As a consequence, vasogenic cerebral edema would represent a cardinal manifestation of decreased viability of the endothelial cells lining the cerebral vessels.

Concluding Remarks

Neuroinflammatory states in Alzheimer disease would constitute an integrative event in the constitutive development of action of nitric oxide and reactive free oxygen molecular species. Such event would further perpetuate the onset dynamics of a process of neuronal injury as manifested not only in dystrophic neurites in plaques but also an impaired blood-brain barrier and progressive injury to cerebral endothelial cells in particular.

References

[1] McLarnon JG, Ryer JK, Walker DG, Choi HB, "Upregulated expression of Purinergic P2X7 Receptor in Alzheimer disease and amyloid-beta peptide-treated microglia and in peptide-injected rat hippocampus" *J Neuropathol Exp Neurol* 2006 Nov;65(11):1090-7.

[2] Morgan TE, Wong AM, Finch CE "Anti-inflammatory mechanisms of dietary restriction in slowing aging processes" *Interdiscip Top Gerontol* 2007;35: 83-97

[3] Hidelgo J, Penkowa M, Espejo C, Martinex-Caceres EM, Carraxo J, Quintana A et al. "Expression of metallothionein-I, -II, and –III in Alzheimer disease and animal models of neuroinflammation" *Exp Biol Med (Maywood)* 2006 Oct;231(9):1450-8.

[4] Sivaprakasam K "Towards a unifying hypothesis of Alzheimer's disease: cholinergic system linked to plaques, tangles, and neuroinflammation" *Curr Med Chem* 2006;13(18):2179-88.

[5] Culbert AA, Skarper SD, Howlett DR, Evans NA, Facci L, Soden PE et al. "MAPK-activated protein kinase 2 deficiency in microglia inhibits proinflammatory mediator release and resultant neurotoxicity. Relevance to neuroinflammation in a transgenic mouse model of Alzheimer disease" *J Biol Chem* 2006 Aug 18;281(33):23658-67.

[6] Okura Y, Miyakoshi A, Kohyama K, Park IK, Stanfenbiel M, Matsumoto Y "Nonviral Abeta DNA vaccine therapy against Alzheimer's disease: long term effects and safety" *Proc Natl Acad Sci USA* 2006 Jun 20;103(25):9619-24.

[7] Vardy ER, Hussain I, Hooper NM "Emerging therapeutics for Alzheimer's disease" *Expert Rev Neurother* 2006 May;6(5):695-704.

[8] Bonifati DM, Kishore U "Role of complement in neurodegeneration and neuroinflammation" *Mol Immunol* 2007 Feb;44(5):999-1010.

[9] Papassotiropoulos A, Fountoulakis M, Dunckley T, Stephen DA, Reiman EM "Genetics, transcriptomics and proteomics of Alzheimer's disease" *J Clin Psychiatry* 2006 Apr;67(4):650-1.

[10] Cheng G, Whitehead SN, Hachinski V, Cechetto DF "Effects of pyrrolidine dithiocarbamate on beta-amyloid (25-35)-induced inflammatory responses and memory deficites in the rat". *Neurobiol Dis* 2006 Jul;23(1):140-51.

[11] Ho L, Qin W, Stetka BS, Pasinetti GM "Is there a future for cyclo-oxygenase inhibitors in Alzheimer's disease?" *CNS Drugs* 2006;20(2):85-98.

[12] Hoozemans JJ, Veerhins R, Rozemuller JM< Eikelenboom P "Neuroinflammation and regeneration in the early stages of Alzheimer's disease pathology" *Int J Dev Neurosci* 2006 Apr-May;24(2-3):157-65.

[13] Walker DG, Link J, Lue LF, Dalsing-Hernandez JE, Boyes BE "Gene expression changes by amyloid beta peptide-stimulated human postmortem brain microglia identify activation of multiple inflammatory processes" *J Leukoc Biol* 2006 Mar;79(3):596-610.

[14] Qin W, Peng Y, Ksiezak-Reding H, Ho L, Stetka B, Lovati E et al. "Inhibition of cyclooxygenase as potential novel therapeutic strategy in N141I presenilin-2 familial Alzheimer's disease" *Mol Psychiatry* 2006 Feb;11(2):172-81.

[15] Ong WY, Farooqui AA "Iron, neuroinflammation, and Alzheimer's disease" *J Alzheimers Dis* 2005 Nov;8(2):183-200.

[16] Streit WJ, Conde JR, Fendrick SE, Flanary BE, Mariani CL "Roleof microglia in the central nervous system's immune system" *Neurol Res* 2005 Oct; 27(7):685-91.

[17] Perevia C, Agostinho P, Moreira PI, Cardoso SM, Oliveira CR "Alzheimer's disease-associated neurotoxic mechanisms and neuroprotective strategies" *Curr Drug Targets CNS Neurol Disord* 2005 Aug;4(4):383-403.

[18] Miao J, Vitek MP, Xu F, Previti ML, Davis J, Van Nostraud WE "Reducing cerebral microvascular amyloid-beta protein deposition diminishes regional neuroinflammation in vasculotropic mutant amyloid precursor protein transgenic mice" *J Neurosci* 2005 Jul 6;25(27):6271-7.

[19] van Muiswinkel FL, Kuiperij HB "The Nrf2-ARE Signaling pathway: promising drug target to combat oxidative stress in neurodegenerative disorders" *Curr Drug Targets CNS Neurol Disord* 2005 Jun;4(3):267-81.

[20] Hu W, Ralay Ranarvo H, Craft JM, Van Eldik LJ, Wattenson DM "Validation of the neuroinflammation cycle as a drug discovery target using integrative chemical biology and lead compound development with an Alzheimer'' disease-related mouse model" *Curr Alzheimer Res* 2005 Apr;2(2):197-205.

[21] Walker DG, Lue LF "Investigations with cultured human microglia on pathogenic mechanisms of Alzheimer's disease and other neurodegenerative diseases" *J Neurosci Res* 2005 Aug 1;81(3):412-25.

[22] Gasparini L, Ongini E, Wilcock D, Morgan D "Activity of flurbiprofen and chemically related anti-inflammatory drugs in models of Alzheimer's disease" *Brain Res Brain Res Rev* 2005 Apr;48(2):400-8.

[23] Ho L, Sharma N, Blackman L, Festa E, Reddy G, Pasinetti GM "From proteomics to biomarker discovery in Alzheimer's disease" *Brain Res Brain Res Rev* 2005 Apr;48(2):360-9.

[24] Koistinaho M, Koistinaho J "Interactions between Alzheimer's disease and cerebral ischemia—focus on inflammation" *Brain Res Brain Res Rev* 2005 Apr;48(2):240-50.

[25] Tuppo EE, Arias HR "The role of inflammation in Alzheimer's disease" *Int J Biochem Cell Biol* 2005 Feb;37(2):289-305.

[26] Deane R, Wu Z, Zlokovic BV "RAGE (yin) versus LRP (yang) balance regulates Alzheimer amyloid beta-peptide clearance through transport across the blood-brain barrier" *Stroke* 2004 Nov;35(11 Suppl 1):2628-31.

[27] Cacquevel M, Lebeurrier N, Cheenne S, Varen D "Cytokines in neuroinflammation and Alzheimer's disease" *Curr Drug Targets* 2004 Aug;5(6):529-34.

[28] Togo T, Katsuse O, Iseki E "Nitric oxide pathways in Alzheimer's disease and other neurodegenerative dementias" *Neurol Res* 2004 Jul;26(5):563-6.

[29] Mhatre M, Floyd RA, Hensley K "Oxidative stress and neuroinflammation in Alzheimer's disease and amyotrophic lateral sclerosis: common links and potential therapeutic targets" *J Alzheimers Dis* 2004 Apr;6(2):147-57.

[30] Versijpt JJ, Dumont F, Van Laere KJ, Decov D, Santens P, Andenaert K et al. "Assessment of neuroinflammation and microglial activation in Alzheimer's disease with radiolabelled PK 11195 and single photon emission computed tomography. A pilot study" *Eur Neurol* 2003;50(1):39-47.

[31] Moore AH, O'Banion MK "Neuroinflammation and anti-inflammatory therapy for Alzheimer's disease" *Adv Drug Deliv Rev* 2002 Dec 7;54(12):1627-56.

[32] Xiang Z, Ho L, Yemul S, Zhao Z, Qing W, Pompl P et al. "Cyclooxygenase-2 promotes amyloid plaque deposition in a mouse model of Alzheimer's disease neuropathology" *Gene Expr* 2002;10(5-6):271-8.

[33] Lam AG, Koppal T, Akama KT, Guo L, Craft JM, Samy B et al. "Mechanism of glial activation by S100B: involvement of the transcription factor NF kappaB" *Neurobiol Aging* 2001 Sep-Oct;22(5):765-72.

[34] Cheon MS, Bajs M, Guleserian T, Cavins N, Lubec G "Evidence for the relation of herpes simplex virus type 1 to Down Syndrome and Alzheimer's disease" *Electrophoresis* 2001 Feb;22(3):445-8.

In: Alzheimer's Disease Research Trends
Editor: A.P. Chan, pp. 253-273

ISBN 978-1-60021-712-8

Chapter XIII

Effects of Dietary Docosahexaenoic Acid on Spatial Cognition of Normal and Alzheimer's Disease Model Rats

Michio Hashimoto[1,*] and Shahdat Hossain[1,2]
[1]Department of Environmental Physiology, Shimane University Faculty of Medicine, Izumo, Shimane 693-8501, Japan;
[2]Department of Biochemistry and Molecular Biology, Jahangirnagar University, Savar, Dhaka-1342, Bangladesh.

Abstract

The n-3 polyunsaturated fatty acids, particularly docosahexaenoic acid (DHA), exert certain effects on the spatial cognition of normal and Alzheimer's disease (AD) model rats. Spatial cognition-related memory refers to the ability to recall previously navigated cues oriented in a specific arrangement in the individual's environment. The ability to navigate the hidden platform in the water maze and to obtain a reward (food-pellet) at the ends of the arms of the radial maze is always greater in DHA-fed rats than in control rats. The enhancement of spatial cognition is associated with both an increase in the molar ratio of DHA to arachidonic acid (AA) and a decrease in the oxidative stress in the hippocampus and cortex regions of the brains of rats administered dietary DHA. Since the hippocampus plays a crucial role in the constitution of the cognitive map and in the concomitant navigation through memory to past events, we demonstrate that DHA exerts a positive effect on accurately constituting the hippocampal map, on the occurrence of related background cellular events at the synapse and on restoring spatial cognition. Moreover, the AD individual characteristically suffers from continued loss of learning and cognitive memory with concomitant neuronal dysfunction attributed to amyloid β (Aβ) peptide-induced formation of neuritic plaques and neurofibrillary tangles.

* Correspondence concerning this article should be addressed to Michio Hashimoto, Ph.D., Department of Environmental Physiology, Shimane University Faculty of Medicine, Izumo, Shimane 693-8501, Japan, E-mail: michio1@med.shimane-u.ac.jp., Telephone: +81 853 20 2112; Fax: +81 853 20 2110.

Therefore, the effects of dietary DHA on memory loss in AD subjects have been estimated. Immunochemical studies on AD model animals produced by infusing $A\beta_{1-40}$ peptide into the cerebral ventricle of rats have revealed that the infusion of the peptide injures the neurons of the hippocampus and cortex and increases the level of DNA fragments. The memory-related performance of AD model rats has been measured in the shuttle avoidance system apparatus or in the eight-arm radial maze. The infusion of the peptide results in the impairment of both active avoidance-related and reference and working memory-related learning abilities, well-known characteristics of AD. The administration of dietary DHA prevents the impairment of active avoidance-related learning ability in the shuttle avoidance system apparatus and ameliorates the impairment of reference and working memory-related learning ability in the radial maze task. Both learning abilities correlate positively with the cortico-hippocampal DHA/AA molar ratio. Oxidative stress, believed to initiate deposition of Aβ peptide and to raise the levels of lipid peroxide and reactive oxygen species in the brains of AD subjects, is significantly lower in DHA-fed AD model rats than in AD model rats. Data suggest that DHA plays a positive role in constituting/restoring memory-retrieving neuro-connections involved in the associative functions of the cortex and the hippocampus, and that animals administered DHA perform better than controls.

Keywords: Docosahexaenoic acid, cognitive memory, Alzheimer's disease.

Introduction

Recently, investigation into the beneficial effects of docosahexaenoic acid (DHA, C22:6n-3), a component of fish oil, on memory-related brain functions has been one of the exciting topics of lipid nutrition in neuroscience [Calon, et al., 2004; Calderon and Kim, 2004; Horroks and Farooqui, 2004; Hirayama, et al., 2004; Hashimoto, et al., 2002, 2005]. Deficiency of brain DHA induces loss of cognition [Sinclair and Crawford, 1973; Messeri, et al., 1975]. In the rat, spatial cognition memory enables it to perceive the location of food at the end of the radial maze or on the hidden platform in the water maze. Studies with animals suggest that an intact hippocampus is requisite for accumulating, processing and storing information about the spatial orientation of the individual's environment, where the hippocampus acts as a cognitive map that enables the subject to recognize navigate the previously cued context [Jeffery and Hayman, 2004]. Damage to the hippocampus causes profound difficulty in forming new memories [Hampton, et al., 2001]. In AD, the hippocampus becomes one of the first regions of the brain to suffer damage [Mortimer, et al., 2004]. Memory problems and disorientation are among the first symptoms and, consequently, AD patients suffer from uncertainty of direction and inability to respond to their surroundings [Pai and Jacobs, 2004]. Histochemically, AD is characterized by the deposition of amyloid beta (Aβ) peptides in the hippocampus as well as in the cerebral cortex, neuronal degeneration and loss of cognition [Selkoe, 2001]. Interestingly, DHA concentration decreases markedly in the hippocampus of patients with AD [Soderberg, et al., 1991]. The AD model rat, artificially produced by the deposition of Aβ peptides into its brain ventricles, mimics many of the behavioral and neurochemical abnormalities of AD patients [Nitta, et al., 1994; Nitta, et al., 1997; Itoh, et al., 1996; Oka, et al., 2000; Hashimoto, et al., 2002, 2005] and amply helps in studying the mechanism of DHA in the spatial cognition of the model and normal rats, and in the associated prognosis of AD.

Over the past several years, the results of longitudinal, epidemiological and large-scale 5-10 years follow-up studies have been successively presented by European [Barberger-Gateau, et al., 2002] and American [Morris, et al., 2003] researchers clarifying that food composition is related to the onset of dementia. In Japan, the findings of an epidemiological study started in 2001 regarding "prevention /a treatment and meal nutrient of dementia" is becoming clear [Ueki, et al., 2004] and has shown similar findings. Taken together, these Japanese and Western findings suggest that fish oil, vegetables and fruits probably are the foods that prevent and/or delay the onset of AD. They do not differ in that the intake of fish oil and its relevance to AD are important in the context of the results accumulated in Japan and abroad.

Docosahexaenoic acid (DHA, 22:6n-3) and eicosapentaenoic acid (EPA, 20:5n-3), n-3 polyunsaturated fatty acids (PUFAs) hardly included in other edible oil sebum, are abundant in fish oil. Animals synthesize saturated (palmitic acid; 16:0) or monounsaturated (oleic acid; 18:1, n-9) fatty acids in vivo, but not the essential n-3 PUFAs such as DHA and EPA. Therefore, DHA and EPA must be taken as dietary nutrients from fishes and vegetable oils such as perilla oil (Perilla ocimoides oil) and rapeseed oil which contain mostly α-linolenic acid (18:2n-3), a precursor of DHA and EPA, to enhance these n-3 PUFAs in the body. The activity of DHA in cerebral neurologic function (Table 1) has been reported; here, we address the effects of dietary DHA and EPA on the spatial cognition of normal and AD model rats.

Table 1. Modulating role of DHA in neurochemical processes in the brain

1. Cognitive function
2. Learning and Memory
3. Neurotransmitter release
4. Membrane-bound enzymes, ion channels, and receptors
5. Immunity and Inflammation
6. Apoptosis
7. Gene expression
8. Blood brain barrier

A modified version of figure by Horroks and Farooqui (2004).

Brain Lipid Profile

About 30-50% of total human cerebral dry weight is lipids containing about 70% phospholipids, and 30-40% of the phospholipids is related to DHA, because the fatty acid is linked by an ester and is present particularly in phosphatidylethanolamine and phosphatidylserine. The cortico-hippocampal fatty acid profiles of young (5 weeks old) and aged (120 weeks old) rats (Table 2) show that the level of DHA and the ratio of DHA to arachidonic acid (20:4n-6) in the hippocampus decrease with rat ageing.

Table 2. Effect of age on cortico-hippocamal fatty acid profiles (μg/mg protein) in male Wistar rats (n=7)

	Young rats (5 weeks old)		Aged rats (120 weeks old)	
	Cortex	Hippocampus	Cortex	Hippocampus
LA, 18:2(n-6)	2.30± 0.1	1.60± 0.1	1.7± 0.1*	1.4± 0.1*
LLN, 18:3(n-3)	0.8± 0.0	0.5± 0.0	0.1± 0.0*	0.1± 0.1*
AA, 20:4(n-6)	36.1± 1.5	29.3± 1.1	20.2± 0.7*	21.9± 1.6*
EPA, 20:5(n-3)	1.7± 0.1	1.2± 0.1	0.3± 0.0*	0.3± 0.0*
DHA, 22:6(n-3)	41.4± 1.8	38.4± 1.4	27.1± 0.7*	23.5± 1.7*
DHA/AA	1.1± 0.0	1.3± 0.0	1.3± 0.0*	1.1± 0.0*

Results are mean ± SE. *P<0.05, compared with young rats.
AA, arachidonic acid; DHA, docosahexaenoic acid; DHA/AA, molar ratio of DHA and AA; EPA, eicosapentaenoic acid; LA, linoleic acid; LLN, linolenic acid.

n-3 PUFAs and Brain Function

(1) Digestion Absorption of n-3 PUFAs and Intracerebral Migration

DHA and EPA in fish oil together with glycerol and phospholipids are degraded to free fatty acids and monoacylglycerol in the intestinum tenue by pancreatic lipase, and absorbed through the microvilli of intestinal epithelial cells. The DHA and EPA are then esterified again as constituent fatty acids of chylomicron and very low density lipoprotein (VLDL), flow into veins or lymph ducts, are carried to the whole body, and taken into each organ. The absorbed fraction of DHA ethyl ester in humans is around 20% [Lawson and Hughes 1988]. Absorption of EPA ethyl ester is good when a lot of bile acid is secreted or immediately after eating. In addition, the n-3 fatty acid linked to the sn-2 position of glycerol is absorbed to a greater extent than that linked to either the sn-1 or the sn-3 position [Christensen, et al., 1995].

DHA secreted from the liver into the bloodstream is transferred to the brain, taken into the phospholipid fraction and promptly carried to the synapses, the mitochondria and the cytoplasmic membranes. It is plentiful in phospholipids such as phosphatidylethanolamine and phosphatidylserine, but little is taken into phosphatidylcholine and phosphatidylinositol [Philbrick et al., 1987]. Dietary alpha-linolenic acid and EPA, n-3 PUFAs, increase the uptake of DHA into cerebral phospholipids [Emken, et al., 1994; Conquer and Holub, 1998; Pawlosky, et al., 2001; Burdge, et al., 2003]. Since the presence of Δ^4 desaturation enzymes in the brain is still unclear [Lauritzen et al., 2001], however, DHA is hard to accept in a system composed α-linolenic acid; therefore, it is assumed that most of the DHA in neuronal cell membranes originates in the liver.

The plasma and brain fatty acid profiles and the quantity of cerebral unsaturated fatty acids of young rats administered DHA for 12 weeks (Table 3) show that AA decreases and DHA increases in the plasma and the liver. The enzyme that limits the rate of AA and DHA generation is Δ^6-desaturation enzyme (Δ^6 desaturase) together; in liver, however, the synthesis of AA is inhibited in the presence of high levels of DHA, n-3 PUFA with a higher affinity for this enzyme than that of the series of n-6 PUFAs [Rodriguez, et al., 1998]. Therefore, in DHA-administered rats, the level of AA decreases in both the plasma and the liver. It is generally accepted that in mature rats the level of cerebral fatty acid is affected not by food lipids. As shown in Table 3 and Table 4, however, dietary DHA and EPA, respectively, increase the levels of the fatty acid in cerebral cortex and hippocampus of rat brain, although clearly at different loci in brain tissue. Aged rats (110 weeks old) administered DHA for 12 weeks show increases of DHA content in both the cortico-hippocampal region and the plasma, whereas no significant change in DHA content is observed in the cerebellum or the brainstem of aged rats [Hossain, et al., 1998]. This site-specific uptake of DHA into the brain may be instrumental in clarifying the role of DHA in spatial cognition.

Table 3. Effects of dietary DHA on plasma, liver and brain fatty acid profiles of young rats

	LA,18:2(n-6)	LLN, 18:3(n-3)	AA, 20:4(n-6)	EPA20:5(n-3)	DHA, 22:6(n-3)	DHA / AA
Plasma						
Control	40.5± 2.8	1.9± 3.80	54.8± 1.9	1.8± 0.1	8.0± 0.3	0.1± 0.0
DHA	46.2± 2.3	2.3± 3.80	30.6± 1.6*	5.6± 0.5*	18.3± 0.7*	0.4± 0.0*
Liver						
Control	29.3± 1.9	0.5± 3.80	34.6± 1.5	0.7± 0.1	10.0± 0.5	0.3± 0.0
DHA	34.1± 1.9	0.6± 0.0	27.0± 1.8*	2.6± 0.2*	18.5± 1.2*	0.7± 0.0*
Cortex						
Control	2.3± 0.1	0.8± 0.0	36.1± 1.5	1.7± 0.1	41.4± 1.8	1.1± 0.0
DHA	3.1± 0.1*	0.8± 0.0	35.6± 1.4	1.8± 0.1	48.2± 2.0*	1.4± 0.0*
Hippocampus						
Control	1.6± 0.1	0.5± 0.0	29.3± 1.1	1.2± 0.1	38.4± 1.4	1.3± 0.0
DHA	2.3± 0.2	0.7± 0.1	32.5± 2.7	1.5± 0.1	49.7± 4.0*	1.6± 0.0*
Cerebrum						
Control	2.7± 0.1	1.0± 0.0	23.5± 1.2	1.7± 0.1	45.1± 2.1	1.9± 0.1
DHA	3.3± 1.0*	0.9± 0.0	23.1± 0.6	1.6± 0.0	47.9± 1.3	2.1± 0.1

Results are mean ± SE. *P<0.05, compared with control.
AA, arachidonic acid; DHA, docosahexaenoic acid; DHA/AA, molar ratio of DHA and AA; EPA, eicosapentaenoic acid; LA, linoleic acid; LLN, linolenic acid.

Compared with that of DHA and AA (Table 4), the cerebral and hippocampal content of EPA is small and hardly changes even if it stands at a high level in the plasma. Since the presence of Δ^4-desaturation enzymes in the brain is still unclear [Lauritzen, et al., 2001], EPA is probably not taken into brain tissue. Nevertheless, in EPA-administered rats, dietary EPA (300 mg/kg/day) significantly increases hippocampal EPA and DHA content with an increase in plasma EPA (Table 4) [Hashimoto, et al., 2004]. ^{14}C-labeled EPA (^{14}C-EPA) is detected in the rat brain one hour after its oral administration to rats, and decreases time-dependently, whereas ^{14}C-docosapentaenoic acid (DPA) and ^{14}C-DHA, metabolites of EPA, increase time-dependently. It is, thus, speculated that in the de novo system each PUFA is metabolized after being taken into cerebral endothelial cells and astrocytes, constituent cells of the blood-brain barrier, that it is released from both cells, and that DHA as the metabolite is taken into neurons. Thus, DHA is taken into neurons from the extracellular medium after its release from glial cells or the capillary endothelium (Figure 1) [Moore, 2001]. Indeed, increased DHA and EPA levels in the plasma raise the fatty acid unsaturation index in rat caudal arteries [Hashimoto, et al., 1998, 1999]. Moreover, lysophosphatidylcholine may be a transporter of DHA in the blood-brain barrier [Spector, 2001].

Table 4. Effects of dietary EPA on plasma and brain fatty acid profiles of rats

	AA, 20:4(n-6)	EPA20:5(n-3)	DPA, 22:5(n-3)	DHA, 22:6(n-3)	DHA/AA	n-6/n-3	USI
Plasma							
Control	431± 16.3	4.14± 0.7	6.87± 1.0	39.0± 3.7	0.09± 0.3	15.3 ± 0.70	201± 6.5
EPA	223± 11.1*	60.9± 6.7*	23.9± 2.8*	32.3± 2.9	0.15± 0.0*	4.28± 0.7*	216± 1.4*
Cortex							
Control	42.1± 3.6	0.21± 0.02	0.29± 0.05	51.1± 3.4	1.23± 0.05	0.91± 0.03	180±1.77
EPA	35.0± 1.5	0.39± 0.02*	0.97± 0.04*	51.8± 3.7*	1.48± 0.09*	0.76± 0.04*	184±2.16
Hippocampus							
Control	40.1± 0.7	0.20± 0.01	0.15± 0.06	44.0± 1.5	1.08± 0.04	1.03± 0.04	178±1.30
EPA	36.9± 0.9*	0.39± 0.01*	0.92± 0.06*	48.9± 1.5*	1.33± 0.04*	0.83± 0.03*	189±3.57*

Results are mean ± SE. *P<0.05, compared with control.
AA, arachidonic acid; DHA, docosahexaenoic acid; DHA/AA, molar ratio of DHA and AA; DPA, docosapentaenoic acid; EPA, eicosapentaenoic acid; USI, unsaturation index, is calculated as [Σ(mol% of each (poly) unsaturated fatty acid X number of double bonds per fatty acid)]/100.

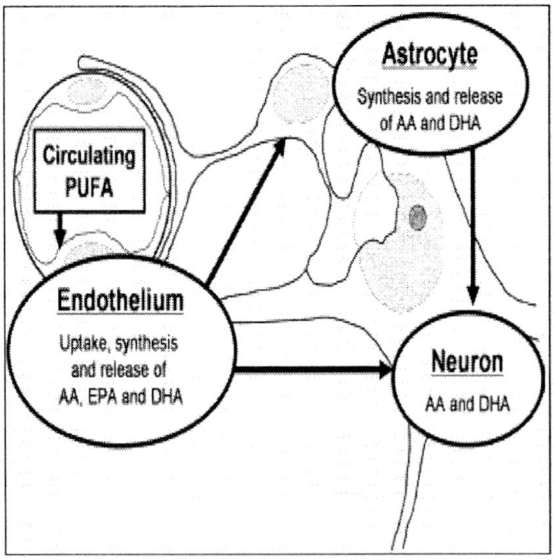

Figure 1. Model of PUFAs uptake and processing by cerebral endothelium and astrocytes. AA, arachidonic acid; EPA, eicosapentaenoic acid; DHA, docosahexaenoic acid; PUFA, polyunsaturated fatty acid. This figure was aggranged from [Moore, 2001].

(2) DHA and Synaptic Function

DHA is abundantly present particularly in the brain, the retina and sperm; in neuronal cells, this fatty acid is present particularly in synaptosomal membranes, synaptic vesicles and auxesis [Scott and Bazan, 1989]. The half-life of cerebral DHA is comparatively short; it is estimated that 2-8 % of phospholipid DHA in the rat brain is replaced daily with DHA from the plasma unesterified fatty acid pool [Rapoprt, 2001]. The level of DHA in the synaptosomal membrane of the cerebral cortex increases significantly, albeit within a small range (17-29%), with an increase in the level of DHA in the plasma of young rats fed DHA for 12 weeks [Hossain, 2004]. These findings suggest that the levels of DHA in the cortico-hippocampal region and in the synaptosomal membranes are influenced by alterations in the level of DHA in the plasma of mature as well as of embryo and neonate of rats.

How does an increase in the level of neuronal DHA affect synaptic functions? Two forms of the synaptic plasticity of neurons, long-term potentiation (LTP) and long-term depression (LTD), are major cellular mechanisms associated with learning and memory processes [Chen and Tonegawa, 1997; Lynch, 2004]. These mechanisms involve depolarization of post-synaptic membranes, calcium entry mediated by N-methyl-D-aspartate (NMDA) receptors, and stimulation of phosphlipase A2. Dietary supplementation with DHA restores neurotransmitter release and impairment in the expression of LTP [McGahon, et al., 1999]. DHA, which is crucial for the induction of LTP and released endogenously during titanic stimulation, triggers the expression of LTP [Fujita, et al., 2001]. In the presence of DHA, the response of NMDA receptor of brain cortex cone cells of juvenile rats is enhanced [Nishikawa, et al., 1994], and the induction of LTD in the hippocampal CA1 region is inhibited [Young, et al., 2000]. Moreover, the impairment in LTP in aged rats is associated with a decrease in membrane PUFAs, specifically AA and DHA, and treatment of aged rats with either of these PUFAs has been shown to reverse age-related decrease in LTP and the decrease in membrane concentration of the fatty acid [McGahon, et al., 1999]. These data suggest that dietary supplementation of DHA modulates long-term potentiation in the hippocampus.

In neuronal cells, DHA influences various receptors, the productivity of neurotransmitters and receptor activity [Horrocks and Faroqui, 2004]. Furthermore, it is an endogenous ligand of the cerebral retinoid X receptor [de Urquiza, et al., 2000], and a ligand of the PPARα receptor [Diep, et al., 2000]. Besides, dietary DHA increases the expression of hippocampal Fos protein [Tanabe, et al., 2004], encoded by the immediate early gene c-fos, which is known to be a transcription factor and a functional marker of neuronal activity. In the awake, but not anesthetized, rats, rapid increase in Fos-related protein is associated with LTP in the dentate gyrus [Abraham, et al., 1991]. These data suggest that DHA directly or indirectly regulates the expression of various genes and may exercise ameliorating effects on brain dysfunction.

Improving Effect of DHA and EPA on Learning Ability

DHA (300mg/kg/day, for ten weeks) administered to young male Wistar rats fed a fish oil-deficient diet through three generations and tested by radial maze tasks demonstrates a decrease in the, number of reference memory errors with a concomitant increase in the level of DHA in the hippocampus [Gamoh, et al., 1999]. DHA administration shows a significantly negative correlation between the number of reference memory errors and the ratio of DHA to AA (DHA/AA) in the cortex and the hippocampus. Reference memory errors represent the number of times that a rat enters unbaited arms, and working memory errors represent repeated entry into arms already visited, within one trial. Thus, reference memory is information that is retained until the next trial, and working memory is information that is lost within a short time. DHA and AA are the main cerebral PUFAs that together contribute to LTP formation, suggesting the influence of synapse on the mechanism of learning ability [Nishikawa, et al., 1994]. Of interest is the significance of the correlation between the DHA/AA ratio and spatial cognition ability in clarifying the beneficial effect of each of these unsaturated fatty acids on brain function. Similarly, dietary administration of DHA to young mice for 4-7 months improves their spatial cognition learning ability [Lim and Suzuki, 2001].

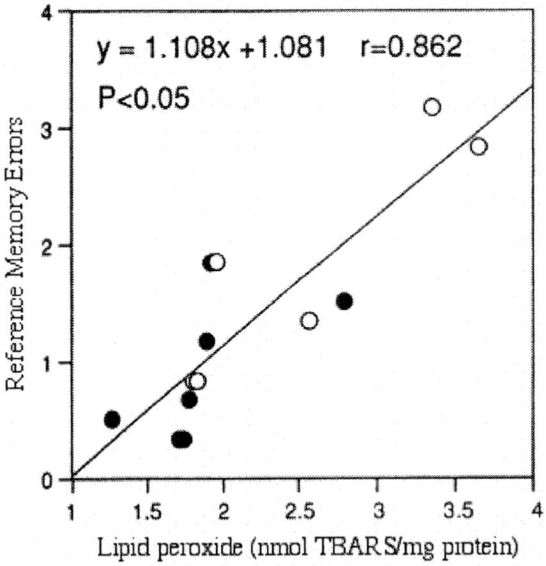

Figure 2. Scatter plots of the relationship between learning ability and the levels of lipid peroxide (LPO) in the hippocampus. Learning ability is expressed as the number of reference memory errors in block 10. The level of LPO is indicated in nmol malondialdehyde/mg protein. (O), control rats; (●), rats administered DHA at 300 mg/kg per day. This figure was arranged from [Gamoh, et al., 2001].

Antioxidative Actio An increase in cerebral lipid peroxidation assumes a disorder of neuronal cells, leading to degradation of brain function [Yatin et al., 1999]. The number of reference and working memory errors declines with an increase in the level of cortico-hippocampal DHA and a decrease in the level of hippocampal lipid peroxidation in DHA-administered aged rats, revealing a significant positive correlation between the level of hippocampal lipid peroxidation and the number of reference memory errors (Figure 2) [Gamoh, et al., 2001]. It is suggested, therefore, that the onset of dementia, which often begins with hippocampal dysfunction, can be prevented or delayed by the prophylactic effect of dietary DHA.

N OF DHA IN BRAIN

Free radical-induced oxidative stress, a normal metabolic event in the homeostatic course of living tissues, plays an important role in cellular physiology. The double bond (-C=C-) undergoes hyperoxidation in the air, and, consequently, lipid peroxidation rises; thus, the presence of PUFA such as DHA would be expected to induce the production of active oxygen and free radicals including lipid radicals, lipid peroxyl radicals and lipid peroxides. The brain is poor in antioxidative enzymes such as catalase, glutathione peroxidase and superoxide dismutase, compared with other organs of the body such as the heart, liver and kidneys [Mizuno and Ohta, 1986; Cohen, 1988]. On the other hand, the brain alone exploits one fifth of the total oxygen demand of the body [Cui, et al., 2004]. Thus, there may remain a theoretical concern that significant DHA incorporation into brain membranes by dietary administration would increase lipid peroxidation, and the brain would remain under the threat of increased oxidation-induced pathogenecity. An increase in the level of DHA in the brain renders more deleterious effects [Eddy and Harman, 1977; Saito and Nakatsugawa, 1994]. Therefore, one might argue that increased levels of cerebral lipid peroxidation with dietary DHA would enhance neuronal cell degeneration [Olanow and Arendash, 1994; Gerlach et al., 1994]. Would the selective accumulation of DHA in the brain be detrimental to neurons and neuronal functions? We speculate that the anticipation of the increases in DHA-induced oxidative stress is applicable to *in vitro* studies, in the absence of adequate antioxidative enzymes, on model membranes such as liposomes [Araseki, et al., 2002], LDL-colesterol particles [van den Berg, et al., 199; Suzukawa, et al., 1995; Nenseter and Drevon, 1996] and cancerous cells including HL-60 cells [Arita, et al., 2001], and an unlikely event in most *in vivo* brain systems. Lipid peroxidation decreases significantly in the cortico-hippocampal synaptosomal fraction, and the activity of cerebral antioxidative enzymes is more enhanced with increased cerebral DHA levels in DHA-administered rats [Hossain, et al. 2004]. These data are consistent with the notion that the brain does not selectively enrich "oxidation-vulnerable lipid molecules" as does DHA. DHA decreases lipid peroxidation and eradicates free radicals in the rat brain [Green, et al., 2001; Yavin, et al., 2002]. DHA protects the brain from traumatic injury-induced oxidative stress, reduced plasticity and impaired learning [Wu et al., 2004]. Biomarkers of peroxidation such as the level of lipid peroxide in rats [Erdogan, et al., 2004] or urinary F2-isoprostanes, which are DHA-specific oxidized derivatives, in men [Mori, et al., 2000] decrease after feeding or consumptions of fish oil diets, respectively. Dietary administration of fish oil to human is also associated with a reduction in the generation of the superoxide anion [Chen, et al., 1994; Luostarinen and Saldeen, 1996]. Retinal neurons exposed to oxidant that generates the superoxide anion and elicits apopototic death are protected by incubation with DHA [Rosenstein, et al., 2003]. These data suggest that brain tissue abundant with DHA protect neuronal cells from oxidative stress and maintain their mechanism.

Now the question that remains to be answered is why the n-3 fatty acid deficient rats exhibit increased lipid peroxidation and how DHA apparently protects neural cells from oxidative stress. An increase in lipid peroxide in ischemic injury is accompanied by higher free fatty acid levels, with the largest increase observed in AA [Rao, et al., 1999; Bazan Jr, 1970]. Oxidation of free AA produces AA-derived free radicals, and subsequent accumulation of peroxidation products in mitochondrial membranes causes the uncoupling of oxidative phosphorylation [Cheremishina and Vladimirou, 1975], disruption of proton gradients and the membrane damage [Wojtczak, 1976]. Dietary n-3 fatty acids, especially DHA and EPA, reduce the amount of AA in phospholipids by a combination of decreasing its synthesis and simple physical replacement [Morita, et al. 1983; Abeywardena, et al. 1991]. Therefore, a high DHA/AA ratio in DHA-administered rats could be one of the major contributors to lower levels of lipid peroxide in the brain.

Superoxide dismutase (SOD), one of the determinant factors in reducing oxidative stress, neutralizes superoxide anion concentration by dismutation to a hydrogen peroxide [Fridovich, 1995]. Hydrogen peroxide also has (modest) oxidative potential and can be converted to hydroxyl radical [Halliwell and Gutteridge, 1999]. Catalase (CAT) and glutathione peroxidase (GPx) next come into action in hydrogen peroxide. DHA significantly increases the activity of these enzymes [Hossain, et al. 1999], although that mechanism remains to be explored with regard to whether these enhanced activities are related to the increased expression of these enzyme proteins or to other factors. Reduced glutathione (GSH), a substrate of GPx and a major water-soluble thiol, plays an important role in maintaining cellular defense mechanisms in multiple ways, including participation in direct reactions with free radicals and in the enzymatic reduction of hydroperoxides [Ishikawa, et al., 1986]. Oxidation of the cysteine sulfhydryl group of GSH produces a disulfide bridge to form glutathione disulfide (oxidized glutathione, GSSG). Depletion of glutathione is, thus, a marker of oxidative stress. DHA administration also increases GSH in rats [Hossain, et al. 1999, Komatsu, et al., 2003, Sekine, et al., 2003]. The relation between the level of antioxidative enzymes and the brain DHA/AA ratio has been examined, because the ratio is considered a marker of host defense capability against oxidative damage. A highly significant positive correlation is observed between CAT or GPx acitivity and the DHA/AA ratio, where an inverse relation is observed between the levels of DHA and AA, suggesting that dietary DHA facilitates the expulsion of cerebral AA, elevates the DHA/AA ratio and potentiates CAT and GPx activity [Hossain, et al., 1999]. Moreover, DHA with its specialized helical conformation [Stubbs, 1992] in the membrane bilayer plays the role of a structural fatty acid [Bazan, 1990; Fonlupt, et al., 1994] and is believed to have a slower turnover rate [Gazzah, et al., 1995], suggesting a lesser probability of its being the substrate for the free radical reaction. In contrast, AA is subject to the AA-cascade and may produce many free radicals, as described above. Therefore, the inverse relation between these polyunsaturated fatty acids offers a possible explanation for the protection of the brain from oxidation. It could be postulated that a DHA-induced decrease in AA with a concomitant increase in the DHA/AA ratio provides a line of defense against peroxidative stress in the brain cerebrum through the activation of antioxidative enzymes (Figure 3).

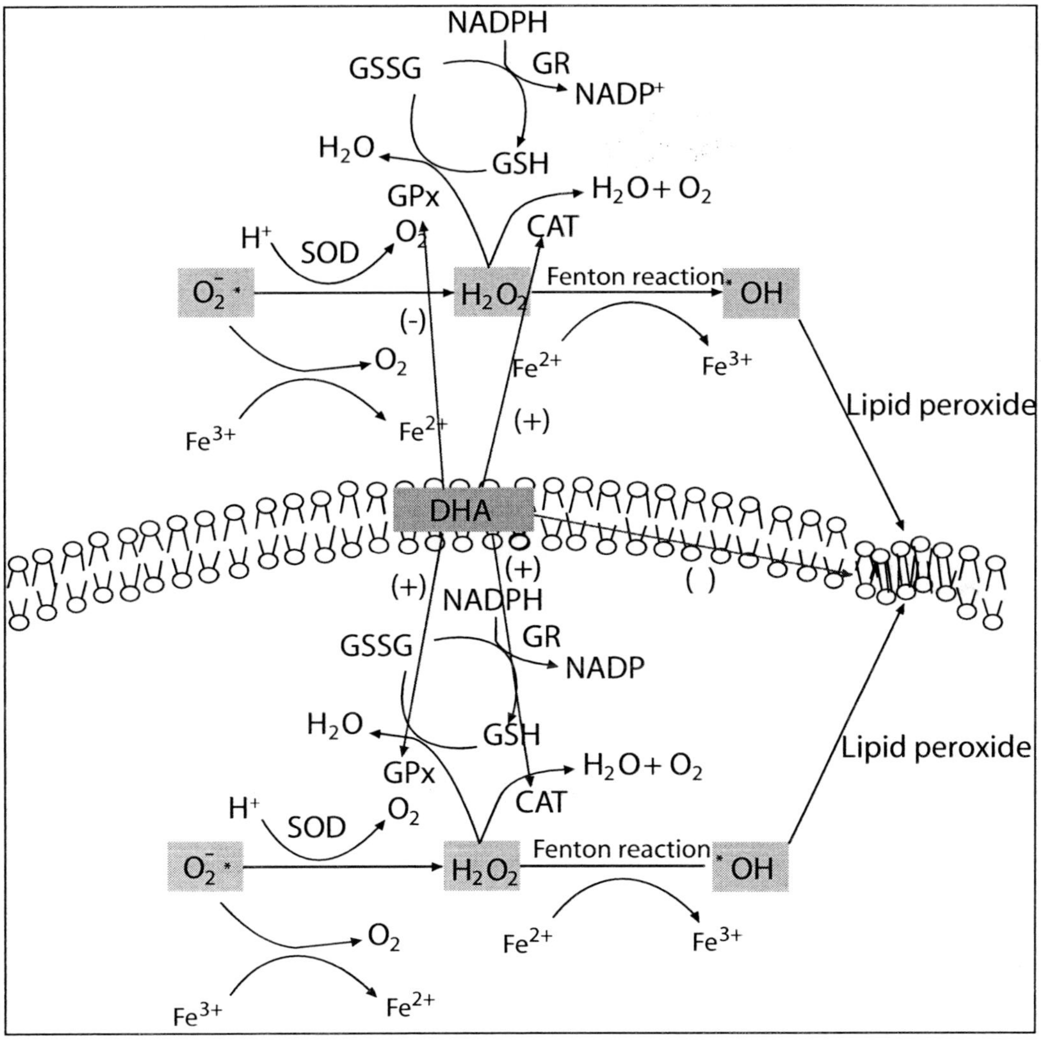

Figure 3. Effects of docosahexaenoic acid are schematized here on the antioxidative enzymes that metabolize the oxidative species of the cytosol and/or mitochondrial matrix. CAT: Catalase, GPx: glutathione peroxidase, GR: Gluthathione reductase, SOD: Superoxide dismutase, GSH: Reduced glutathione: GSSG, Oxidized glutathione, LPO: Lipid peroxide, H_2O_2: Hydrogen peroxide, O_{-2}: Superoxide anion, OH: Hydroxyl radical. The brain is abundant in iron-rich hemoglobin. The ferrous iron produced by the reduction of O_{-2}. reacts with H_2O_2 and produces OH. The superoxide anion, which is produced by single electron reduction, and H_2O_2 which is produced by the dismutation O_{-2} by SOD, can further be transformed to OH by the so called Fenton reaction. The membrane polyunsaturated fatty acids are particularly, arachidonic acid, vulnerable to oxidation by OH radicals and gives rise to extensive production of LPO. For more details, refer to the text.

Does Antioxidative Action by DHA Affect Brain Function?

A large-scale epidemiological study in Europe and USA shows that an increased intake of dietary antioxidative substrates can regulate the onset and development of AD [Grant, 1997]. It is also suggested that the potency which neuronal cells achieve by the antioxidative action of DHA prevents lipid peroxidation from contributing to the accelerated accumulation of the β-amyloid, one of the critical causal proteins in AD [Pratico, et al., 2001]. Since AD impairs memory, and infusion of β-amyloid protein into the rat cerebral ventricle reduces learning ability, an investigation of the effect of dietary administration of DHA on spatial cognition learning ability in β-amyloid–produced AD model rats has demonstrated that in DHA pre-administered AD model rats both lipid peroxidation, induced by the deposition of amyloid-β protein, and apoptosis are inhibited by the pre-administration associated with the enhanced antioxidative effect of DHA in the cortex and the hippocampus [Hashimoto, et al., 2002]. Furthermore, dietary administration of DHA to AD-model rats improves the spatial cognition learning ability (which deteriorates by the deposition of amyloid-β peptide) and increases antioxidant activity in the hippocampus (Figure 4) [Hashimoto et al., 2005].

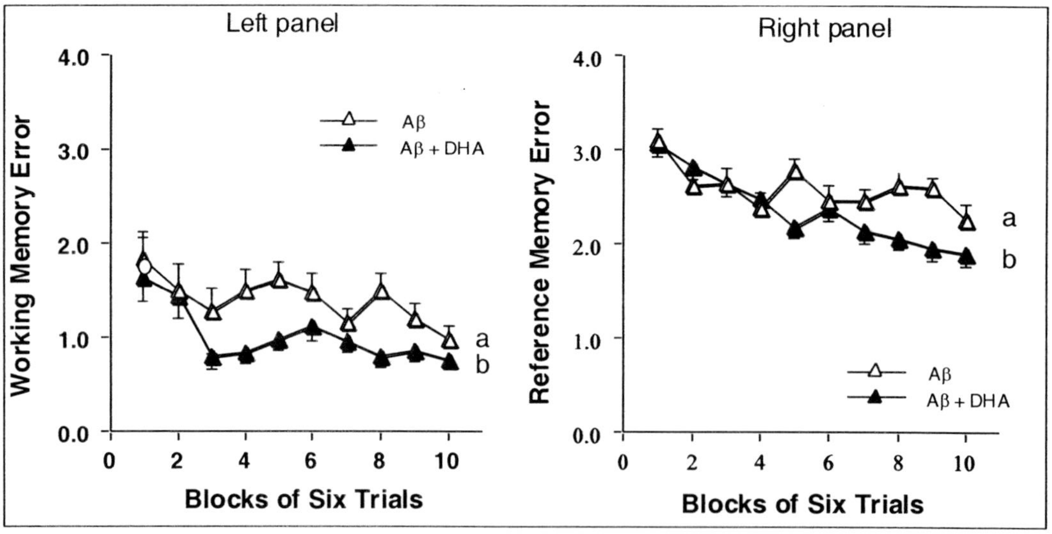

Figure 4. Effect of docosahexaenoic acid (DHA) administered to the amyloid-β (Aβ) peptide (1-40)-infused rats on working (left panel) and reference (right panel) memory-related learning ability in the radial maze task. Each value represents the number of working and reference memory errors as the mean ± SEM in each block of six trials. Aβ = Aβ-infused rats (n=9); Aβ+DHA = DHA-administered Aβ-infused rats (n=10). Groups without a common letter for the main effects of groups are significantly different at $P < 0.05$. This figure was arranged from [Hashimoto, et al., 2005].

DHA significantly cleares amyloid beta peptide$_{1\text{-}40}$ and concomitantly decreases cholesterol from detergent-insoluble membrane fractions [Hashimoto et al., in press]. After excision of the amyloid precursor protein (APP) by β and γ-secretase, amyloid β peptides are harbored in the detergent-insoluble, cholesterol plus glycolipid-enriched membrane domains, or the so-called lipid rafts [Lee, et al., 1998], wherefrom they are believed to start the seeding of the process of amylogenesis in the neurons of AD individuals. We speculate that DHA directly or indirectly induces a mechanism by which the amyloid peptides are cleared, probably by means of the induction of the microglial cell activity that is noted for phagocytic effects in the brain. Amylogenesis is also known to be dependent on cholesterol [Simons, et al., 1998; Simons, et al., 2001], and antihypercholesterolemic drugs like statins significantly decrease Aβ production [Ehehalt, et al., 2003]. Thus it is reasonable to also speculate that DHA ameliorates the cognition memory by reducing the harboring of membrane raft-residing cholesterol (Figure 5).

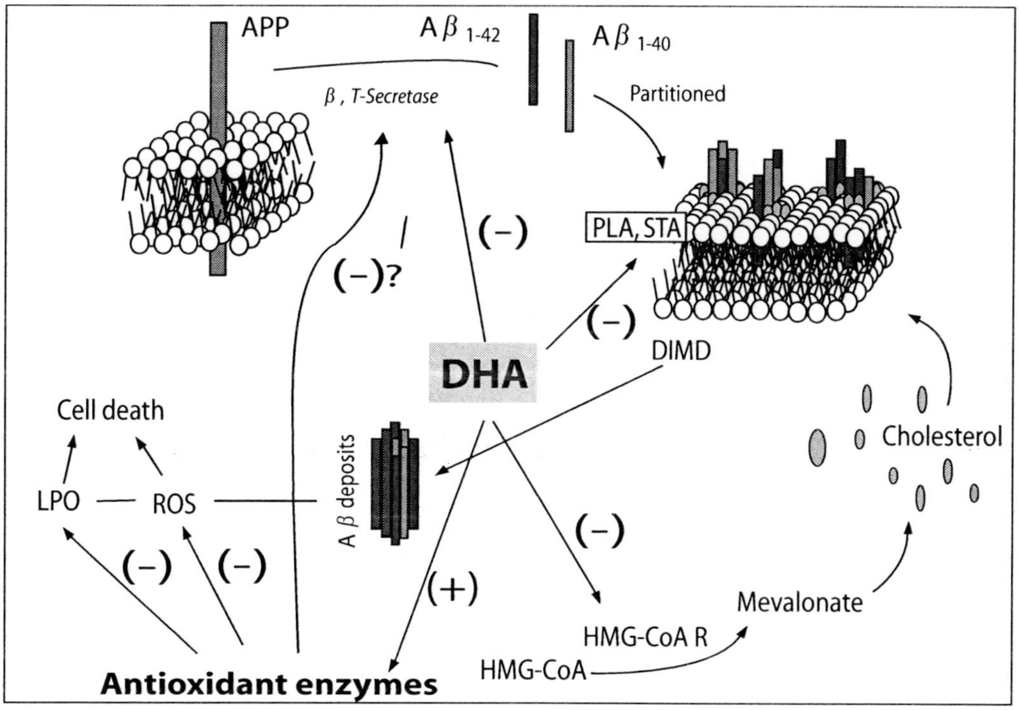

Figure 5. Schematized figure for the roles of docosahexaenoic acid (DHA) on the A□$_{1-40}$-induced neurotoxicity and cell death. The Aβ_{1-40} after in vivo infusion (or in vivo sequential cleavage by β, γ-secretase enzymes) partitioned into the cholesterol-glycosphinglipids-enriched detergent-insoluble membrane microdomains (DIMD). DHA inhibits the harboring of Aβ_{1-40} into DIMDs by decreasing their cholesterol, probably by inhibiting the cholesterol biosynthesizing enzyme 3-hydroxy-3-methylglutaryl coenzyme A reductase (HMGCoA-R), and palmitic (PLA) and steric acid (STA) levels. DHA, by activating antioxidative defenses, scavenges the Aβ_{1-40}-induced oxidative stress ((lipid peroxide (LPO) and reactive oxygen species (ROS)) and protects neuronal death. DHA directly inhibits the β, γ-secretase enzyme and/or, DHA-induced antioxidative enzymes shields the cleavage sites of amyloid precursor protein (APP), wherein the protease enzymes (β, γ-secretases) cuts to produce Aβ_{1-40} and Aβ_{1-42}. For more details, refer to the text.

Cognition learning ability decreases with age, and its impairment is a major symptom of AD. In the hippocampus, DHA levels are found to be extremely low in patients with AD compared with those in age-matched brains of human controls [Söderberg et al., 1991]. In the mouse model of AD, a DHA-enriched diet produces a 40-50 % reduction in amyloid-β protein deposition in the hippocampus and the parietal cortex [Lim, et al., 2005]. Short-term feeding of fish oil to aged rats induces the expression of numerous genes in the hippocampus. Transcription of transthyretin, a protein involved in the transport of thyroxin, increases 10-fold [Puskas, et al., 2003]. This protein also acts as an amyloid-β protein scavenger. Interestingly, moreover, DHA affects amyloid precursor protein (APP) processing by β- and γ-secretase activity [de Wilde et al., 2003]. Thus, DHA supplements provide neuroprotection against the deposition of amyloid-β protein without significant toxic effects.

Conclusion

Dietary administration of DHA improves cognition memory of normal young and aged rats, as well as that of AD model rats. The improvement in these cases is associated with cortico-hippocampal accumulation of DHA with a concomitant increase in the DHA/AA ratio, antioxidative defense, and decreases in lipid peroxide, apoptotic-like death and detergent-insoluble membrane-resident cholesterol. Taken together, all this evidence suggests that dietary DHA enhances cognitive memory and ameliorates the deterioration of learning ability-related memory, oxidative stress and apoptosis-like cell death in AD-model animals. Further studies are needed not only to understand DHA-induced improvement of cognitive function but also to elucidate both the mechanism of preventing AD and the outcome of treatment with DHA.

References

Abeywardena, M. Y., McLennan, P. L., & Charnock, J. S. (1991) Differential effects of dietary fish oil on myocardial prostaglandin I2 and thromboxane A2 production. *Am J Physiol*, 260(2 Pt 2): H379-385.

Abraham, W. C., Dragunow, M., and Tate, W. P. (1991) The role of immediate early genes in the stabilization of long-term potentiation. *Mol. Neurobiol.* 5: 297-314.

Araseki, M., Yamamoto, K., Miyashita, K. (2002) Oxidative stability of polyunsaturated fatty acid in phosphatidylcholine liposomes. *Biosci Biotechnol Biochem.* 66(12): 2573-2577.

Arita, K., Kobuchi, H., Utsumi, T., et al. (2001) Mechanism of apoptosis in HL-60 cells induced by n-3 and n-6 polyunsaturated fatty acids. *Biochem Pharmacol.* 62: 821-828.

Barberger-Gateau, P., Letenneur, L., Deschamps, V., Peres, K., Dartigues, J. F., & Renaud, S. (2002) Fish, meat, and risk of dementia: cohort study. *BMJ*, 325(7370): 932-933.

Bazan, N. G., Jr. (1990) *Nutrition and the Brain,* Wurtman, R. J. and Wurtman, J. J. (eds): 1-24. Ravan Press, New York.

Bazan, N. G., Jr. (1970) Effects of ischemia and electroconvulsive shock on free fatty acid pool in the brain. *Biochim Biophys Acta*, 218(1): 1-10.

Barberger-Gateau, P., Letenneur, L., Deschamps, V., Peres, K., Dartigues, J.F., Renaud, S. (2002) Fish, meat, and risk of dementia: cohort study. *BMJ.* 325(7370): 932-3.

Burdge, G. C., Finnegan, Y. E., Minihane, A. M., Williams, C. M., Wootton, S. A. (2003) Effect of altered dietary n-3 fatty acid intake upon plasma lipid fatty acid composition, conversion of [13C] α-linolenic acid to longer-chain fatty acids and partitioning towards β-oxidation in older men. *Br J Nutr*. 90(2): 311-21.

Calon, F., Lim, G. P., Yang, F., Morihara, T., Teter, B., Ubeda, O., Rostaing, P., Triller, A., Salem, N., Jr., Ashe, K. H., Frautschy, S. A., & Cole, G. M. (2004) Docosahexaenoic acid protects from dendritic pathology in an Alzheimer's disease mouse model. *Neuron*, 43(5): 633-645.

Calderon, F., Kim, H. Y. (2004) Docosahexaenoic acid promotes neurite growth in hippocampal neurons. *J Neurochem*. 90(4):979-88.

Chen, L. Y., Lawson, D.L., Mehta, J. L., (1994) Reduction in human neutrophil superoxide anion generation by n-3 polyunsaturated fatty acids: role of cyclooxygenase products and endothelium derived relaxing factor. *Thromb. Res.* 76, 317–322.

Chen, C., & Tonegawa, S. (1997) Molecular genetic analysis of synaptic plasticity, activity-dependent neural development, learning, and memory in the mammalian brain. *Annu Rev Neurosci*, 20: 157-184.

Cheremishina, Z. P., & Vladimirou, Y. A., (1975) Effect of endogenous lipid peroxides on respiration in rat liver. *Biokimiia* 40: 242-247.

Christensen, M. S., Hoy, C. E., Becker, C. C., & Redgrave, T. G. (1995) Intestinal absorption and lymphatic transport of eicosapentaenoic (EPA), docosahexaenoic (DHA), and decanoic acids: dependence on intramolecular triacylglycerol structure. *Am J Clin Nutr*, 61(1): 56-61.

Cohen, G. 1988. Oxygen radicals and Parkinson's disease, in, *Oxygen Radicals and Tissue Injury* (Haliwell B., ed), pp. 130-135. Federation of American Societies for Experimental Biology, Bethesda, Maryland.

Conquer, J. A., and Holub, B. J. (1998) Effect of supplementation with different doses of DHA on the levels of circulating DHA as non-esterified fatty acid in subjects of Asian Indian background. *J. Lipid Res.* 39:286-292.

Cui, K., Luo, X., Xu, K., Ven Murthy, M.R. (2004) Role of oxidative stress in neurodegeneration: recent developments in assay methods for oxidative stress and nutraceutical antioxidants. Prog. Neuro-Psychopharmacol. *Biol. Psych.* 28:771-799.

de Urquiza, A. M., Liu, S., Sjoberg, M., Zetterstrom, R. H., Griffiths, W., Sjovall, J., & Perlmann, T. (2000) Docosahexaenoic acid, a ligand for the retinoid X receptor in mouse brain. *Science*, 290(5499): 2140-2144.

de Wilde, M. C., Leenders, I., Broersen, L. M., et al., (2003) The omega-3 fatty acid docosahexaenoic acid (DHA) inhibits the formation of beta amyloid in CHO7PA2 cells. *Soc Neurosci Program* No. 730: 11 (Abstract).

Diep, Q. N., Touyz, R. M., & Schiffrin, E. L. (2000) Docosahexaenoic acid, a peroxisome proliferator-activated receptor-alpha ligand, induces apoptosis in vascular smooth muscle cells by stimulation of p38 mitogen-activated protein kinase. *Hypertension*, 36(5): 851-855.

Eddy, D. E., & Harman, D. (1977) Free radical theory of aging: effect of age, sex and dietary precursors on rat-brain docosahexanoic acid. *J Am Geriatr Soc*, 25(5): 220-229.

Ehehalt, R., Keller, P., Haass, C., Thiele, C., & Simons, K. (2003) Amyloidogenic processing of the Alzheimer β-amyloid precursor protein depends on lipid rafts. *J Cell Biol*, 160(1): 113-123.

Emken, E. A, Adlof, R. O, Gulley, R. M. (1994) Dietary linoleic acid influences desaturation and acylation of deuterium-labeled linoleic acid and linolenic acids in young adult males. *Biochim Biophys Acta* 1213: 277-288.

Erdogan, H., Fadillioglu, E., Ozgocmen, S., Sogut, S., Ozyurt, B., Akyol, O., Ardicoglu, O. (2004) Effect of fish oil supplementation on plasma oxidant/antioxidant status in rats. *Prostaglandins Leukot. Essent. Fatty Acids* 71(3): 149-52.

Fonlupt, P., Croset, M., & Lagarde, M. (1994) Incorporation of arachidonic and docosahexaenoic acids into phospholipids of rat brain membranes. *Neurosci Lett*, 171(1-2): 137-141.

Fridovich, I. (1995) Superoxide radical and superoxide dismutases. *Annu Rev Biochem*, 64: 97-112.

Fujita, S., Ikegaya, Y., Nishikawa, M., Nishiyama, N., & Matsuki, N. (2001) Docosahexaenoic acid improves long-term potentiation attenuated by phospholipase A(2) inhibitor in rat hippocampal slices. *Br J Pharmacol*, 132(7): 1417-1422.

Gamoh, S., Hashimoto, M., Hossain, S., & Masumura, S. (2001) Chronic administration of docosahexaenoic acid improves the performance of radial arm maze task in aged rats. *Clin Exp Pharmacol Physiol*, 28(4): 266-270.

Gamoh, S., Hashimoto, M., Sugioka, K., Shahdat Hossain, M., Hata, N., Misawa, Y., & Masumura, S. (1999) Chronic administration of docosahexaenoic acid improves reference memory-related learning ability in young rats. *Neuroscience*, 93(1): 237-241.

Gazzah, N., Gharib, A., Croset, M., Bobillier, P., Lagarde, M., & Sarda, N. (1995) Decrease of brain phospholipid synthesis in free-moving n-3 fatty acid deficient rats. *J Neurochem*, 64(2): 908-918.

Gerlach, M., Ben-Shachar, D., Riederer, P., Youdim, M. B. (1994) Altered brain metabolism of iron as a cause of neurodegenerative diseases? *J Neurochem*. 63(3): 793-807.

Grant, W. B. (1997) Dietary links to Alzheimer's disease. *Alzheimer's disease Review*, 2: 42-55.

Green, P., Glozman, S., Weiner, L., & Yavin, E. (2001) Enhanced free radical scavenging and decreased lipid peroxidation in the rat fetal brain after treatment with ethyl docosahexaenoate. *Biochim Biophys Acta*, 1532(3): 203-212.

Halliwell, B., Gutteridge, J. M. C. Oxidative stress and antioxidant protection: some special cases. In: Halliwell B, Gutteridge JMC, editors. Free Radicals in Biology and Medicine. 3rd ed. Oxford: Clarendon Press; 1999. p. 530-533.

Hampton, R. R., Hampstead, B. M., & Murray, E. A. (2004) Selective hippocampal damage in rhesus monkeys impairs spatial memory in an open-field test. *Hippocampus*, 14(7): 808-818.

Hashimoto, M., Hossain, M. S., Haqu, A., & Shido, O. (2006) Docosahexaenoic acid-induced amelioration on impairment of memory learning in amyloid β-infused rats relates to the decreases of amyloid β and cholesterol levels in detergent-insoluble membrane fractions. *Biochim Biophys Acta - Mol. Cell Biol. Lipids,* in press.

Hashimoto, M., Tanabe, Y., Fujii, Y., Kikuta, T., Shibata, H., & Shido, O. (2005) Chronic Administration of Docosahexaenoic Acid Ameliorates the Impairment of Spatial Cognition Learning Ability in Amyloid β-Infused Rats. *J Nutr,* 135(3):549-55.

Hashimoto, M., Yano, Y., Tanabe, Y., Fujii, Y., Harada, T., Kawashima, A., Kawakita, E., Mizuguchi, K., Ueki, A., & Shido, O. (2004) An improvement effect of spatial cognitive functions with dietary eicosapentaenoic acid in young rats. *J Nutr Health Aging* 8: 430 (Abstract)

Hashimoto, M., Hossain, S., Shimada, T., Sugioka, K., Yamasaki, H., Fujii, Y., Ishibashi, Y., Oka, J., & Shido, O. (2002) Docosahexaenoic acid provides protection from impairment of learning ability in Alzheimer's disease model rats. *J Neurochem*, 81(5): 1084-1091.

Hashimoto, M., Shinozuka, K., Gamoh, S., Tanabe, Y., Hossain, M. S., Kwon, Y. M., Hata, N., Misawa, Y., Kunitomo, M., & Masumura, S. (1999) The hypotensive effect of docosahexaenoic acid is associated with the enhanced release of ATP from the caudal artery of aged rats. *J Nutr*, 129(1): 70-76.

Hashimoto, M., Shinozuka, K., Hossain, MS., Kwon, Y. M., Tanabe Y., Kunitomo, M., Masumura, S. (1998) Antihypertensive effect of all-cis-5,8,11,14,17-icosapentaenoate of aged rats is associated with an increase in the release of ATP from the caudal artery. *J Vasc Res,* 35: 55-62.

Hirayama, S., Hamazaki, T., & Terasawa, K. (2004) Effect of docosahexaenoic acid-containing food administration on symptoms of attention-deficit/hyperactivity disorder - a placebo-controlled double-blind study. *Eur J Clin Nutr*, 58(3): 467-473.

Horrocks, L. A., & Farooqui, A. A. (2004) Docosahexaenoic acid in the diet: its importance in maintenance and restoration of neural membrane function. *Prostaglandins Leukot Essent Fatty Acids*, 70(4): 361-372.

Hossain, M. S., Hashimoto, M., Gamoh, S., & Masumura, S. (1999) Antioxidative effects of docosahexaenoic acid in the cerebrum versus cerebellum and brainstem of aged hypercholesterolemic rats. *J Neurochem*, 72(3): 1133-1138.

Hossain, M. S., Hashimoto, M., & Masumura, S. (1998) Influence of docosahexaenoic acid on cerebral lipid peroxide level in aged rats with and without hypercholesterolemia. *Neurosci Lett*, 244(3): 157-160.

Hossain, M. S., Hashimoto, M., Shimada, T., & Shido, O. (2004) Synaptic plasma membrane-bound acetylcholinesterase activity is not affected by docosahexaenoic acid-induced decrease in membrane order. *Life Science*, 74: 3009-3024.

Ishikawa, T., Akerboom, T. M. P., & Sies, H. (1986) Role of key defense systems in target organ toxicity. *in Target Organ Toxicity*, Vol. Ⅰ: 129-143. CRC Press, Boca Raton, Florida.

Itoh, A., Nitta, A., Nadai, M., Nishimura, K., Hirose, M., Hasegawa, T., & Nabeshima, T. (1996) Dysfunction of cholinergic and dopaminergic neuronal systems in β-amyloid protein-infused rats. *J Neurochem*, 66(3): 1113-1117.

Itokazu, N., Ikegaya, Y., Nishikawa, M., & Matsuki, N. (2000) Bidirectional actions of docosahexaenoic acid on hippocampal neurotransmissions in vivo. *Brain Res*, 862(1-2): 211-216.

Jeffery, K. J., & Hayman, R. (2004) Plasticity of the hippocampal place cell representation. *Rev Neurosci*, 15(5): 309-331.

Komatsu, W., Ishihara, K., Murata, M., Saito, H., & Shinohara, K. (2003) Docosahexaenoic acid suppresses nitric oxide production and inducible nitric oxide synthase expression in interferon-γ plus lipopolysaccharide-stimulated murine macrophages by inhibiting the oxidative stress free radical biology & medicine, vol. 34, no. 8, pp. 1006-1016.

Lauritzen, L., Hansen, H. S., Jorgensen, M. H., & Michaelsen, K. F. (2001) The essentiality of long chain n-3 fatty acids in relation to development and function of the brain and retina. *Prog Lipid Res*, 40(1-2): 1-94.

Lawson, L. D., & Hughes, B. G. (1988) Absorption of eicosapentaenoic acid and docosahexaenoic acid from fish oil triacylglycerols or fish oil ethyl esters co-ingested with a high-fat meal. *Biochem Biophys Res Commun*, 156(2): 960-963.

Lee, S. J., Liyanage, U., Bickel, P. E., Xia, W., Lansbury, P. T., Jr., & Kosik, K. S. (1998) A detergent-insoluble membrane compartment contains Aβ in vivo. *Nat Med*, 4(6): 730-734.

Lim, G. P., Calon, F., Morihara, T., Yang, F., Teter, B., Ubeda, O., Salem, N. Jr., Frautshy, S. A., & Cole, G. M. (2005) A diet entiched with the omega-3 fatty acid docosahexaenoic acid reduced amyloid burden in an aged Alzheimer mouse model. *J Neurosci*, 25: 3032-3040.

Lim, S. Y., & Suzuki, H. (2001) Intakes of dietary docosahexaenoic acid ethyl ester and egg phosphatidylcholine improve maze-learning ability in young and old mice. *J Nutr*, 130(6): 1629-1632.

Luostarinen, R., & Saldeen, T. (1996) Dietary fish oil decreases superoxide generation by human neutrophils: relation to cyclooxygenase pathway and lysosomal enzyme release. *Prostaglandins Leukot Essent Fatty Acids*, 55(3): 167-172.

Lynch, M. (2004) Long-term potentiation and memory. *Physiol Rev*. 84(1):87-136.

McGahon, B. M., Martin, D. S., Horrobin, D. F., & Lynch, M. A. (1999) Age-related changes in synaptic function: analysis of the effect of dietary supplementation with omega-3 fatty acids. *Neuroscience*, 94(1): 305-314.

Messeri, G. P., Oliverio, A., Paoletti, R., & Galli, C. (1975) Deficiency of essential fatty acids during pregnancy and avoidance learning in the progeny. *Pharmacol Res Commun*, 7(1): 71-80.

Mizuno, Y., & Ohta, K. (1986) Regional distributions of thiobarbituric acid-reactive products, activities of enzymes regulating the metabolism of oxygen free radicals, and some of the related enzymes in adult and aged rat brains. *J Neurochem*. 46:1344 1352.

Moore, S. A. (2001) Polyunsaturated fatty acid synthesis and release by brain-derived cells in vitro. *J Mol Neurosci*, 16(2-3): 195-200; discussion 215-121.

Mori, T. A., Puddey, I. B., Burke, V., Croft, K. D, Dunstan, D. W., Rivera, J. H., Beilin, L. J. (2000) Effect of omega 3 fatty acids on oxidative stress in humans: GC-MS measurement of urinary F2-isoprostane excretion. *Redox Rep*. 5: 45–46.

Morita, I., Takahashi, R., Saito, Y., & Murota, S. (1983) Effects of eicosapentaenoic acid on arachidonic acid metabolism in cultured vascular cells and platelets: species difference. *Thromb Res*, 31(2): 211-217.

Morris, M. C., Evans, D. A., Bienias, J. L., Tangney, C. C., Bennett, D. A., Wilson, R. S., Aggarwal, N., & Schneider, J. (2003) Consumption of fish and n-3 fatty acids and risk of incident Alzheimer disease. *Arch Neurol*, 60(7): 940-946.

Mortimer, J. A., Gosche, K. M., Riley, K. P., Markesbery, W. R., & Snowdon, D. A. (2004) Delayed recall, hippocampal volume and Alzheimer neuropathology: findings from the Nun Study. *Neurology*, 62(3): 428-432.

Nenseter, M. S., & Drevon, C. A. (1996) Dietary polyunsaturates and peroxidation of low density lipoprotein. *Curr Opin Lipidol.* 7: 8-13

Nishikawa, M., Kimura, S., & Akaike, N. (1994) Facilitatory effect of docosahexaenoic acid on N-methyl-D-aspartate response in pyramidal neurones of rat cerebral cortex. *J Physiol*, 475(1): 83-93.

Nitta, A., Fukuta, T., Hasegawa, T., & Nabeshima, T. (1997) Continuous infusion of β-amyloid protein into the rat cerebral ventricle induces learning impairment and neuronal and morphological degeneration. *Jpn J Pharmacol*, 73(1): 51-57.

Nitta, A., Itoh, A., Hasegawa, T., & Nabeshima, T. (1994) β-Amyloid protein-induced Alzheimer's disease animal model. *Neurosci Lett*, 170(1): 63-66.

Oka, J., Suzuki, E., & Kondo, Y. (2000) Endogenous GLP-1 is involved in β-amyloid protein-induced memory impairment and hippocampal neuronal death in rats. *Brain Res*, 878(1-2): 194-198.

Olanow, C. W., & Arendash, G. W. (1994) Metals and free radicals in neurodegeneration. *Curr Opin Neurol.* 7(6): 548-58. Review.

Pai, M. C., & Jacobs, W. J. (2004) Topographical disorientation in community-residing patients with Alzheimer's disease. *Int J Geriatr Psychiatry*, 19(3): 250-255.

Pawlosky, R. J., Hibbeln, J. R., Novotny, J. A., Salem, N. Jr. (2001) Physiological compartmental analysis of α-linolenic acid metabolism in adult humans. *J Lipid Res.* 42: 1257-1265.

Philbrick, D. J., Mahadevappa, V. G., Ackman, R. G., & Holub, B. J. (1987) Ingestion of fish oil or a derived n-3 fatty acid concentrate containing eicosapentaenoic acid (EPA) affects fatty acid compositions of individual phospholipids of rat brain, sciatic nerve and retina. *J Nutr*, 117(10): 1663-1670.

Pratico, D., Uryu, K., Leight, S., Trojanoswki, J. Q., & Lee, V. M. (2001) Increased lipid peroxidation precedes amyloid plaque formation in an animal model of Alzheimer amyloidosis. *J Neurosci*, 21(12): 4183-4187.

Puskas, L.G., Kitajka, K., Nyakas, C., Barcelo-Coblijn, G., & Farkas, T. (2003) Short-term administration of omega 3 fatty acids from fish oil results in increased transthyretin transcription in old rat hippocampus. *Proc Natl Acad Sci USA*. 100: 1580-1585.

Rao, A. M., Hatcher, J. F., Kindy, M. S., & Dempsey, R. J. (1999) Arachidonic acid and leukotriene C4: role in transient cerebral ischemia of gerbils. *Neurochem Res*, 24(10): 1225-1232.

Rapoport, S. I., Chang, M. C., & Spector, A. A. (2001) Delivery and turnover of plasma-derived essential PUFAs in mammalian brain. *J Lipid Res*, 42(5): 678-685.

Rodriguez, A., Sarda, P., Nessmann, C., Boulot, P., Leger, C. L., & Descomps, B. (1998) Δ6- and Δ5-desaturase activities in the human fetal liver: kinetic aspects. *J Lipid Res*, 39(9): 1825-1832.

Rosenstein, E. D., Kushner, L. J., Kramer, N., & Kazandjian, G. (2003) Pilot study of dietary fatty acid supplementation in the treatment of adult periodontitis. *Prostaglandins Leukot Essent Fatty Acids*, 68(3): 213-218.

Saito, M. & Nakatsugawa, K. (1994) Increased susceptibility of liver to lipid peroxidation after ingestion of a high fish oil diet. *Int. J Vitam Nutr Res.* 64: 144-151.

Scott, B. L., & Bazan, N. G. (1989) Membrane docosahexaenoate is supplied to the developing brain and retina by the liver. *Proc Natl Acad Sci U S A*, 86(8): 2903-2907.

Selkoe, D. J. (2001) Alzheimer's disease: genes, proteins, and therapy. *Physiol Rev*, 81(2): 741-766.

Sekine, S., Kubo, K., Tadokoro, T., Maekawa, A., & Saito, M. (2003) Dietary docosahexaenoic acid-induced production of tissue lipid peroxides is not suppressed by higher intake of ascorbic acid in genetically scorbutic Osteogenic Disorder Shionogi/Shi-od/od rats. *Br J Nutr.* 90(2):385-94.

Simons, M., Keller, P., De Strooper, B., Beyreuther, K., Dotti, C. G., & Simons, K. (1998) Cholesterol depletion inhibits the generation of β-amyloid in hippocampal neurons. *Proc Natl Acad Sci U S A*, 95(11): 6460-6464.

Simons, M., Keller, P., Dichgans, J., & Schulz, J. B. (2001) Cholesterol and Alzheimer's disease: is there a link? *Neurology*, 57(6): 1089-1093.

Sinclair, A. J., & Crawford, M. A. (1973) The effect of a low-fat maternal diet on neonatal rats. *Br J Nutr*, 29(1): 127-137.

Soderberg, M., Edlund, C., Kristensson, K., & Dallner, G. (1991) Fatty acid composition of brain phospholipids in aging and in Alzheimer's disease. *Lipids*, 26(6): 421-425.

Sosenko, I. R. (1995) Do polyunsaturated fatty acids protect against oxidant-induced lung damage? *J Nutr*, 125(6 Suppl): 1652S-1656S.

Spector, A. A. (2001) Plasma free fatty acid and lipoproteins as sources of polyunsaturated fatty acid for the brain. *J Mol Neurosci*, 16(2-3): 159-165; discussion 215-121.

Sutubbs, C. D. (1992) *Essential Fatty Acids and Eicosanoids: 3rd International Congress*, Sinclair, A. and Gibson, R. (eds) 116-121. America Oil Chemists Society Press, Champaign, IL.

Suzukawa, M., Abbey, M., Howe, P. R., Nestel, P. J. (1995) Effects of fish oil fatty acids on low density lipoprotein size, oxidizability, and uptake by macrophages. *J. Lipid Res.* 36: 473-48.

Tanabe, Y., Hashimoto, M., Sugioka, K., Maruyama, M., Fujii, Y., Hagiwara, R., Hara, T., Hossain, S. M., & Shido, O. (2004) Improvement of spatial cognition with dietary docosahexaenoic acid is associated with an increase in Fos expression in rat CA1 hippocampus. *Clin Exp Pharmacol Physiol*, 31(10): 700-703.

Ueki, A., Otsuka, M., Sato, T., & Sasaki, S. (2004) Nutritional approach for prevention and treatment of Alzheimer's disease-The Japanease study- *J Nutr Health Aging* 8: 432 (Abstract).

van den Berg, J.J, de Fouw, N. J., Kuypers, F. A., Roelofsen, B., Houtsmuller, U. M., Op den Kamp J. A. (1991) Increased n-3 polyunsaturated fatty acid content of red blood cells from fish oil-fed rabbits increases in vitro lipid peroxidation, but decreases hemolysis. *Free Radic Biol Med.* 11(4):393-399.

Wojtczak, L. (1976) Effect of long-chain fatty acids and acyl-CoA on mitochondrial permeability, transport, and energy-coupling processes. *J Bioenerg Biomembr*, 8(6): 293-311.

Wu, A., Ying, Z., & Gomez-Pinilla, F. (2004) Dietary omega-3 fatty acids normalize BDNF levels, reduce oxidative damage, and counteract learning disability after traumatic brain injury in rats. *J Neurotrauma*, 21(10): 1457-1467.

Yatin, S. M., Aksenov, M., & Butterfield, D. A. (1999) The antioxidant vitamin E modulates amyloid β-peptide-induced creatine kinase activity inhibition and increased protein oxidation: implications for the free radical hypothesis of Alzheimer's disease. *Neurochem Res*, 24(3): 427-435.

Yavin, E., Brand, A., Green. P. (2002) Docosahexaenoic acid abundance in the brain: a biodevice to combat oxidative stress. *Nutr Neurosci.* 5:149-157.

Young, C., Gean, P. W., Chiou, L. C., & Shen, Y. Z. (2000) Docosahexaenoic acid inhibits synaptic transmission and epileptiform activity in the rat hippocampus. *Synapse*, 37(2): 90-94.

In: Alzheimer's Disease Research Trends
Editor: A.P. Chan, pp. 275-288

ISBN 978-1-60021-712-8

Chapter XIV

NAVIGATIONAL DISORDERS IN PATIENTS WITH ALZHEIMER'S DISEASE

Ming-Chyi Pai[1,*] and W. Jake Jacobs[2]

[1]Division of Behavioral Neurology, Department of Neurology, National Cheng Kung University Hospital, Tainan, Taiwan;
[2]Department of Psychology, the University of Arizona, Tucson, USA.

ABSTRACT

Normal episodic memory and navigation require intact hippocampi and surrounding structures. Both are damaged in the early stages of Alzheimer's disease (AD). Specific cognitive dysfunction during early stage AD and the progressive course of AD offer an opportunity to understand the neural bases of higher cortical function and dysfunction both in human memory and in human spatial cognition. Understanding how residual cerebral functions compensate and cope with the progressive neural compromise – and associated cognitive impairment – also helps us to pinpoint the neural substrates of complex cognitive processes.

After a brief review of the literature concerning navigational disorders in patients with AD, we introduce our previous and current studies.

First, we describe a study investigating navigational skills in community-residing early AD patients. Following an average 37 months of disease duration, more than 50% of the participants had easily detected navigational problems, and 18% reported getting lost (GL) – a complete spatial disorientation requiring escort from others to return home – at least once. Second, we describe results from interviews of individuals caring for AD patients who had been lost at least once. These interviews focused on the settings in which GL occurred. Most of the patients first got lost in the early stage of AD in familiar places. Most had a definite destination at the beginning of the GL episode; some exhibited stereotypical search behaviors shortly after becoming disoriented. Third, we

* Correspondence concerning this article should be addressed to Dr. Ming-Chyi Pai, 138 Sheng Li Road, Tainan 704, Taiwan. Tel: 886-6-235-3535-5534, Fax: 886-6-208-8036; pair@mail.ncku.edu.tw.

describe results from three experiments designed to test a retrogenetic account of navigational capacities in early AD patients. These theoretically driven experiments included measures of learning and recognition of novel landmarks, egocentric route learning, and allocentric map formation. The results confirm that navigational disorder appears in early stage AD and follows a sequence reverse to the topographic abilities a human develops over childhood.

We conclude that specific forms of navigational problems appear early in the clinical course of AD. Whether these demonstrable failures in cognitive mapping are based on progressive hippocampal damage, and whether we are studying a variant of AD in which navigational disorder manifests an incipient symptom, remain open questions.

Keywords: Navigation, human, Alzheimer's disease, memory, hippocampus, topographical disorientation, cognitive map.

A. Introduction

Patients in the early stages of Alzheimer's disease (AD) often exhibit cognitive deficits other than episodic amnesia. These deficits include impairment in solving problems and reasoning, loss of previously expert skills, difficulty in competent communication, and the appearance of navigational disorders (Perry 1999; Cherrier 2001; Mapstone 2003; Pai 2002, 2004). The present paper focuses on the appearance and course of navigational disorders in early AD.

Navigational disorders such as topographical disorientation (impaired navigation in the real world or TD) are often marked by hesitation or confusion and almost always produce a loss of spatial autonomy. TD is primarily characterized by deficits in the ability to learn spatial layouts and to follow specific routes to specific destinations in both unfamiliar and familiar environments (Barrash 2000). Although upon leaving home AD patients with TD may become lost, they sometimes use methods, such as making a phone call or hiring a taxi, to return home. As the disease progresses, however, patients with AD will require help from others to relocate their home, and, eventually, will either confine themselves or be confined to places in which their travels may be safely managed. Wandering may also appear. Obviously, TD not only worries the patient, but also casts a heavy burden on the family.

The idea that the hippocampus and related structures are important for spatial cognition, and hence to navigational abilities, is based on the discovery of place cells in the rodent hippocampus (O'Keefe 1971), the documentation of impaired spatial learning in humans with surgically placed lesions to right, but not left hippocampus (Thomas 2001), demonstrations of profound spatial deficits in animals with hippocampal damage (O'Keefe 1978; Redish 1999; Burgees 2002), and neuroimaging studies of topographical memory (Aguirre 1998).

Early in the course of the disease, patients with AD incur bilateral damage to hippocampal structures, structures that appear essential for normal declarative memory (Vargha-Khadem 1997, Eichenbaum 2001, Burgess 2002) and some forms of spatial navigation (McNamara 2003; Burgess 2002). Thus, in addition to increasingly dense episodic amnesia, these patients should experience a progressive loss of cognitive maps, formed recently or long ago, and should become lost in both novel and familiar environments.

Studies of deficits in way-finding behaviors (a form of spatial navigation) in patients with AD, however, are scant. This may be due to the fact that many researchers regard AD as involving global cognitive impairments – which makes TD an inevitable result. This belief has been changing, because over the past few years, the number of studies addressing wayfinding in early Alzheimer's has increased (Liu 1991; Passini 1995; McShane 1998; Tetewsky 1999; Cherrier 2001; Pai 2003; Monacelli 2003; Mapstone 2003; Kavcic 2003; Pai 2004; Chiu 2004; Rosenbaum 2005; Kalova 2005; Cherrier 2005).

B. The Background

For successful travel from one point in space to another, it is necessary to (i) identify origin and destination, (ii) determine turn angles, (iii) identify segment lengths and direction of movement, (iv) recognize on route and distant landmarks, and (v) embed the route to be taken in some large frame of reference (Golledge 1999). Each step in this process can be further subdivided into components involving perception, central processing, and execution.

The term wayfining, defined as spatial problem solving, imposed itself as a complementary notion to spatial orientation (Passini 1995). Cognitive maps, in this conceptualization, are one source of information used in decision processes underlying navigation (wayfinding) itself. From the viewpoint of environmental psychology purposeful mobility encompasses perceptuo-cognitive and decision making abilities, and motor planning, not merely the cognitive map (Passini 1995).

C. Previous Papers

C1. Studies of TD in Patients with Focal Brain Damages

Recently, Aguirre (1999) classified impaired navigation in the real world into four types, (see Table 1). Patient with right lingual gyrus lesion, for example, may become unable to recognize familiar or novel landmarks (Pallis 1955; Paterson 1944). Patients with right posterior parietal lesion may lose the ability to navigate by egocentric orientation at a ground level (Stalk 1996), while patients with lesion in right parahippocampus may experience anterograde TD (Pai 1997; Lin 2000), a condition in which the individual no longer learns new environments or new routes. Rare patients may suffer from a navigational disorder called head disorientation, which occurs after a lesion in retrosplenial structure or posterior cingulate gyrus. These patients cannot imagine a view from a specific location in space (Suzuki 1996, Suzuki 1998). The syndrome is called head disorientation because, in rodents, a group of cells in the subiculum (called head direction cells) activate when the head is oriented in a specific direction in a specific environment (Taube 1990).

In short, these clinical cases, and the classification scheme driven by them, provide evidence that successful navigation depends on various combinations of a number of components; deficit in any one of which may produce disorientation or navigational problems. These cases also suggests that, patients who have experienced TD may, at first, use unique combinations of spatial skills strategies to compensate (Habib 1987).

Table 1. Four syndromes of topographical disorientation after focal cerebral damage

Disorders	Lesion location
Landmark agnosia	Right lingual gyrus
Egocentric disorientation	Right posterior parietal cortex
Head disorientation	Right retrosplenial cortex
Anterograde disorientation	Right parahippocamus

To our knowledge, no one has yet described a syndrome that might be characterized as a cognitive map impairment or allocentric representation failure. Given the extensive literature on relations between hippocampus and cognitive mapping (Brandeis 1989; Jacobs 2003) and no reports of cases with TD due to an isolated hippocampal injury, this surprising gap in the literature raised a question regarding the role of hippocampus in human navigation.

The unquestionable role of hippocampus in some forms of spatial navigation originates from study on rodents and the discovery of place cells (O'Keefe 1978). Although Barrash (2000), after reviewing the human literature examining TD and its neuroanatomcal correlates, stressed the equal contribution of bilateral hippocampi to human navigation, studies based on neuropsychological measures, e.g., recognition-based tests of spatial memory, including the recognition of landmarks (Whiteley 1978) and topographical scenes (Warrington 1996), have pointed toward parahippocampus as a structure critical to spatial cognition. This disparity was resolved when it became apparent that parahippocampal areas are required for iconic representation of scenes, with hippocampus being required in addition only when memory for location in 3D space is required (Burgess 2002).

In contrast to lesion studies, which demonstrate the critical role of various parietal and temporal sites for a specific topographical function, functional imaging studies demonstrate that hippocampus proper is active in normal individuals when they are navigating a virtual spatial environment (Burgess 2002). Moreover, studies using imaging methodology have demonstrated that areas such as bilateral medial parietal cortex, right inferior parietal cortex, posterior cingulum, parts of basal ganglia, left prefrontal cortex, bilateral medial temporal regions (including parahippocampus) and hippocampus proper become more active when humans perform a navigation task, usually in virtual settings,. These areas are compatible with the neurosubstrates classified in Aguirre's paper (1999).

C2. Studies of TD in Patients with AD

Many cerebral regions outside of the hippocampus are also vulnerable to the effects of AD at different stages, although the particular neuropathogical – and the cognitive – trajectory of the disease often varies from one patient to another. Some patients experience GL in the early part of the disease, while others retain full navigational abilities even when episodic memory shows severe deficits. Hence, AD is heterogeneous in clinical and cognitive manifestation.

Liu (1991), who examined relations between different types of spatial skills, concluded that AD patients in the early stage were impaired on all tasks measuring higher cognitive spatial orientation. Proper performance on these tasks requires spatial planning, spatial memory, decision making, and mental representation. McShane (1998), who described five-year follow up data on 104 patients, reported that up to 41% of these patients reported both TD and GL. The occurrence of one or more episodes of GL in such patients increases the likelihood of them being placed in a nursing home.

Many patients with AD experience visuospatial disorientation accompanied by prominent deficits in judging spatial relations and in constructional capacities early in the course of the disease. Such deficits prevent these individuals from monitoring their own movements through a spatial environment. Factors affecting GL in AD patients are complex, but practically GL requires contributions from two major sources, the patients and environments, see Table 2. Contributions from the patients come through sensory, motor and personal characteristics.

Table 2. The factors affecting successful navigation in daily life

Sources	Divisions	Components
Patients	Sensory	Visual acuity, familiar landmarks recognition, new landmarks learning, egocentric orientation, head orientation
	Motor	Problem solving ability, tactics used, ambulation
	Personal characteristics	Education level, gender, age, geographical knowledge
Settings and Situations		Novel or familiar, daytime or night, simple or complex, crowded or not

Most research into this matter tends to focus on sensory impairments, such as visual impairment, agnosia to old landmarks, inability to learn new landmarks, egocentric disorientation, and inability to form and recover cognitive maps (Aguirre 1999). Little is known about the contribution of motor components to solving spatial problems when an individual is lost. Passini (1995), who studied wayfinding in AD patients, considered wayfinding in everyday life a problem-solving task and suggested it is misleading to ascribe wayfinding difficulties in AD patients only to difficulties with mental representation or memory. Personal characters are also important, including gender, age, educational level, geographical knowledge, and the disease severity (Cherrier 2005).

The contexts in which the patients may get lost are also important. Is the place familiar or novel to the patient, simple or complex, crowded or not and in daytime or night (Tu 2006)?

Some argue that GL associated with early AD involves a failure to encode/recall the spatial layout or unique landmarks that aid in orientation; still others argue the problem occurs at the level of perception. For example, the research group lead by Duffy at Rochester University argues that patients with AD become lost because of impairments in visual perception rather than forgetting route or location. This group emphasizes relations between parietal impairment and optic flow as an explanation of TD in patients with AD (Tetewsky 1999; O'Brien 2001; Mapstone 2003; Monacelli 2003; Kavic 2003). One variant of this proposal is that older adults with isolated spatial deficits have a spatial variant of mild cognitive impairment (MCI) (Mapstone 2003). Mono-symptomatic syndromes such as this may help to identify patients at risk for developing AD, and who may be good candidates for focused monitoring and possible treatment (Monacelli 2003). In the same way, isolated perceptual impairment in some normal older adults suggests that mono-symptomatic presentations of pre-AD states are not limited to the isolated memory impairment of MCI.

One mechanism by which this variant of MCI may be linked to spatial disorientation is via extrastriate visual cortical analysis of the orienting information in optic flow, the visual changes experienced by an individual as s/he moves through space. Early-stage AD patients with TD represent a specific-variant group, one that experiences an impairment in optic flow processing. This concept is compatible with results described by de Leon and colleagues (1984). These authors found that nursing-home patients with AD who wandered and became lost (even in familiar surroundings) differed from other patients on tests of parietal function (visuoconstruction, right/left orientation, clock reading, finger writing, and identification), but not on tests measuring general mental strengths and weaknesses. They suggested that wandering in AD patients may be an indication of a specific parietal lobe involvement.

Other authors stress the role of landmark recognition in TD and GL. Cherrier (2001) tested the performance of AD patients on several navigation tasks and found that the patients performed poorly, as predicted (see also Ranville 2002). More recently, Cherrier (2005) reported that testosterone supplements improves spatial memory in men with AD and MCI.

The debate regarding the role (if any) of hippocampus and cognitive maps in TD and GL experienced by early AD patients continues. Teng & Squire (1999) described an individual with extensive bilateral damage to the medial temporal lobes, but with preserved memory for remote spatial information. Moreover, this individual could accurately navigate detours or short-cuts when a point in a familiar path was blocked. Teng & Squire (1999) proposed that parietal and retrosplenial cortices, rather than the hippocampus and associated temporal structures, are the brain regions that maintain long-term spatial maps (Pai 1997). Rosenbaum et al. (2000) also described an amnesic person with extensive bilateral hippocampal lesions but with preserved remote spatial memory. More recently, Rosenbaum et al. (2005) examined a retired taxi driver of 40 years who developed AD. These authors reported the driver had preserved memory for well-known landmarks, their locations, and the spatial relations among them despite significant hippocampal atrophy. Kalova et al. (2005) used a Morris Water Maze modified for human use in patients with AD. The results of this study showed the AD patients lost their ability to relocate an invisible target using relations among distal cues, but their ability to relocate a visible target remained comparable to that of normal subjects.

D. Studies from our Group

We interviewed family members of 155 patients with AD visiting a behavioral neurology clinic in a medical center located in southern Taiwan. The family members were asked questions regarding the onset of incipient symptoms of AD (Pai 2002). The results showed that 7% of the patients had experienced TD as an incipient symptom.[1] Moreover, patients with TD as an incipient symptom, compared to those with other incipient symptoms such as memory impairment, delusions, personality change and executive dysfunction or apraxia, were brought to hospital earlier.

We further studied 112 community-residing early AD patients recruited from the same clinic (Pai 2004). These individuals had an average disease duration of 37 months at the completion of the study. Fifty-five percent of the participants had documented navigational disorders, and 18% had experienced GL and required an escort from others to return their home. The caregivers reported that the AD patients with TD were confined to a more restricted safety range than those without TD, and the patients with a history of change in residence over the past five years are at a higher risk of GL. No correlation was found between the AD patients' performance on neuropsychological tests and the extent of their navigational disorders.

One fourth of the family members interviewed agreed that TD was one of the incipient symptoms exhibited by the individual under their care. Hence, the occurrence of TD in these patients was associated with TD as an incipient symptom, a history of change in residence, the presence of a small 'territorial range', and longer disease duration. GL with a requirement of an escort from others to return home was associated with TD as an incipient symptom, a small "territorial" range, and relatively worse cognitive abilitites, TD, and indoor disorientation. These results again demonstrate the prevalence of TD in patients with AD, even during early stage, and further demonstrate this cognitive deficit is not related to global mental states as measured by neuropsychological tests.

Like patients with damage to the left medial temporal lobe, who have concomitant declarative amnesia but can recognize what they learned before the damage occurred, early AD patients might recognize familiar landmarks, such as their homes and neighborhood. To examine this possibility we interviewed the caregivers of 19 AD patients who had experienced GL. We focused on the context in which the episodes had occurred (Tu 2006). Of these 19 cases, 18 experienced their first GL in a place they had been familiar with for a decade or more. Seventeen of the nineteen cases experienced GL when they had a definite destination. Finally, these patients experienced more difficulty navigating toward their home than away from it.

Although these data are important for caregivers, we interpret them cautiously because the range these patients were permitted to navigate was increasing restricted as the disease progressed. For such patients, being lost in novel environments was no longer a novel experience. Nevertheless, it is possible that these patients initially experienced a perceptual impairment of familiar landmarks. By that we mean that, although the patients may recognize landmarks, the landmarks or scene may no longer evoke a feeling of familiarity. Experiments to examine this possibility are underway.

Pai, Gia, & Jacobs (2005) are now conducting an experiment examining the ability of patients with AD to recognize familiar landmarks. We used landmarks that fall into four categories of familiarity to test recognition and familiarity in patients and their spouses: personally familiar, regionally familiar, nationally familiar, and internationally familiar.

[1] We accepted report when at least one member of the family provided an appropriate description and another

Personally familiar landmarks include pictures of the individual's home and neighborhood (familiarity was determined during an extensive interview designed to elicit the appropriate information). The preliminary results showed that the patients recognize these familiar landmarks as well as their spouses[2]. This result raises a question: Why are AD patients lost in familiar surroundings? The result is similar those obtained by Cherrier (2001) who reported that AD participants, while walking a specified route, correctly identified landmarks but deviated from the route specified by them. These deviations require a correction or cue from the examiner to return the participants to the correct route (Cherrier 2001). The idea that these patients may recognize familiar landmarks but fail to use them appropriately receives some support from a case study reported by Mendez (2003), in which a patient who developed TD after a stroke involving right medial occipitotemporal lobes could not recognize a scene without prominent landmarks in it even though he could recognize familiar landmarks and use them appropriately. His inability to find his way in familiar environments was due to the visuospatial difficulty of integrating spatial relationships or his inability to access or retrieve adequate mental maps (Mendez 2003).

E. The Retrogenetic Hypothesis of Human Navigation

To contextualize this discussion, we must first provide an overview of navigational capacities as they develop in children. A famous and compelling theory was proposed by Piaget (1960) and his followers. In his view, children develop various navigational capacities hierarchically. They can recognize landmarks first, they then develop the capacity to set up egocentric routes, and finally they develop the ability to form allocentric representations. This development of navigational capacities fits recent findings in the neuropsysiological development literature well.

Reisberg (1999) described retrogenesis or a loss of cognitive or life function which, in adults, occurs in a sequence exactly opposite of that described by Piaget (1960). Applying this idea, we predicted that AD patients will lose navigational capacities in a sequence that is the reverse of that acquired in early life. Although the clinical manifestation of AD is heterogeneous, a large proportion of AD patients experience a sequence of progressive cognitive deficit which mirror underlying neural pathology (Braak 1996). Basically, the pathology begins from medial temporal structures, and spreads to parietal and other neocortical cerebral cortex. The primary cortices are the last to be involved.

This retrogenesis-based description of navigation ability in AD (see Figure 1) predicts that patients with AD will lose allocentric map or internal spatial representation first, followed by egocentric route learning ability, and finally the recognition of landmarks. We designed three experiments to test this prediction. These experiments examined learning and recognition of novel landmarks, and novel route learning dependent on egocentric or allocentric map formation after exploration of a novel environment (Pai 2003). We found that navigation abilities do not decline in parallel. Although not perfectly fitting the predictions,

independently confirmed it.

[2] We have not yet analyzed the data related to regional, national, and international familiarity

there were discrepancies in functional loss as the disease progressed. MCI patients were impaired in egocentric route learning, while their ability to recognize landmarks and to perform path integration, measured by pointing to starting point, was comparable to normal older adults.

	Piaget's ontogenesis					Retrogenesis		
Way-finding steps	LR	→	ERL	→	ISR	→	ERL	→ LR
Neuro-anatomy	LG		PPC		H/paraH	→	PPC	→ LG
						Braak's stages		

Figure 1. Retrogenetic hypothesis of human navigation, LR: landmark recognition; ERL: egocentric route learning' ISR: internal spatial representation; LG: landmark agnosia; PPC: posterior parietal cortex; LG: lingual gyrus; H: hippocampus.

Given that SPECT scans revealed that the majority of these MCI patients had hypoperfusion in temporal regions, representing pre-AD, the observed preservation of cognitive maps in these individuals is inconsistent with cognitive map theory (O'Keefe 1978), which claimed that hippocampus is required for the formation of cognitive maps. Deficits caused by progressive degenerative disorders, such as AD, are quite different from those by acute insults, such as traumatic brain injury or stroke, which represent the majority of case studies on TD. AD, as a slowly progressive disease, may permit changes in the neural networks, permitting compensation through as-yet poorly understood neuroplasticity. Hence it is possible that, although their hippocampi were structurally impaired, MCI patients preserve their ability to represent allocentric space through mechanisms permitting cerebral cortex to compensate for the loss.

Several other interpretations of this data pattern remain viable. It is possible that the damage observed through SPECT did not involve hippocampal tissue critical to the formation of cognitive maps. Another possibility is that AD patients may lose the abilities they acquired early in life only at the terminal stage of the disease. Children develop navigation abilities within the first few years of life, a period representing only a small fraction of a normal life span (Laurance 2003). If the children have more abilities, or develop them more quickly than Piaget predicted (Newcombe 2003), then, retrogenesis predicts that it would be difficult for us to observe the progressive loss of these abilities during late stage. We do not have much confidence in the latter account because navigational abilities do not parallel the development of other motor or daily-living skills.

F. Questions to be Answered

F1. Hippocampus, Cognitive Map, and Alzheimer Disease

The results of the studies reviewed above move us to ask: Is GL in a familiar setting, which is a relatively common occurrence in early AD, caused by a failure to form or retrieve appropriate cognitive maps? If yes, is the failure caused by hippocampal damage?

Damage to hippocampus in early AD impairs learning about new spaces; being lost in novel places is the rule for AD patients, they are extremely deficient at acquiring new spatial knowledge. Conversely, patients with hippocampal damage can navigate familiar neighborhoods and reproduce accurate sketch maps of familiar locations such as floor plans of houses (Rosenbaum 2005). This data patterns suggests that hippocampus is crucial for the acquisition of cognitive maps but not for the maintenance and retrieval of maps acquired and used extensively long before the injury (Rosenbaum 2005).

Furthermore, patients with AD first get lost in familiar places (Tu 2006). Although cognitive maps are important navigational aids under some conditions, they are not necessary for all forms of navigation in either normal individuals or patients with AD. The environments in which we live are full of visual cues such as buildings and landmarks, all of which may be used to form cognitive maps, to link landmarks-to-landmarks as a route, or to aid in integrating a series of paths. Hence, hippocampal patients may show deficits in tasks designed to detect allocentric representations, but not experience TD in the real life. Perhaps these patients rarely go out alone, seldom experience novel places, and most certainly never encounter places free of landmarks. Given this, while cognitive mapping may be lost in AD patients, they are not necessarily impaired in day-to-day navigation. This is because they can use landmarks and sequences of landmarks in series to follow a path.

Finally, the quality of cognitive maps may slowly – and perhaps gracefully – degrade. In this case, patients with AD may use schematic, course-grained, cognitive map to guide them to a place near their home (see e.g., Rosenbaum 2005). To reach their home, however, they may need more detailed knowledge to differentiate their house from the neighbors'. The grain of the map, by this thinking, relies on the quality of hippocampal function. This view suggests that, in AD patients, GL in familiar places is not due to inability to retrieve an old map, no matter whether this function is dependent on hippocampus or not, instead it is due to the quality of the maps formed by these individuals (see Laurance 2002).

F2. If not Damage to Hippocampus, what Causes AD Patients to Become Lost?

If the patients with early AD still preserved cognitive maps of old settings, or at least schematic versions of a cognitive map, then the simple possession of a cognitive map is not enough for successful navigation of familiar space. Some other cognitive deficits must be involved in AD-associated TD. As many investigators have noted, in addition to the presence of internal spatial representation of the environments, one must recognize key landmarks to navigate successfully. From clinical observation and our studies, however, patients with early

AD can recognize familiar landmarks as well as their spouses (Pai 2005). Hence, the recognition of familiar landmarks is not involved.

Patients with AD had been reported to have difficulty inhibiting useless information or impulses. This may manifest as irritability, confusion, or an inability to make correct choices (e.g., to make appropriate decisions at choice-points when navigating a path, Chiu 2004). Here, we should notice the information that permits such patients to make appropriate choice-point decisions, and where distracters might come from. Obviously, distracters may come from the environment within which the navigator is walking. This proposal is weakened somewhat by the fact that some individuals who experienced GL claimed that they could recognize major landmarks but somehow lost the ability to determine which way to go next. In addition, they report becoming lost after taking a wrong turn and being unable to trace their route back to the point where they became lost. None of the patients could explain why or how this phenomenon occurred.

Although spatial memory and episodic memory decline in parallel in older adults (Newman 2000), people with an impaired ability to form spatial representations or path integration do not report TD. It is possible that older adults form cognitive maps slowly, or the maps that are formed are course (e.g., Laurance 2002) and, as a result, may rely more on landmarks and egocentric route learning than on allocentric representations. It is also possible that in modern life, humans rely more heavily on verbal, written, or symbolic information (e.g., directions, street signs, addresses, iconic traffic signs) to guide their way than on path integration or internal spatial representation just as mammals that stay and move in group may rely less on independent navigation than signals coming from conspecifics. For humans under most circumstances, the ability to recognize landmarks and to remember the sequences of them is enough to permit accurate navigation through most of the environment. This fact may help us understand why amnesic Alzheimer's patients with bilateral damages to their hippocampi do not get lost.

G. Summary

Bilateral hippocampi are demonstrably damaged in early AD. Theoretically, these patients should get lost because of an inability to learn new route and spatial orientation and, unless old maps are stored in hippocampus, they should not become disoriented in familiar places. Although the data are consistent with the first prediction, they are inconsistent with the second. Some (perhaps many) AD patients are prone to become lost, even in highly familiar territory. Moreover, patients with damage to the right temporal lobe may experience disrupted abilities to form cognitive maps, they may do poorly on route learning tests, but they are not often lost. In the same way, the quality of cognitive maps in normal older adults is often degraded, but they do not get lost. These facts set intriguing puzzles regarding relationships among AD, TD, cognitive mapping, and temporal lobes structures, including the hippocampus. Understanding these relations more clearly may help us identify early AD, permit us to offer early therapeutic interventions, and, perhaps most importantly, may help individuals afflicted with AD prolong their functional independence.

H. Acknowledgements

This work was supported in part by the National Science Council (Taiwan) grants NSC 90-2341-B-006-095 and NSC 93-2314-B-006-102.

I. References

Aguirre GK, Zarahn E, D'Esposito M. Neural components of topographical representation. *Proc Natl Acad Sci* 1998; 95: 839-46.

Aguirre GK, D'Esposito M. Topographical disorientation: a synthesis and taxonomy. *Brain* 1999; 122: 1613-28.

Barrash J, Damasio H, Adolphs R, Tranel D. The neuroanatomical correlated of route learning impairment. *Neuropsychologia* 2000; 38: 820-36.

Braak H, Braak E. Evolution of the neuropathology of Alzheimer's disease. *Acta Neurolol Scandinav* 1996; 165(suppl), 3-12.

Brandeis R, Brandys Y, Yehuda S. The use of the Morris water maze in the study of memory and learning. *Int J Neurosci* 1989; 48: 29-69.

Burgess N, Maguire EA, O'Keefe J. The human hippocampus and spatial and episodic memory. *Neuron* 2002; 35: 625-41.

Cherrier MM, Mendez M, Perryman K. Route learning performance in Alzheimer's disease patients. *Neuropsychiatry Neurolpsychol Behav Neurol* 2001; 14: 159-68.

Cherrier MM. Matsumoto AM, Amory JK, Asthana S, Bremner W, Peskind ER, Taskind MA, Craft S. Testosterone improves spatial memory in men with Alzheimer disease and mild cognitive impairment. *Neurology* 2005; 64: 2063-8.

Chiu YC, Algase D, Whall A, Liang J, Liu HC, Lin KN, Wang PN. Getting lost: directed attention and executive functions in early Alzheimer's disease patients. *Dementia Geriatr Cogn Disord* 2004; 17: 174-80.

Cipolotti L, Maguire EA. A combined neuropsychological and neuroimaging study of topographical and non-verbal memory in semantic dementia. *Neuropsychologia* 2003; 41: 1148-59.

de Leon MJ, Potegal M, Gurland B. Wandering and parietal signs in senile dementia of Alzheimer's type. *Neuropsychobiology* 1984; 11: 155-7.

Eichenbaum H, Cohen NJ. *From Conditioning to Conscious Recollection.* Oxford: Oxford University Press, 2001.

Golledge RG. Human wayfinding and cognitive map. In: Colledge RG ed. *Wayfinding Behavior*. Baltimore: The Johns Hopkins University Press, 1999: 5-45.

Habib M, Sirigu A. Pure topographical disorientation: a definition and anatomical basis. *Cortex* 1987; 23: 73-85.

Jacobs LF, Schenk F. Unpacking the cognitive map: The parallel map theory of hippocampal function. *Psychol Rev* 2003; 110: 285-315.

Kalova E, Vlcek K, Jarolimova E, Bures J. Allothetic orientation and sequential ordering of places is impaired in early stages of Alzheimer's disease: corresponding results in real space tests and computer tests. *Behav Brain Res.* 2005; 159: 175-86.

Kavcic V, Duffy CJ. Attentional dynamic and visual perception: mechanisms of spatial disorientation in Alzheimer's disease. *Brain* 2003; 126: 1173-82.

Laurance, H. E., Learmonth, A. E., Nadel, L., & Jacobs, W. J. (2003). Maturation of spatial navigation strategies: Convergent findings from computerized spatial environments and self-report. *Journal of Cognition and Development, 4,* 211-238.

Laurance H E, Thomas KGF, Newman MC, Kaszniak AW, Nadel L, Jacobs WJ. Older adults map novel environments but do not place learn: Findings from a computerized spatial task. *Aging Neuropsychol Cogn* 2002; 9: 85-97.

Lin CC, Pai MC. Transient topographical disorientation as a manifestation of cerebral ischemic attack. *J Formosan Med Assoc* 2000; 99: 653-5.

Liu L, Gauthier L, Gauthier S. Spatial disorientation in persons with early senile dementia of the Alzheimer type. *Am J Occup Ther* 1991; 45: 67-74.

Mapstone M, Steffenella TM, Duffy CJ. A visuospatial variant of mild cognitive impairment. Getting lost between aging and AD. *Neurology* 2003; 60: 802-8.

McNamara TP, Shelton AL. Cognitive maps and the hippocampus. *Treads Cogn Sci* 2003; 7: 333-5.

McShane R, Gedling K, Keenw J, Fairgurn C, Jacoby R, Hope T. Getting lost in dementia: a longitudinal study of a behavioral symptom. *Int Psychogeriatr* 1998; 10: 253-60.

Mendez MF, Cherrier MM. Agnosia for scenes in topographagnosia. *Neuropsychologia* 2003; 41: 1387-95.

Monacelli AM, Cushman LA, Kavcic V, Duffy CJ. Spatial disorientation in Alzheimer's disease. *Neurology* 2003; 61: 1491-7.

Newcombe NS, Huttenlocher J. *Making Space.* MIT Press, 2003.

Newman MC, Kaszniak AW. Spatial memory and aging: performance on a human analog of the Morris Water Maze. *Aging Neuropsychol Cogn* 2000; 7: 86-93.

O'Brien HL. Tetewsky SJ, Avery LM, Cushman LA, Makous W, Duffy CJ. Visual mechanisms of spatial disorientation in Alzheimer's disease. *Cerebral Cortex* 2001; 11: 1083-92.

O'Keefe J, Dostrovsky J. The hippocampus as a spatial map: preliminary evidence from unit activity in the freely-moving rat. *Brain Res* 1971; 34: 171-5.

O'Keefe J, Nadel L. 1978. *The Hippocampus as a Cognitive Map.* Oxford University Press; Oxford.

O'Keefe J. A review of the hippocampal place cells. *Prog Neurobiol* 1979; 13: 419-39.

Pai MC, Gai PS, Jacobs WJ. Early Alzheimer's patients recognize familiar landmarks well enough. *Soc. Neurosci Abstr.* 2005.

Pai MC, Hsiao S. Incipient symptoms of Alzheimer disease and effect of education on the onset age: a study of 155 Taiwanese patients. *Acta Neurol Taiwan* 2002; 11: 66-9.

Pai MC, Hsiao S. Navigation ability in advancing Alzheimer's disease patients. *Soc. Neurosci. Abstr.* 2003.

Pai MC, Jacobs WJ. Topographical disorientation in community-residing patients with Alzheimer disease. *Int J Geriatric Psychiatry* 2004; 19: 250-5.

Pai MC. Topographic disorientation: Two cases. *J Formosan Med Assoc* 1997; 96: 660-3.

Pallis CA. Impaired identification of faces and places with agnosia for colour. Report of a case due to cerebral embolism. *J Neurol Neurosurg Psychiatry* 1955; 18: 218-24.

Passini R, Rainville C, Marchand N, Joanette Y. Wayfinding in dementia of the Alzheimer type: planning abilities. *J Clin Exp Neurospsychol* 1995; 17: 820-32.

Paterson A, Zangwill OL. Disorders of visual space perception associated with lesions of the right cerebral hemisphere. *Brain* 1944; 67: 331-58.

Perry RJ, Hodges JR. Attention and executive deficits in Alzheimer's disease. *Brain* 1999; 122: 383-404.

Piaget J, Inhelder B, Szeminska A. *The Child's Conception of Geometry*. New York: Basic Books, 1960.

Rainville C, Marchand N, Passini R. Peformances of patients with a dementia of the Alzheimer type in the Standardized Road-Map test of Direction Sense. *Neuropsychologia* 2002; 40: 567-73.

Redish AD. *Beyond the cognitive map. From place cells to episodic memory*. Cambridge: The MIP Press, 1999.

Reisberg B, Kenowsky S, Franssen EH, Stefanie RA, Souren LEM. Toward a science of Alzheimer's disease management: a model based upon current knowledge of retrogenesis. *Int Psychogeriatr* 1999; 11: 7-23.

Rosenbaum RS, Gao FQ, Richards B, Black SE, Moscovitch M. "Where to?" Remote memory for spatial relations and landmark identity in former taxi drivers with Alzheimer's disease and encephalitis. *J Cogn Neurosci* 2005; 17: 446-62.

Stark M, Coslett HB, Saffran EM. Impairment of an egocentric map of locations: implications for perception and action. *Cogn Neuropsychol* 1996; 13: 481-523.

Suzuki K, Yamadori A, Hyakawa Y, Fujii T. Pure topographical disorientation related to dysfunction of the viewpoint dependent visual system. *Cortex* 1998; 34: 589-99.

Suzuki K, Yamadori A, Takase S, Nagamine Y, Itoyama Y. Transient prosopagnosia and lasting topographical disorientation after the total removal of a right occipital arteriovenous malformation [Japanese]. *Rinsho Shinkeigaku* 1996; 36: 1114-7.

Taube JS, Muller RU, Ranck JB. Head direction cells recorded from the presubiculum in freely moving rats. I. Description and quantitative analysis. *J Neurosci* 1990; 10: 420-35.

Teng E, Squire LR. Memory for places learned long ago is intact after hippocampus damage. *Nature* 1999; 400: 675-7.

Tetewsky SJ, Duffy CJ. Visual loss and getting lost in Alzheimer's disease. *Neurology* 1999; 52: 958-65.

Thomas KGF, Hsu M, Laurance H E, Nadel L, Jacobs WJ. Place learning in virtual space III: Perceptive learning. *Behav Res Methods Instrum Compt* 2001; 33: 21-37.

Tu MC, Pai MC. Getting lost for the first time in patients with Alzheimer's disease. *Int Psychogeriatr* 2006; 18: 67-70.

Vargha-Khadem F, Gadian DG, Watkins KE, Connelly A, Paesschen WV, Mishkin M. Differential effects of early hippocampal pathology on episodic and semantic memory. *Science* 1997; 277: 376-80.

Warrington EK, Shallice T. Word-form dyslexia. *Brain* 1980; 103: 99-112.

Whiteley AM, Warrington E. Selective impairment of topographical memory: a single case study. *J Neurol Neurosurg Psychiatry* 1978; 41: 575-8.

INDEX

A

B

C

D

E

H

I

O

P

Q

R

S

T

U

V